Palliative Care

PALLIATIVE CARE

The 400-Year Quest for a Good Death

Harold Y. Vanderpool

McFarland & Company, Inc., Publishers

Jefferson, North Carolina

ISBN 978-0-7864-9799-7 (softcover : acid free paper) ∞
ISBN 978-1-4766-1971-2 (ebook)

LIBRARY OF CONGRESS CATALOGUING DATA ARE AVAILABLE

British Library cataloguing data are available

On the cover: *clockwise from top left* hospice nurse with patient
(Stockbyte/Thinkstock); Doctor Onstine, medical doctor,
making an examination, 1943 (Library of Congress); Doctor and
nurse examining patient in hospital room (Digital Vision/Thinkstock);
The doctor's office on Transylvania Project, Louisiana, 1940
(Library of Congress); Intensive Care Unit (iStock/Thinkstock)

Printed in the United States of America

*McFarland & Company, Inc., Publishers
Box 611, Jefferson, North Carolina 28640
www.mcfarlandpub.com*

For Jan

Table of Contents

Acknowledgments

Research on the topics in this history began when I wrote the first of two master's degree theses as a Kennedy fellow in medical ethics and the history of medicine at Harvard University. Upon becoming an assistant professor in the history and philosophy of medicine in the Institute for the Medical Humanities at the University of Texas Medical Branch (UTMB) in Galveston, my research continued in the form of publishing a number of articles and book chapters; teaching courses on death, dying, and human suffering; and walking medical wards (including those for oncology) with senior physicians and medical residents. Physician friends, colleagues, and authors have been my teachers.

When I became an associate and then a full professor in UTMB, I enjoyed greater opportunities to conduct research in the United States and abroad. My appointment as James Wade Rockwell Professor in the History of Medicine furthered those opportunities. This book reflects how I profited immensely from working at different times with the staffs and archival holdings of the Wellcome Library in London, the Royal Physicians of Edinburgh Library, the University of Edinburgh Library, the Royal College of Physicians of London Library, the British Library in London, the Countway Library of Medicine in Boston, and the main University of Texas Library in Austin.

Beyond these institutions and their invaluable resources, I profited from extensive research for long periods of time in the Moody Medical Library of UTMB, especially research in its outstanding Truman Blocker History of Medicine Collections. I can hardly convey my great fortune in working with one of the Blocker Collections' stellar archivists, Robert O. (Bobby) Marlin IV. As I searched through card catalogs to find promising historical sources, Bobby retrieved numerous volumes for me to explore. He then enabled me to secure copies of the valuable sources. He also readily contacted archivists elsewhere to secure copies of books and articles from other institutions. In addition to Bobby's assistance, staff members of the Moody Medical Library enabled me to identify and secure hundreds of articles from medical and other journals, past and present, through UTMB's superb article retrieval services.

With respect to the topics in this book, the term *research* is open-ended. It includes visiting and counseling with dying patients, doing rounds in internal medicine, having back-and-forth exchanges with medical students and graduate students in the medical humanities, and spending countless hours searching out web resources. It also includes talking and exchanging emails with friends and family members struggling with the deaths of loved ones. On occasion I confess to putting on the mantle of Samuel Taylor

Coleridge's ancient mariner, who stopped a man going to a wedding feast to speak of matters the stranger resisted hearing. The motivation to undertake this quest surely also arises from the deaths of my parents—the tragic death of my father at the end of my sophomore year in high school and the peaceful passing of my mother late in life.

Beyond all other acknowledgments, I am indebted to my beloved wife Jan, to whom I dedicate this book. Together we traveled to the libraries I've listed, all surrounded by intriguing cities filled with museums, restaurants, and historical sites. Within and outside the cities are stunning natural settings travelers like ourselves are lured to walk and ride carts through—golf courses. Beyond these attractions, however, are Jan's patience and expertise. She has not only responded to my time-consuming questions—and surely, at times, off-putting obsessions—but also, based on her professional expertise in English, edited all four drafts of this book. ("Edit" is shorthand for accurate writing, deletions of repetition, and questions that call for answers.) As soulmate and helpmate, she is an abiding source of inspiration.

Preface

The 400-year quest of palliative care is a living story about dying. (The term *palliative care* refers to the use of medical measures to ease or palliate the symptoms of critically ill and dying persons, combined with personalized and respectful caring.)

This history brings to life the centuries-long quest for good death with the aid of physicians, nurses, clergy, social workers, and other healthcare professionals. The last parts of the story focus on the nature of palliative care at the present time—descriptions of the types of care available in homes, hospices, and hospitals; the duties of various healthcare professionals; symptom-easing care for patients with non-fatal conditions; the various choices seriously and terminally ill patients and family members are ethically and legally empowered make; the difficulties accompanying differing options; and ways of dealing with these difficulties.

This 400-year quest serves as an empowering resource for grappling with death and dying at the present time. It is also intriguing, in that it displays all the features of classic quests: treasured goals, daunting obstacles, travels through unfamiliar domains, and conflicts between protectors and abusers.

Unlike mythological quests, however, this story is rooted in history. It relies upon a vast number of sources and wide experiences that ensure historical accuracy. It traverses centuries of the past and persists in the present. It pursues the treasured goal of enabling persons to experience peaceful dying, to experience death as good by means of medical and other measures from skilled caregivers who assuage oppressive symptoms and provide emotional and spiritual comfort grounded in moral respect.

Daunting obstacles include centuries of struggle with humankind's greatest enemy—death. The struggle encompasses fighting against the use of punishing and futile medical treatments for persons approaching the end of life, finding ways to ease pain and other physical symptoms, overcoming widespread neglect, liberating dying persons from loneliness and isolation in hospitals, changing entrenched cultural dynamics of modern hospitals, and securing patient rights of choice.

Travels through strange cultural settings include journeys through eras far removed in time from our own and separated from ordinary life experiences in recent decades. Bygone medical cures that radically differ from modern modes of treatment are explained and explored. Readers are also taken inside modern hospitals and introduced to technologically sophisticated ways of saving and sustaining human life. Life-sustaining technologies are magnetically attractive to patients and family members, and understanding their benefits and harms is imperative for end-of-life decision making.

Protectors and *abusers* refer to shapers of this history, many of whom are immensely admirable, inventive, caring, brave, and protective. In opposition, others manifest insensitivity, single-mindedness, and shocking obliviousness to the suffering of dying persons, the agonies of families, and the moral dimensions of respectful human relationships.

Coinciding with its personal value and historical intrigue, this study is crafted with a devotion to scholarly accuracy. I have drawn upon a vast literature on clinical medicine, medical research, palliative care practices and advocacy, personal testimonials, biomedical ethics, death and dying, the law, and the history of medicine and culture. My identification and securing of primary sources included funded research in notable archival collections, such as the Wellcome Library in London, the Royal Physicians of Edinburgh Library, the Royal College of Physicians of London Library, the Countway Library of Medicine in Boston, the main University of Texas Library in Austin, and the Truman Blocker History of Medicine Collections at the University of Texas Medical Branch in Galveston. The foundations for this work include my study during a fellowship at Harvard; counseling with dying patients at the side of a resident physician oncologist; publications on topics within this story; national and international lectures; and courses for medical and nursing students on medical ethics, terminal care, and human suffering.

This history is also innovative. No existing study has explored the comprehensive and sustained history of palliative care (dying with medical and personal support of healthcare professionals).[1] None has identified how the beginning point of the history of palliative care is chronologically clear—how it originated over 400 years ago and has continued as an unbroken tradition to the present time. The story of medically assisted palliative care began in 1605, when Sir Francis Bacon challenged physicians to accept the new responsibility of easing the pangs of dying persons so they could expire with greater tranquility. For centuries, physicians directly appealed to Bacon's legacy, which, like the small beginnings of a great river, has now become a powerful current of specialized caring.

Although countless academic books and articles have been written about death, dying, and palliative care, none steadfastly focuses on the history of palliative care in its chronological and conceptual fullness, with an abiding concern for its relevance to patients, family members, and healthcare professionals. A recent study, for example, claims to be a history of the care of dying patients in America. In fact, except for pages in its conclusion, the study only extends from the 1860s to the mid–1960s—the point in time when the palliative care movement began to flourish. While it gives little attention to the interactions between dying persons and caregivers, the book does explore contributions of social workers and the ways religious and spiritual concerns enable persons to grapple with terminal disease.[2] Other authors maintain that the movement to improve end-of-life care began in the 1960s, 1970s, or even the 1990s.[3]

Several recent studies dwell on aspects of the broader cultural background of the history of palliative care, not the practices and voices of those giving and receiving that care. One history impressively chronicles Americans' emotional and intellectual responses to death as conveyed in popular magazines, newspapers, and a variety of scholarly sources from the 1920s to the present.[4] Another typologizes the history of dying into three overarching eras without attending to their ongoing interconnections: religious dying in the 18th century, dying according to medical technique in the 19th century, and dying in accordance with law and public policy beginning in the 20th century. That study also focuses on the history of doctor-induced death (euthanasia in its modern sense), which was fervently and systematically opposed by the vast majority of palliative caregivers.[5] A third 21st-century history dwells on political, economic, scientific and ideological factors, leading its author to claim that hospital and hospice palliative care are reactionary responses to the reductionism of modern medicine. It also includes a lengthy discussion of modern euthanasia, as well as valuable sections on the care of dying patients by Catholic nuns and Protestant deaconesses, information regarding palliative care services in five English-speaking nations, and a chapter on pain control.[6] At relevant points in the chapters that follow, these and other histories of death and dying will be discussed and, when pertinent, utilized.

Why this book's historical narrative has been neglected is not altogether clear. The neglect is due in part to its lacking a common name—indeed, its being identified with names and phrases that fracture its historical identity. Francis Bacon coined the Greek term *euthanasia* (*eu* for good, and *thanatas* for death) to summarize his palliative care challenge to physicians. The pursuit of euthanasia described by Bacon continued to be advanced in the medical literature through the 1880s. But after that, the meaning of the word *euthanasia* changed to its present-day definition—the practice of physicians actively ending the lives of terminally ill persons. Opposed to euthanasia in its modern sense, caregivers devoted to peaceful dying used a variety of other terms to describe their goal—natural dying, medically managing death, dying with dignity, and care for the dying. By the last decades of the 20th century, the term *good death*, the English equivalent of Bacon's Greek term *euthanasia*, summarized the essence of this goal. The motivating power and inner tensions of the term *good death* command attention.

Exceeding all other names, the term *palliative care* began to designate—and now officially designates—the *means* or *methods* by which both symptomatic relief from severe illnesses and good or better deaths are made possible. Palliative care is not cure-intended care, even though studies show that it often extends life. To better convey its meaning with respect to the care of dying persons, palliative care will sometimes be referred to as comfort care, comfort-directed care, end-of-life care, and occasionally quality-of-life or supportive care. Studies show that numerous non-physicians and physicians do not understand what palliative care is. This book aims to remedy that deficiency.

Earlier chapters invite readers to stand at the bedsides of dying persons in former eras. Surrounded by family members, neighbors, and clergy, these persons received kind and steadfast attention from physicians whose interventions were limited, but whose ministrations were honed by dedication and years of first-hand experience. During eras when cure-directed medical practices radically differed from modern modes of curing, physicians upheld the tradition of peaceful dying first advanced by Francis Bacon.

Later chapters take us inside early modern and contemporary hospitals with ever-changing and increasingly complex means of saving and sustaining human life. These chapters bring to life the personalities and convictions of physician and nurse traditionalists and reformers, as well as clergy, bioethicists, lawyers, and concerned citizens. They tell of persons suffering at the hands of medical enthusiasts, whose offenses against patients led to calls for extensive reform. They also take us inside hospices and relate stories of good dying in hospitals, hospices, and homes.

This study fully appreciates the great career of Dame Cicely Saunders in the formation and flourishing of modern hospice care beginning in the late 1950s. At the same time, it counters the common view that palliative medical care began with Dr. Saunders.[7] Expert and sensitive end-of-life care became an essential component of medical practice as early as 1772, and at times Dr. Saunders praised several of her predecessors.

This book displays profound appreciation for the amazing and effective advances of curative medicine and those who discovered and perfected these cures. Nevertheless, it focuses on diverse reformers who held that the living should faithfully keep company with grievously ill and dying persons. It gives special attention to present-day alternatives of choosing palliative care during life's final chapters or opting for life-sustaining medical treatments as long as possible. It travels through multiple eras and inside the major movements and controversies that have enabled severely and fatally ill persons to have choices.

The multifaceted cultural dimensions of this history include the following:

- The wisdom of persons over the centuries who were deeply acquainted with dying and death
- First-hand narratives of the experiences of dying persons, family members, and caregivers
- Summaries of historical and contemporary types of life-prolonging medical advancements
- The inner workings of the medical system and the respective powers and responsibilities of physicians, nurses, administrators, and others
- Discussions and debates over vitally important ethical issues
- State and federal enactments and judicial rulings over choosing or refusing medical interventions
- The origins, growth, and inner dynamics of hospice care
- Government coverage of hospice care
- The ways patients and family members have secured rights to choose the type of care they want
- Physician-assisted suicide
- Descriptions of recently developed and developing initiatives that enhance choice

These themes are visited, revisited, and interwoven into a sweeping and living story. They rise from the contexts of time—from the persons who set them forth, gave the best years of their lives to them, and fought those perceived as adversaries. The subjects of this quest have been suppressed and denied, but they will not go away.

This history walks through the shadows of death. It neither runs nor hides. It explores, reveals, exposes, disturbs, and guides. Against the background of the historical past, the last chapter on developments in the 21st century poses the question, "How shall I face life-threatening illness and the end of my earthly existence?" For caregivers in hospitals, hospices, and homes, it asks, "How should critically ill and dying persons be treated and cared for in ways befitting the worth of each human being and the character, virtues, and capabilities of the healthcare professions?"

1

From Proclamation to Recognition

1605–1772

Long in the womb, the fundamental features of medical palliation—its fetal DNA, so to speak—were fashioned by Francis Bacon (1561–1626). Over the ensuing 165 years, Bacon's proclamation that physicians should enable persons to pass peacefully out of life became a standard, widely recognized feature of medical practice. The fact that "making death easy" would become installed and promoted as a medical imperative by 1770 in one of the premier medical schools of the time attested to its future importance.

Francis Bacon's Revolutionary Proclamation: 1605–1623

Rightly praised for his wide-ranging scholarship and pivotal contributions to philosophy and science, Sir Francis Bacon was the first person in history to commission physicians with the duty to offer and continually improve palliative medical care and treatment for dying persons. His insights regarding death and the components of peaceful dying are prophetic and comprehensive, arising from his impressively conceived intellectual agenda.

With his political fortunes on the rise, Francis Bacon, commonly referred to historically as Lord Verulam,[1] secured his intellectual fame by publishing *Two Books on the Proficiency and Advancement of Learning* in 1605. *Advancement* displayed Bacon's passionate desire to bring about a revolution in human reasoning that would progressively reveal the hidden processes of nature. The dates 1605–1623 indicate that Bacon's convictions with respect to end-of-life care remained intact when he published a greatly expanded edition of *Advancement* in 1623.[2]

Astonishingly, but accurately, Bacon remarked in the concluding paragraph of *Advancement* that he had "made as it were a small Globe" out of "the Intellectual World" of his time.[3] For almost twenty years, Bacon circumnavigated that intellectual world. His explorations extended from the writings of ancient authors to those of notable contemporaries. Upon purging that world from hearsay, faulty reasoning, unsound experiments, and displays of pompous verbosity, he fashioned a globe suited to his "contemplative ends"—the generation of "grounded conclusions" that would bring forth new and profitable discoveries for the good of humanity.[4]

Advancement highlights the dignity and excellence of learning and the manifold ways in which Bacon's reformation of human thought would benefit humankind, relieve the human condition, and abound to the glory of the Creator.[5] The reformation Bacon advanced embraced philosophical logic, the sciences, medicine (physic), mechanical arts, government, the law, theology, rhetoric, athletics, and other divisions of learning such as cosmetics.

For each of the areas he analyzes, Bacon demonstrates that he knows his topics. He exercises his role as a transformative thinker by identifying the "deficiencies" of each of his subject areas. He construes these as omissions, deficits, and inadequacies that should be improved upon and/or remedied by human effort and industry.[6] He adds that some persons will regard these deficiencies as too difficult, if not virtually impossible, to rectify. To such persons, he replies that some of the changes he foresees may have to be accomplished in "a succession of ages ... not within the hour-glass of one man's life." Quoting from the biblical book of Proverbs credited to King Solomon, Bacon adds that only "the slothful person says there is a lion in the path" that makes travel impossible.[7]

In *Advancement* Bacon is not vain or pompous. He is not writing for purposes of glory, pleasure, profit, and superiority, but rather for the purpose of endowing "the human family with new mercies" motivated by charity.[8]

On the Deficiencies of Medicine

The practice of medicine receives detailed attention in Book Two of *Advancement*. Bacon's "perambulation" in that book consists of walking around and sizing up all the areas he explores.[9] His catalogs of deficiencies constitute obligatory programs of action that should be undertaken within all of the areas of human endeavor that he analyzes. His identification of the deficiencies of medicine sets forth an inventory of Bacon's admonitions to physicians—his judgments regarding faults and oversights that should be rectified.

Bacon does not mince words about the deficiencies of the theory and practice of medicine in his time. He begins with sweeping criticisms, the first of which charges physicians with resting on their laurels because they know their desperate patients have no other reasonable treatment alternatives:

> [Physicians] find that mediocrity and excellency in their own art makes no difference in profit or reputation: for men's impatience of diseases, the solicitations of friends, the sweetness of life, and the inducement of hope, make them depend upon physicians with all their defects. But when this is seriously considered, it turns rather to the reproach and the excuse of physicians, who ought not hence to despair, but to use greater diligence.[10]

Other criticisms follow. Physicians profess loyalty to their craft, but do not diligently labor to change it. The efforts of physicians are circular, rather than progressive. "I find great repetition" in what they do, Bacon charges. There is "little new matter" in the books on physic.[11]

Bacon divides physic, or medicine, into three parts, or "offices." For Bacon, the term "office" refers not to a place of business but to a professional duty. The first duty pertains to the preservation of health, the second to the cure of diseases, and the third to the prolongation of life. The first involves how to remain healthy and fend off disease. Bacon charges physicians with writing "unskillfully" about how to do that. No physician, for example, has accented the preservation of health by exercise that protects persons from becoming sick—like walking, horseback riding, and shooting arrows with longbows for maintaining healthy lungs and digestion.[12]

Bacon also writes extensively about the third part of medicine—the prolongation or lengthening of life and resisting "the wasting of age." Prolongation of life at this stage in the history of medicine pertained to extending natural life through better health habits and other matters, not to life prolongation by medical interventions designed to extend life in the face of catastrophic illness and injuries.

Physicians, he charges, confound this third part of medicine with the other two parts due to the false assumption that if diseases are cured, "long life must follow." To rectify the commonly held assumption that lengthening human life is "no capital part of medicine," Bacon published *Historia Vitae et Mortis* (*History of Life and Death*) in 1623. *Historia* thoroughly surveys the healthy effects of foods, drink, exercise, coolness, heat, moisture, dryness and other factors that increase or decrease health and longevity.[13] He regards the duty of doctors in this area as so new and vastly important that he summarized *Historia* in his 1623 expansion of *Advancement of Learning*.[14]

Bacon then turns to the division of medicine that consumed most of the attention of the physicians of his time—their "great pains bestowed" on the cure of diseases. He says that their deficits, faults, and inadequacies are so numerous in this area that he will focus on the "more remarkable" of these deficiencies[15]:

1. The loss of the tradition of Hippocrates, the "father" of the art of medicine, on writing exacting narratives of particular cures associated with particular disease states.
2. A lack of attention to comparative anatomy—the exploration of internal organs in search of the marks and influences of various diseases, which serves as a critical addendum to the profession's grasp of "simple anatomy" respecting the location of organs, muscles, nerves, and bones.
3. Too quickly pronouncing that various diseases are incurable, which delivers patients over to death and can be rectified by searching for cures within the constraints of nature.
4. Mitigation of "the pains and tortures of diseases" (the discussion of which will follow).
5. The deficiency of not having particular medicines for the cure of particular diseases, which should replace the existing practice of using general concoctions for general purposes, such as "opening obstructions."
6. The absence of chemically made medicines that will match the effects of springs and waters impregnated with sulfur, iron, and other compounds.
7. The irrational, vain, and flattering notion that brief and single attempts to

cure—rather than an exacting, carefully observed, and rationally discovered series of curative efforts—will be effective against the power and perseverance of natural diseases.[16]

Near the end of this discussion, Bacon voices another broadside criticism:

To see the daily labors of physicians in their visits, consultations, and prescriptions, one would think that they diligently pursued the cure, and went directly in a certain beaten track about it; but whoever looks attentively into their prescriptions and directions, will find, that the most of what they do is full of uncertainty, wavering, and irresolution, without any certain view or foreknowledge of the course of the cure.[17]

Bacon's Historic Proclamation Concerning Physicians' Care for Dying Persons

In the middle of this list of medicine's major deficiencies—number 4 in the above listing—Bacon issues a historic proclamation concerning the duty of physicians to attend to the needs of dying persons. His text is so laden with meaning and has been so seriously misinterpreted that it is given here in full[18]:

I esteem it likewise to be clearly the office of a physician, not only to restore health, but also to mitigate the pains and torments of diseases; and not only when such mitigation of pain, as of a dangerous symptom, helps and conduces to recovery; but also when, all hope of recovery being gone, it serves only to make a fair and easy passage from life. For it was no small felicity which Augustus Caesar was wont so earnestly to pray for. That same **Euthanasia** was likewise observed in the death of Antoninus Pius, which was not so much like death as like falling into a deep and pleasant sleep.[19] And it is written of Epicurus, that he procured the same for himself. For after his disease was judged desperate, he drowned his stomach and senses with a large draught and ingurgitation of wine; whereupon the epigram was made, "hinc Stygias ebrius hausit aquas" ("He drowned in wine the bitterness of the Stygian water.")[20]

But physicians of our times make a kind of scruple to stay with the patient after the disease is thought past cure, whereas in my judgment, if they would not be wanting to their profession and indeed to humanity, they ought both to acquire the skill, and to bestow the attention whereby the dying person may pass more easily and quietly out of life. This part I call the inquiry concerning outward Euthanasia, or the easy dying of the body (to distinguish it from that Euthanasia regarding the preparation of the soul); and set it down as a desiderata.[21]

The historic significance of these admonitions by Bacon can hardly be overstated. Here he is commissioning physicians to fulfill an office or duty that they are failing to do. They should be mitigating the pains and torments of the diseases of their patients. They should be giving what is now called palliative or comfort care. They should do that for the purposes of enabling some patients to recover from their painful diseases and enabling others with hopelessly fatal diseases "to make a fair and easy passage from life." Bacon focuses on the second of these purposes, and so shall we.

Instead of acquiring the skill and giving due attention to dying persons that will allow them to "pass more easily and quietly out of life," physicians, Bacon charges, are standing at the beds of terminally ill patients scrupulously—that is, properly, cautiously, and reservedly.[22] They ought to get past their scruples and began to do things that will contribute to their profession and "indeed to humanity" itself. They should, Bacon said in 1605, be "assuaging the pains and agonies of death."[23]

The newness of Bacon's proclamation regarding terminal care is underlined by two accents in the above text. First, Bacon constantly appealed to renowned physician writers such as Hippocrates and Galen as he explicated the deficiencies of medicine. But he could not appeal to them as proponents of palliative care for dying persons. So to emphasize the great value of that care, he turned to famed historical figures—Augustus Caesar, Antoninus Pius, and Epicurus[24]—to secure the credibility and beauty of his revolutionary proclamation. These famous persons teach us that dying peacefully is a source of happiness, something to earnestly pray for, something to be sought after with sedatives like wine.

Second, the newness of Bacon's proclamation is registered by his assigning it a Greek name—outward or physical *euthanasia* (*eu for* good or noble, and *thanatos for* death), which he distinguishes "from that *Euthanasia* regarding the preparation of the soul." Francis Bacon thereby introduces the word "euthanasia" into the English language as a fitting and memorable title for calm and suffering-free death for fatally ill persons.[25] The text of *Advancement* Bacon wrote in 1605 shows that he adopted the term "euthanasia" from Augustus Caesar, who used it to refer to an easy death to be longed for.[26]

Bacon is a world removed from the modern meaning of euthanasia, which refers to physicians taking steps to actively end human life.[27] One might try to argue that Bacon's reference to Epicurus' drinking a large draught of wine indicated an act of suicide. That's not found in his text, however, which says Epicurus used wine to drown out the bitterness of his feelings when he knew his disease was desperate. The modern meaning of euthanasia did not emerge until after the 1870s, 250 years after Francis Bacon.[28] The chapters that follow will indicate how Bacon's understanding of the phrase "outward euthanasia" defined the purpose of palliative care over the ensuing two and a half centuries.

Euthanasia Regarding the Preparation of the Soul

Neither in the preceding text nor, apparently, in any of his other writings does Bacon discuss the "euthanasia" or calm dying associated with the preparation of the soul. Indeed, his brief reference to that dimension of peaceful dying at the end of the above extract appears to assume that his readers already knew what that preparation included. In fact, books full of counsel about proper and peaceful spiritual dying filled the shelves of homes and bookshops in Bacon's age. These books describe and promote deathbed rituals and experiences of Roman Catholics, Calvinists, and members of the Church of England (Anglicans).[29] Two notable best sellers included the Calvinist counsels of Thomas Becon, *Sycke Mans Salve*, first published in 1561 and published in 18 editions from 1561 to 1632,[30] and William Perkins' *A Salve for a Sick Man, or a Treatise of ... the Right Way to Die*, published in 1595, followed by subsequent editions.[31]

Importantly, Bacon's personal religious beliefs reflect how he prepared his soul for calm dying. Bacon's mother, Lady Anne Bacon, actively supported the Puritan or Calvinist Reformation tradition of her time, and Bacon remained loyal to the Anglican church.[32] He believed that all human hope should be "bestowed upon the heavenly life to come." Upon discussing "felicity, beatitude, or the highest good," he says, instructed by the Christian faith, that persons should "embrace the felicity" of hope in the world to come.[33] The last paragraph of Bacon's long, carefully crafted "A Confession of Faith" describes the eternal blessings of faithful believers. While his confession draws upon previous Protestant confessions, it bears the marks of Bacon's natural philosophy, especially his interest in the cosmic order and laws of nature. First published in 1641, it was declared by his personal chaplain to be representative of "the Faith wherein he resigned his [last] breath."[34]

How do these perspectives about "euthanasia regarding the preparation of the soul" relate to the "outward euthanasia" provided by physicians? Bacon does not discuss their connections. He also does not discuss what should be included in the attention physicians should give to patients without hope of recovery. He nevertheless maintains that physicians' attention, combined with their medical skills to enable patients to die peacefully, will both enhance the profession of medicine and contribute to the human good. He also appears to believe that easing physical anguish and granting personal attention to patients without hope of recovery are essential preconditions for enabling them to depart life in spiritual peace.

Yet Bacon explicitly links the physical and spiritual dimensions of good dying together under the term "euthanasia" and thereby views both as essential components of good and peaceful dying for persons beset with fatal diseases. He thereby depicts the roles of physicians, clergy, and family members as complementary, a vision that would also be prophetic for ensuing centuries.

Bacon fervently believed that good deaths are possible. He coined the term "euthanasia" to indicate that death can and should be good if, when persons are approaching the end of life, their distressing symptoms are eased and their souls are at peace.

The Naturalness of Death

Francis Bacon knew that calm dying is undermined if death is feared. Not one to leave this essential component of peaceful dying unexplored and undefended, Bacon reflected at length on the meaning of death in human life. In 1612 he crafted an essay titled "Of Death," which he expanded in 1625. As opposed to unwarranted fear, he maintains in this essay that death should be accepted as natural and explores why death is feared and why that fear is unwarranted. He begins with often-quoted words[35]:

> Men fear Death, as children fear to go into the dark, and as that natural fear in children is increased with tales, so is the fear of death. Certainly the contemplation of death, as the wages of sin[36] and passage into another world, is holy and religious; but the fear of it, as a tribute due to nature is weak.

Two fascinating topics are found in this quote—that the fear of death is "increased with tales" and that attributing the fear of death to the natural order is rationally weak, not strong. The tales Bacon has in mind are many. Some are superstitious stories found in friars' books on punishing one's body for greater holiness.[37] According to Bacon, one of these books calls for pressing and torturing the ends of one's fingers for the purpose of imagining what the pains of death are like. Other tall tales are found in "the trappings of death that scare us more than death itself": the groans and convulsions, discolored faces, weeping friends, and black mourning clothes of funerals that "make death seem terrible."[38] These tales haunt unschooled and unreflective persons who are incapable of discovering ways to counter overwhelming fears of death.[39]

Bacon brings his learning to bear on the second of these topics—his contention that the fear of death "as a tribute due to nature is weak." What he means by that phrase is that only a rationally weak case can be made for the notion that the fear of death is an inherent and dominating force in natural human experience. Many other passions and feelings, Bacon argues, far outweigh fears of death. Revenge puts the fear of death to flight. Love often slights death. "Honor aspireth to it. Grief flieth to it." Even pity, the weakest or most delicate of human affections, has provoked many to kill themselves. Numerous subjects of Ortho the emperor,[40] for example, killed themselves out of compassion for their emperor's slaying himself. Other persons wish to die out of weariness of having to do the same thing over and over again.[41]

Furthermore, courageous persons often face approaching death with little or no alteration in the way they have always felt and lived:

> They appear to be the same till the last instant. Augustus Caesar[42] died with a compliment: "Livia, conjugii nostri memor, vive et vale" ["Fairwell, Livia, and forget not our married life."] Vespasian[43] in a jest, sitting upon the toilet, "Ut puto Deus fio" ["I suppose I am on the point of becoming a god."] Galba[44] with a sentence: "Feri, siex re sit pouuli Romani" ["Strike if it be for the benefit of the Roman people"], holding forth his neck. And the like.

Bacon contends that historical knowledge, courage, and wisdom teach us that death is not terrible. Indeed, death may be counted as a gift of nature that "opens the gate to good fame and extinguishes envy." Persons who live in fear of death end up suffering continually. We can choose to live in fear and misery or accept death as inescapable in full knowledge that "it is as natural to die as to be born." This awareness commissions us to set aside irrational and overplayed fears for greater things:

> He that dies in the pursuit of some great cause is like one that is wounded in the heat of battle; who, for the time, scarce feels the hurt. And therefore a mind fixed and bent upon something that is good averts the pangs of death. But above all, believe it, the sweetest song is, "Nunc dimittis" ["Lord, now let thy servant depart (in peace)."][45]; when a man has attained worthy ends and expectations.[46]

In conclusion, Sir Francis Bacon believed that physicians should assist persons approaching the end of life to experience "a fair and easy passage from life." Accomplishing that aim rests on three conditions: that physicians accept and fulfill the professional duty of providing skilled and attentive care to free dying persons from pain and other distressing symptoms; that patients, with help from clergy, family members, and personal contemplation, should prepare their souls for calm dying; and that persons must overcome irrational fears of death that undermine peaceful dying. Predicated on these three essential and achievable goals, death will be experienced as good, in accord with the original meaning of euthanasia, which Bacon coined, described, and defended.

Doctors at Deathbeds

The historical record regarding physicians' care for dying persons during the first 165 years after Francis Bacon's initial proclamation is episodic but nevertheless forward moving. The examples that follow make clear that certain generalizations about the history of palliative care during these years are questionable. These generalizations include assertions that only clergy attended to persons who were deemed to have incurable diseases and that physicians would shun such care[47]; that the notion that care of dying persons "became a medical concern" only in the 19th century[48]; and that persons did not begin to name a spiritually triumphant passage from life "euthanasia" until the early 19th century.[49]

In addition to the historical discussion that follows, these generalizations are refuted by the recent study of Ian Mortimer, which shows that "religious and medical strategies for coping with severe and terminal illness coexisted with and complemented one another throughout the seventeenth century."[50] They are also proven erroneous by the popular, frequently reprinted, earlier-mentioned 17th- and 18th-century religious manuals filled with spiritual and practical guidance on holy and peaceful dying. In *A Salve for a Sick Man*, William Perkins argues against the widely used practice that the physician "is first sent for, and the minister comes when a man is half dead."[51] In *The Saint's Everlasting Rest*, first published in 1650, Richard Baxter says, "Physicians are much about dying men." And he urges physicians to teach those nearing death "both how to live and how to die, and give them some physic for their souls, as you do for their bodies."[52] In *The Afflicted Man's Companion*, John Willison says that physicians should indeed be called, but that elder church members and ministers should not be called "in the last place" when the sick person is "at the point of death; and scarce capable to speak or hear." It is necessary to employ physicians, but they "must not be trusted to the exclusion of God."[53]

Searches in history of medicine collections enable us to identify two especially notable 17th-century physicians—Thomas Browne and Theophile Bonet—who take us to the beds of dying persons, introduce us to the ways dying persons were treated and cared for, and speak forthrightly about death.

Thomas Browne's Care of a Dying Patient and Contemplations About Death: 1643–1672

Thomas Browne graduated from Pembroke College in Oxford University in 1626, after which he studied medicine in a number of Continental universities and received his MD from Leiden University in Holland in 1633. He began practicing medicine in Norwich, England, in 1637 and continued his medical career until his death in 1682. His reputation was such that when King Charles II, accompanied by the Royal Court, visited Norwich in 1671, the king honored Browne with a knighthood.

Browne's renown rests on his consummate crafting of English literature, his philosophical and theological deliberations on human life and death, and his lifetime of reflection on what is now called the medical humanities—the interconnections among medicine, literature, theology, philosophy, and social custom. Eighteenth- and 19th-century literary romantics such as Samuel Taylor Coleridge and Ralph Waldo Emerson embraced Browne as a kindred spirit. One of the great founders of modern medicine, Sir William Osler (1849–1919), kept Browne's *Religio Medici* (*The Religion of a Physician*) ever available. A copy of the book was even placed on the purple pall covering Osler's coffin at his funeral.[54]

Extending the tradition of Francis Bacon, but without Bacon's intellectual acuity and power, Browne held that humans cannot "properly believe" what they hold to be true without reasoned arguments and empirical experiments.[55] Browne's widely purchased and re-edited *Enquiries* made lengthy excursions into what is now regarded as popular science in the form of exposing and debunking false and dubious beliefs of his time. Drawing upon a vast number of authors from antiquity to his own era, he refuted beliefs and myths about gold, ashes, stones, ginger, mistletoe, almonds, horses, beavers, wolves, deer, storks, pigeons, toads, vipers, spiders, human anatomy, swimming, sneezing, and other matters. He also conducted experiments with static electricity and magnetism.[56]

In a beautifully crafted letter Browne first mentions that, like other "consumptive persons," his patient did not feel that he was dying. Not wanting to upset his patient, he says that when he visited him,

> I was bold to tell [his friends] who had not let fall all hopes of his Recovery, That in my sad Opinion he was not likely to behold a Grasshopper, much less to pluck another Fig; and in no long time after seemed to discover that odd mortal Symptom in him not mentioned by Hippocrates, that is, to lose his own Face and look like some of his near Relations; for he maintained not his proper Countenance, but looked like his Uncle.

With gifted language Brown is saying that the young man would probably not live long enough to experience summer. Demonstrating his observation skills, he also notes an additional sign or precursor of death not mentioned in Hippocrates'[57] classic list of the signs of impending death, called *facies Hippocratica* (Hippocratic face). Francis Bacon had summarized them well:

> The immediate signs which precede death are great restlessness and tossing of the body, fumbling of the hands, hard clutching and grasping, teeth firmly set, a hollow voice, trembling of the lower lip, pallor of the face, and confused memory, loss of speech, cold sweats ... alternation of the whole countenance (as the nose becomes sharp, the eyes hollow, and the cheeks sinking in) ... coldness of the extremities ... thick breathing, falling of the lower jaw, and the like.[58]

Browne correctly predicted his patient's early death. And he voiced his regret at not being able to extend the young man's life. Yet Browne and all those surrounding the young man's bedside were comforted by

> his soft Departure, which was scarce an Expiration; and his End not unlike his Beginning, when the salient Point [of death] scarce affords a sensible motion, and his Departure so like unto Sleep, that he scarce needed the civil Ceremony of closing his Eyes ... his Departure was so easy, that we might justly suspect his Birth was of another nature.[59]

Browne does not describe what he had done to contribute to his patient's "soft Departure." But Browne knew that describing the young man's peaceful death to his friend was comforting, and he is personally pleased that his attendance at the bedside contributed to a shared ideal of peaceful dying.

In accordance with widely held convictions of the time and with the admonitions of Francis Bacon, this patient with consumption had prepared for the euthanasia of his soul. Browne's description reveals how he intimately knew his patients:

> Not to fear Death, nor desire it ... to be dissolved, and be with Christ, was his dying ditty.... To be content with Death may be better than to desire it: a miserable Life may make us wish for Death, but a virtuous one to rest in it; which is the advantage of those ... who looking on Death not only as the sting, but as ... the Horizon and Isthmus between this Life and a better ... do contentedly submit unto.... Necessity.[60]

At the end of his letter Browne offers a window into his personal views of death, in keeping with how he counseled others. Time flees like a shadow, so "live like a neighbor unto Death." By thoughts and actions, unite life here with that which is to come, for "He who thus ordereth the Purposes of this Life, will never be far from the next; and is in some manner already in it."[61]

Browne's greatest work, *Religio Medici*, first published in 1643, is a book of wide-ranging contemplation, musings, and confessions about his religious, philosophical, medical, and personal beliefs and experiences. He wears his feelings about these and other topics on his sleeve. He does not hide behind cloaks of professionalism, religious orthodoxy, or conventional cultural mores.

Browne is thoroughly acquainted with death, and the pages of *Religio* are filled with his musings about it. He writes candidly about the structures and frailty of the human body, the limits and flaws of medical practice, and ways to overcome fears of death. Concerning the body's frailties, he says, "I ... have examined the parts of man, and know upon what tender filaments that Fabrick hangs ... and considering the thousand doors that lead to death doe thanke my God that we can die but once."[62] He has raked through the bowels of the deceased and continually observed anatomies, skeletons, and cadavers. As a physician, he is "not only ashamed, but heartily sorry" that so many diseases are incurable and therefore beyond the reach of his medical art, to which he is loyal for the sake of humanity.[63] He distances himself from the "sordid and un–Christian desires" of members of his profession who "secretly implore and wish for" plagues, famines, malignant influences, and unseasonably cold winters that will enable them to profit by treating expanding numbers of sick persons. He'd rather become sick himself than wish sicknesses upon others. When he cannot cure his patients, he shuns the thought that he is making an "honest living" by accepting payment for his endeavors.[64]

Browne's medical practice made him so intimate with death that he continually strove to come to terms with human mortality. Death molded Browne's understanding of the world, which he says is not an inn to be lived in, but a hospital to die in. When we labor against death, "we all labour against our owne cure, for death is the cure of all diseases. There is no ... universall remedy I know of but [death]; which, though nauseous to queasier stomachs, yet to prepared appetites is Nector ... a pleasant portion of immortality."[65]

Browne is more ashamed of death than afraid of it—ashamed because it can disgrace our natures. In a brief period of time dying can disfigure us to the point of startling our nearest friends, our spouse, and our children. Showing no respect for human death, birds and beasts of the field will prey upon the mortal remains of human beings. He is not ashamed, he says, "of the anatomy of my parts," and he cannot "accuse nature for playing the bungler in any part of me," or accuse himself "for contracting any shameful disease." Like all mortal beings, Browne considers himself as a "wholesome a morsel for the wormes as any."[66]

Concerning dying and death, Thomas Browne was not given to euphemisms or words found in contemporary sympathy cards. More than any other influence, his unorthodox religious convictions enabled him to wrestle openly with the haunting realities of human sickness and mortality that he dealt with in his medical practice. As stated earlier, those with queasy stomachs will fear death, but those who possess the "pleasant potion of immortality" will view death as sweet nectar. Brown asserts that he does not "dote on life or convulse and tremble at the name of death."[67]

Browne did not think that death is merely the inescapable final chapter of life. He believed, rather, that death was ever-present within life—within life because by sleeping we experience half of what it means to die. Through sleep we experience "a middle and moderating point between life and death." So when Browne lay down to sleep, he bid "halfe adiew to the world."

> Sleepe is a death, O make me try,
> By sleeping [know] what it is to die.[68]

Theophile Bonet's Guidelines for Palliative Care: 1683

Except for his historic contributions to pathology, Theophile Bonet (1620–1689) is scarcely appreciated. He came from a medical family, received his MD from Bologna at the age of 23, became renowned as a medical practitioner in the Republic of Geneva, and, even after becoming deaf at about the age of 50, produced an impressive number of medical works.[69] Based on 30 years of medical practice, and some 3,000 postmortem examinations by himself and other physicians, Bonet published his 1,700-page *Sepulchretum sive anatomia*, which Geovanni Battista Morgagni (1682–1771), the founder of modern anatomical pathology, praised as extremely useful.[70] Breaking with medical tradition, Bonet's postmortem dissections enabled him to classify diseases in relation to particular anatomical pathologies. This contributed to a rational system of diagnosis and treatment, which became revolutionary when Morgagni and others linked pathological findings to the symptoms of patients suffering from specific disease conditions.

Far less known and appreciated is Bonet's *Mercurius compitalitius*, named for Mercury, the right-guiding Roman god, and published in Latin in 1683 and then in English in 1684 and 1686 under the title *A Guide to the Practical Physician*. Book XX of that English publication is titled "The Office of a Physician," which discusses 63 topics on medical ethics and decorum; patient behavior; and medical diagnosis, prognosis, and practice guidelines. Based on Bonet's spending some forty years in curing the sick and drawing upon the writings of notable physician authors, "The Office" is a captivating window into the practice of medicine. It describes in detail the remedies being used, the importance of empirical experience combined with knowledge of the curative treatments of the age, and recommendations for how to relate to patients in all matters—from the frequencies of physician visits to rules of consultation, to how the medicines of the times should be used, to stories about determining when patients are faking sickness.[71]

In many respects, Bonet's *Guide* is a precursor to the historic Code of Medical Ethics composed by Thomas Percival in 1803. The fact that Bonet's *Guide* was quickly translated into other languages, as well as republished, testifies to its widely valued use as a manual of advice for medical practitioners.

Momentously, Theophile Bonet set forth his carefully considered views about how fatally ill persons should be related to, cared for, and treated. He first notes that many physicians of his time "bid adieu to their Patients" when patients display "the Hippocratical Signs of Death" (described in the discussion of Thomas Browne above). According to Bonet, physicians commonly abandon patients who manifest late stages of dying because practitioners fear they will expose their art and medicines as ineffective.[72]

Bonet disagrees with such abandonment. First, he has witnessed "several [patients] at the point of death, who have been given over by Physicians [as dead], and yet have recovered."[73] The strength of nature manifest in the human body is admirable. Oftentimes when physicians believe that patients are oppressed by disease, such that they appear to be "knocked down dead" and unable to defend themselves, for mysterious reasons they will rally against death, the "Triumphant Enemy" of humankind. These "Unexpected Events have convinced us, that as long as there is Life, there may be hopes, [so] we ought not to despair." It follows that the physician should be doubtful of his prognosis, "unless there be most certain and infallible signs of death. Let him be moderate in his promises: Yet let him always give hopes [for] Health, than foretell certain Death."[74]

Second, one must consider the physician's reputation with respect to his soundness of judgment. If the practicing physician gives up on the care and treatment of dying patients, and the patient recovers, "as he often does either by chance or Nature, the Physician incurs infamy." But "if he give hopes of Health, and Death does follow, the Disgrace is not so great; because many things might happen," including the patient's contracting some new disease.[75]

Third, physicians should not abandon dying patients out of concern for their own religious reputations. To abandon the bedsides of dying persons can disgrace the physician with a reputation of "impiety," the displaying of a lack of faith, hope, and charity to religious patients and their kindred. In contrast, "it is a Pious thing ... though death, or some incurable Disease be upon a Man, while the Patient has his Understanding entire, to comfort him, put him in hopes, and, as much as may be [possible], to assuage his Disease by Remedies."[76]

And fourth, attending to dying patients—even those who appear to be close to death—is in keeping with the physician's duty to prolong human life. For Bonet, the key to prolongation is found in the last phrase of the previous quote: the assuaging of the patient's fatal disease condition by means of remedies. The remedies he has in mind are mostly palliative measures that will ease terminally ill patients' symptoms and suffering and, by so doing, extend their lives. That is little short of revolutionary and takes us beyond the attention and care of dying persons advanced by Francis Bacon. Indeed, Bonet's association of palliative measures with extending human life has been welcomed as a surprising finding in the 21st century—over 325 years after Bonet discussed it at length.[77]

Theophile Bonet's discussion of remedies that are both life-extending and palliative is found in Book I of his *A Guide to the Practical Physician* under the subtitle "Agonia, or Pangs of Death: How persons at the point of Death are to be Revived." Warm baths and potions of spirituous liquors will soothe and extend the lives of patients with consumption, scurvy and other diseases. Persons "choked by suffocating inflammations" or whose lungs are "choaked by a cold viscidity, glutinuous or sticky matter" should be turned on their sides in order for the phlegm or mucous to run out of their mouths. The patient's head must be raised and shaken a little to make viscid matter descend. When death "agony" (that is, a rattling in the throat) occurs and is accompanied by scarcely any breathing, poultices (medicated mushes) or hot sand can be applied to the throat and chest. A small draught of warm spirit of wine with oil of almonds restored a man of seventy, Bonet testifies.[78]

Bonet also spoke plainly about ethical guidelines for physician's relationships with dying patients. Convinced that his young patient with consumption would soon die, Thomas Browne revealed that prognosis not to his patient, but rather to his patient's friends. In contrast, Bonet instructs his readers with a differing set of ethical duties. If a physician is convinced that the patient is manifesting "most certain and infallible signs of death,"

> I make no question, but a Physician ought plainly to foretell the Patient of his Death, when he desires to know the Event of his Disease. For there are both Political and Theological Reasons, for which I think it good that the Patient should know the event of his Disease: And a Physician has no reason, to deceive his Patient, especially when [the patient] is sincere, and willing to know the truth.[79]

These are powerful, unquestioned convictions on Bonet's part. The contrast between Browne's and Bonet's practices foreshadow clashing convictions over the ethics of truth telling to dying patients that would continue for another 275 years.

Equally noteworthy, Bonet holds that "it is the duty of an ingenuous Physician to instruct his Patient, and not to order him, what must be done, till by informing [the patient] he had persuaded him" about what "is expedient to be done." Bonet adds that persuasion based on information imparted to the patient makes the patient "more willingly obey" the physician's recommended course of action.[80] He could never have known that his convictions concerning the duty of physicians to inform and persuade their patients to accept practitioners' recommendations would not become officially recognized for centuries, when they were finally preserved in laws requiring the patient's fully informed consent and emphasized in courses on medical ethics.

Samuel Bard's *Discourse on the Duties of a Physician* (1769)

Samuel Bard (1742–1821), one of the most notable American physicians during and after the years of the American Revolution, delivered his *Discourse on the Duties of a Physician* to the first-ever MD graduates of King's College in New York. The Medical School of King's College was largely established through Bard's zeal and devotion. He served as its first professor in the theory and practice of physic (medicine). Having received his MD from the University of Edinburgh in 1765, Bard brought the ideals of systematic medical education back to America, where the "prevailing ignorance" of too many medical practitioners "cannot be contested."[81] By an act of Congress, King's College was rechartered as Columbia College in 1784.[82]

Bard's *Discourse* has been identified as the first tract on medical ethics in America.[83] He celebrates the establishment of a sorely needed medical school, outlines the duties and moral virtues of physicians, and ends with a plea for the establishment of a public hospital. This hospital will treat workers and their families who live on subsistence wages, contribute to the safety and welfare of the whole New York community, and become a training ground for future physicians.

His discussion of end-of-life care is situated within a broad vision of the duties of doctors: a life-long commitment to learning, the preeminent value of preserving life, sentiments of tenderness and humanity, the "unspeakable Pleasure of doing good," avoidance of secret nostrums and panaceas, and opposition to multiplying prescriptions for personal gain.[84]

Samuel Bard does not single out palliative care as a special or neglected physician's duty. He assumes, instead, that it is a regular feature of medical practice and that the new graduates have been taught how to care for dying patients, including what to do to relieve their painful symptoms. Surely part of symptom relief included opium, because Bard's MD graduation thesis argued that opium was a sedative, not (according to received opinion) a stimulant.[85]

He speaks about some of the moral questions inherent in attentive care for dying patients and their family members. Physicians should display their apprehensions of the mortal dangers that patients face through assiduous attention to the relief of their symptoms. They should not utter "any harsh or brutal expressions" about the patient's danger of dying. Nor should they ever seek to "buoy up a dying Man with groundless Expectations of Recovery." At best, the latter is well-intended deception, but too often it is a groundless expression of optimism that arises from "baser Motives of Lucre and Avarice." These motives are cruel and criminal, because the stroke of death is always felt most severely when it is not expected, which leaves families confused and distressed.[86] These moral guidelines by Bard manifest indirect truth-revealing.

Lastly, Bard holds that "the grim Tyrant" of death can usually be "disarmed of his Terrors." Even for timid and apprehensive persons, the key to the disarming is familiarity. Fears of death can be eased by frequent meditation on its meaning and certitude, by arguments of philosophy, and by the hopes and promises of religion. Bard lists these methods cryptically, and present-day readers are left to wonder what Bard would say about the respective (and possibly interconnecting) roles of physicians, family members, and clergy who seek to ease the fears of persons facing the end of life.

While we are not privy to details of Samuel Bard's personal care of dying patients, nor to what he taught medical students, we can be sure that Bard and the generations of students he taught offered symptomatic relief and tender care for these patients and their family members. Perhaps he inherited this palliative care tradition from his father, a famous, well-healed New York physician who passed his practice to his son. Perhaps his views were shaped by his MD training at the University of Edinburgh, which, as we will soon see through the work of John Gregory, became a beacon for the convictions of Francis Bacon.

Bard became the personal physician of George Washington, was associated with King's College/Columbia College for forty years, served for ten years as the president of the College of Physicians and Surgeons in the City of New York, authored several medical publications, and received honorary degrees and memberships from Princeton College and the College of Physicians in Philadelphia.[87] His *Discourse* shows that palliative care for dying patients received attention from physicians in the American colonies.

John Gregory on "Making Death Easy": A Medical Imperative by 1770

John Gregory (1724–1773) received an MD from King's College in Aberdeen, Scotland, in 1746 and became professor of the practice of medicine first in Aberdeen (1754–1764), and then in Edinburgh from 1766 (the year after Samuel Bard graduated) through 1773. Gregory's philosophical pedigree included continued intellectual and personal engagement with the great Scottish Enlightenment figures of the time—Thomas Reid (1710–1796), Francis Hutcheson, David Hume (1711–1776) and others.[88]

In his influential *Lectures on the Duties and Qualifications of a Physician*, first published in 1770, Gregory divided the practice of medicine into four parts, or branches: "the art of preserving health, of prolonging life, of curing diseases, and making death easy."[89] These four branches are expressly drawn from Francis Bacon's three parts of medicine. Bacon had incorporated Gregory's fourth branch (making death easy) within his discussion of the third division of medicine—the curing of diseases. By separating "making death easy" from "curing diseases," Gregory took the liberty of reordering Bacon's analysis. Gregory's outline clearly reflects the spirit and content of Bacon's divisions, but highlighting "making death easy" as its own, distinct area of medical practice further underlines the importance of palliative care.

Gregory's lectures to medical students display his profound indebtedness to and virtual awe-struck admiration for Bacon, whom Gregory thought surely had to have been a physician:

> Let me take this opportunity of recommending to your serious study the writings of Lord Bacon, who of all men possessed, perhaps, the most enlarged and penetrating genius. He has explained the method of acquiring knowledge, and promoting science, with incomparable judgment and perspicuity. He has likewise left us some beautiful specimens of true philosophical induction. Lord Bacon has enlarged views of medicine, and of its deficiencies, and of the proper method of supplying them, as perhaps any physician who ever wrote.[90]

Gregory's *Lectures* reflect a changing era of medical practice, an era that included new hospitals devoted to the treatment of the sick in England, Europe, and their colonies; new medical societies and periodicals; and hospital-related medical schools with lectures in anatomy, chemistry, botany, materia medica, and clinical medicine. His lectures were carefully written, then read to his medical audiences.[91] For many years Gregory and his influential physician colleague William Cullen (1710–1790) alternated chairs in the theory and practice of medicine at the University of Edinburgh.[92]

The therapies used throughout the 18th century were eclectic—traditional reliance on bloodletting, purging, and blistering; milder therapeutic schemas that objected to these practices; increased use of opium; and the discovery of a few effective remedies, such as citrus fruit juices for scurvy and digitalis for heart conditions.[93]

Like Theophile Bonet, John Gregory criticized physicians who abandoned dying patients. "Let me here exhort you," he said, "against the custom of some physicians, who leave their patients when their life is despaired of, and when it is no longer decent to put them to farther expense." Doing that even when death is certain betrays a duty of doctors that is equal to the duty of their curing diseases: "It is as much the business of a physician to alleviate pain, and to smooth the avenues of death, when [death is] unavoidable as [it is] to cure diseases."[94]

This assertion that "making death easy" is just as important as the curing of diseases is a staggering association by Gregory. It manifests his profound humanitarianism, whereby the values of human beings are intrinsic to their status as living and feeling creatures, not to their social or financial or political or professional status and fame. It also reflects what many physicians of the time were either doing or believed they should be doing and thereby evoked wide sympathy and agreement on the part of students and practitioners. It illustrates Gregory's belief that renewed medical attention should be given to the ways palliative treatments and opiates can be used to alleviate pain, thirst, wakefulness, and other symptoms, and, by doing so, extend human life.[95]

Unlike Francis Bacon, Gregory does not compartmentalize the good death of the physical body on the part of physicians as separate from the good death of the soul. He argues that physicians should contribute to the emotional care of patients and their families. "Even in cases where his skill as a physician can be of no further avail, his presence and assistance as a friend may be agreeable and useful, both to the patient and his nearest relations."[96] Physicians should not withdraw when a clergyman is called to assist the patient in his spiritual concerns. Indeed, "it is decent and fit that they should mutually understand one another and act together" to enable persons to die peacefully.

> The conversation of a clergyman of cheerful piety and good sense, in whom a sick man confides, may sometimes be of much more consequence in composing the anguish of his mind, and the agitation of his spirits, than any medicine; but a gloomy and indiscrete enthusiast[97] may do great hurt, may terrify the patient, and contribute to shorten a life that might otherwise be saved.

So, for Gregory, the overarching aim of making death easy and extending life as long as possible calls for prescribed duties on the part of both physicians and clergy working together.[98]

While Gregory harshly judges emotionally and theologically unbridled clergy, he is equally critical of what he deemed anti- or a-religious excesses of physicians who foist their beliefs on dying patients. Physicians who disbelieve in an afterlife are as duty-bound to conceal their beliefs from patients as they are obligated to keep from infecting patients with some mortal disease. It is particularly "barbarous" to seek to deprive expiring patients of their last emotional and spiritual support and thus "blast the only surviving comfort of those who have taken a last farewell of every sublunary [terrestrial] pleasure." Actually, that was the mild side of Gregory's criticisms of practitioners who lack sensitivity with respect to their patients' faith. He asserted that their insensitivity "proceeds from an ungovernable levity, or criminal vanity, that forgets all the ties of morals, decency, and good Manners."[99]

John Gregory struggled with the ethics of telling or not telling dying patients about the seriousness of their medical conditions. Thomas Browne did not seem to worry about the rightness or wrongness of keeping his prognosis of early death from his young patient while revealing that prognosis boldly to his friends. Theophile Bonet defended the wisdom of plainly telling dying patients when he thought they would die if they wanted to know the truth. But fearful that such news would prove to be fatal to dangerously and terminally ill patients, Gregory viewed what should or should not be said as a "painful office ... one of the most disagreeable duties of the profession."[100]

To alleviate some of that pain, Gregory sets forth several options depending on the patient's and family's circumstances. If the doctor thinks that telling an extremely ill patient about the dangerousness of his conditions may keep the patient from recovering, lying or fudging on the truth can be "both justifiable and necessary." If the doctor knows that a dangerously sick man has not yet made out his will, which is pivotal to the "future happiness of his family," the physician should "in the most prudent and gentle manner ... give a hint to the patient of his real danger," as well as encourage him to make out his will. But in all cases the physicians must reveal "the real situation" to the patient's relatives, giving them the chance to call upon the assistance of others to help the man fulfill his duties to his family.[101]

Gregory's options are predicated on medical paternalism—the duty of physicians to make decisions for patients and family members based on physicians' moral duties to protect persons from harm and to display beneficence so as to maximize well-being. That authority is inseparable from the practitioners' experience and expertise in presaging the signs of death, palliating distressing and painful symptoms, possessing skills that can prolong human life, and believing that emotional terrors will shorten life.[102] Gregory held that the "government of a physician over his patient should undoubtedly be great."[103]

To put Gregory's medically paternalistic directives into historical and ethical perspective, he believed that the emotional-psychological bonds between physicians and patients are great enough for physicians to influence the health of patients by their presence and counsel. On the one hand, physicians can have what is now called a positive, curative placebo effect on their patients. On the other hand, their communication can produce a negative, nocebo effect that will undermine a patient's health and longevity of life.

John Gregory's attention to palliative care and his devotion to teaching and inspiring generations of students to attend to the needs of dying persons and their families were symbolized by his own death. Upon dying, probably during his sleep and without any sign of discomfort, Gregory's death was described as "a perfect *Euthanasia*."[104]

Concluding Perspectives

The 400-year quest for a good death began momentously in 1605 when Francis Bacon first challenged physicians with the duty of enabling dying persons "to make a fair and easy passage from life." The long journey over the ensuing 165 years displays how Bacon's initial challenge became a legacy in the thinking and practices of Thomas Browne, Theophile Bonet, Samuel Bard, and John Gregory. Gregory in particular emerged as a pivotal figure who expanded upon Bacon's proclamation and then, as if it were a torch, passed it on to future generations of physicians.

Bacon's prophetic genius became the foundation upon which many would build. By the mid–1770s some physicians were linking treatments that would mitigate the pains and torments of terminal illness with remedies that were also life-prolonging. By that time physician caregivers recognized that end-of-life care raised ethical concerns about truth telling versus concealing and deception. In addition, physicians recognized the importance of dying persons' relatives. Gregory also expressly combined Bacon's two types of euthanasia—the physical and spiritual dimensions of good death. Palliative care and comfort now included emotional care on the part of physicians, as well as interconnected relationships between physicians and clergy.

The legacy of physician-assisted peaceful dying has been interpreted by some as a means by which physicians secured greater power and prestige, whereby "From womb to tomb, the empire of medicine was steadily extending itself."[105] That intent betrays the story of the search for a good death in this chapter. Francis Bacon, Thomas Browne, Samuel Bard, and Theophile Bonet spoke and acted out of compassion for the pains and plights of dying persons. They spoke of death as natural and inevitable, and they considered palliative care a professional duty that would ease physical symptoms as a precondition for peaceful dying.

Because Gregory believed that the "government" of physicians over patients should be great, he might be charged with seeking power and prestige. That charge is questionable. Gregory held that the governance of physicians is often disagreeable and painful—one that should be shouldered for the purpose of extending the lives of dangerously ill patients and protecting them from the shock of learning about impending death. Gregory also believed that physicians should share deathbed responsibilities with clergy and patients' family members. He and other physicians of the time were seeking to abide by the vision of Francis Bacon: peaceful death is something worth praying for and assisting persons to experience good death promotes the good of humanity.

2

Minute Details and Codified Conduct

1789–1825

Comparable to how explorers sometimes discover strikingly new places and peoples, physicians in quest of enabling persons to die peacefully discovered new features of palliative care during the fifty-five years after John Gregory first published his *Lectures.* Gregory held that medical care toward the end of life should be a fourth dimension of medical practice. Left unexplored was the early mapping of that dimension.

The story of these fifty-five years begins with the American physician Benjamin Rush (1746–1813), whose fame matches or exceeds that of any other physician-professor-politician-social reformer in American history. It then proceeds to John Ferriar (1761–1815), a prominent physician and social reformer in Manchester, England, who published the first full-scale article on care for terminally ill persons. Ferriar recognized the importance and rarity of his article titled "Of the Treatment of the Dying." He says, "There is hardly any subject … more impressive … than the consideration of death," but "perhaps there is none less studied in its minute details."[1]

This era ends with the contributions of Ferrier's colleague, Thomas Percival (1740–1804), whose carefully crafted *Code of Medical Ethics* was published in 1803. Percival's enormously influential code established the care of dying persons as a full-fledged moral duty of physicians.[2] Within his code, he outlined essential components of physicians' palliative care duties. One of those components required the physician to become a "minister of hope," which, to Percival, meant that physicians should not only not tell patients about their grim prognoses but also, at times, deceive patients who ask about the severity of their medical conditions.[3] Percival's friend, the Reverend Thomas Gisborne (1758–1846), sought to convince Percival to alter his position. Their differing positions on truth telling rested on reasoned debate, not just position-taking. Their disagreements foreshadow how end-of-life care and treatment would be laden with contentious ethical concerns.

Benjamin Rush on Duties of Physicians with Patients Struggling Between Life and Death

Benjamin Rush's medical career unfolded in the midst of a remarkable number of accomplishments, any one of which would have secured his fame. He wrote and campaigned against slavery and for women's education. Through additional publications and activities he advanced public school education, humane reforms in the treatment of imprisoned criminals, revolutionary changes with respect to the causes of insanity and the treatment of mentally ill persons, and temperance in drinking spirited liquors and using tobacco. Rush also served as surgeon general of the Continental Army during the American Revolution. Beyond those accomplishments, he served in the Continental Congress from its inception to the signing of the Declaration of Independence and even to the ratification of the U.S. Constitution.[4]

Young Benjamin secured a classics education before he became an apprentice to enter the practice of medicine under the tutelage of Dr. John Redman. Gifted in languages, Rush translated the Greek aphorisms attributed to Hippocrates when he was seventeen. Before and after the American Revolution, including after the first medical schools in the United States were founded, many licensed American physicians became certified to practice medicine through apprenticeships. Lower down on the social ladder were numerous "empirics" who lacked professional training, but often became skilled in the use of botanical herbs and called themselves doctors when they switched from shoemaking and other trades to cure-intended activities. The ranks of empirics were supplemented by midwives and bonesetters.[5] Educated practitioners during (and for many years after) America's colonial period could rarely depend on the practice of medicine as a full-time vocation. As late as 1789, Benjamin Rush advised students who planned to practice in rural areas to supplement their incomes with farming.[6]

Like Samuel Bard and over one hundred other wealthier American students between 1749 and 1812, Rush traveled to the University of Edinburgh to receive medical training. He entered Edinburgh in 1766, the year John Gregory began lecturing on the theory and practice of medicine, and received his MD in 1768. Heeding the advice of Ben Franklin, he spent a summer in Paris before he returned to Philadelphia to practice medicine and become professor of chemistry in the newly established Medical Department of the College of Pennsylvania. Rush became professor of the theory and practice of medicine in that medical department in 1789.

Benjamin Rush's instructions about palliative care are primarily found in the bookend lectures from his course on the theory and practice of medicine—his carefully written and clearly delivered "The Vices and Virtues of Physicians" at the beginning and "Duties of a Physician" at the end. Rush held that undertaking the care of sick persons and then neglecting them thereafter is a vice akin to "a malignant dye" within a physician. "The most important contract" that can be made "is that which takes place between a sick man and his doctor." The subject of the contract is human life, and the breach of that contract "by willful negligence ... followed by death, is murder," which should be charged as a crime against physicians guilty of such negligence.[7]

"Equally criminal is the practice among some physicians of encouraging patients to expect a recovery" when their diseases have arrived at the incurable stage. "The mischief done by falsehood in this case, is the more to be deplored, as it often prevents the dying from settling their worldly affairs." False encouragements also keep patients from spending their last hours in spiritual preparation. When physicians discover that their standard efforts to cure patients are of no avail, they should be prepared to express a word of religious hope when patients are experiencing depression and grief. There is, he says, "no substitute for this cordial in the materia medica."[8]

In his closing lecture on the "Duties of a Physician," Rush expands on these themes. Because it is often impossible to tell when life will end and death will begin, physicians should avoid pronouncing that patients—including those struck with acute diseases— are incurable. To the disgrace of the profession, too many physicians who say that patients' diseases are incurable will witness a patient's recovery. Worse still, some physicians predict danger and death in order to increase profits from their prescriptions. This mode of acting is sometimes due to a physician's overconfidence. More often it is "mean and illiberal."[9]

Rush contends that in the face of dread disease, physicians should display a composed or cheerful countenance in order "to inspire as much hope of recovery as you can, consistent with truth, especially in acute diseases." For patients "struggling between life and death," physicians should also utilize "the powers of the mind" by the use of placebo treatments. Rush confesses, "I have frequently prescribed remedies of doubtful efficacy in the critical stage of acute diseases, but never till I had worked up my patients into a confidence, borrowing upon certainty, of their probable good effects."[10] So at times Rush used standard remedies of purging, blistering, and bleeding patients with the expectation and success of contributing to their eventual recovery.[11] Fortunately, many dying patients under Rush's care were not subjected to heroic treatments until they were nearly dead. He weighed the probable effects of his commonly used remedies in light of the recuperative powers of the mind. In keeping with the other duties he set forth, he also expected his students to know when patients' diseases were incurable and, therefore, when to cease all efforts to cure.

John Ferriar on the Details
of Palliative Care: 1798

After receiving his MD from Edinburgh in 1781, John Ferriar settled in Manchester, England, in 1785 and joined the literary and philosophical society that had been co-founded by his elderly and life-long friend Thomas Percival. Along with Percival, Ferriar became a pioneer in public health and better living conditions for factory workers and the poor. In 1789 he was appointed a physician of the Manchester Infirmary, after which the infirmary became the nucleus of a professional community dedicated to the advancement of medicine.[12]

Ferriar established an isolation or "fever" ward for persons with infectious diseases, contributed to the use of digitalis for heart conditions, and became one of the first to argue that the ghostly apparitions experienced by some persons were signs of mental disturbance, not supernatural visitations.[13] His remarkable career included fervent efforts to abolish the slave trade. He even rewrote a stage play for the purpose of awakening audiences to the evils of slavery.[14]

John Ferriar published 31 of his medical essays in four volumes titled *Medical Histories and Reflections*, the first three of which were published separately between 1792 and 1798. Along with other essays, these volumes were combined into one volume in 1809, which was published as an American edition in 1816.[15] His essays were notable and highly sought after.[16]

His essay on the treatment of dying persons was first published in 1798 in Volume III of his essays. This apparently first-ever full essay on palliative care is tightly reasoned and carefully crafted—an innovative classic in the literature that attests to years of first-hand experience in the care of gravely ill and dying persons. He titled his essay "Of the Treatment of the Dying: Disturb him not—let him pass peaceably."[17]

Unlike Theophile Bonet, John Gregory, and Benjamin Rush, Ferriar does not criticize practitioners for abandoning dying patients. His concerns are different, but perhaps even more serious. He observes that many physicians are present at deathbeds, but for the wrong reasons. Ignorant of palliative care, they "torment" dying persons "with unavailing attempts to stimulate the dissolving system, from the idle vanity of prolonging the flutter of the pulse for a few more vibrations."[18] Ferriar believed such physicians ought to know better, and they would know better if they learned about how dying occurs and how fatally ill persons could be treated and comforted. Ignorant of John Gregory's fourth branch of medicine (making death easy), many physicians, Ferriar argues, rely on Gregory's third branch of medical practice (curing disease) to treat dying patients. In keeping with the medical treatments of the late 18th century, they were using stimulants to prolong life—or, more accurately, to prolong signs of continuing life to the doors of death.

John Ferriar calls these physicians "ignorant practitioners," because they avoid learning about the details of palliative care for fatally ill persons. Instead of mastering details, they shun the "terrible" subjects of death and dying. Even "wise" doctors overlook those details, and "inconsiderate" doctors escape thinking about dying and death altogether.[19]

Ferriar critiques these escapists. Since dying is "a scene through which we must all pass," one might expect that dying and death "should excite closer attention" by physicians. Attention to the physical process of dying will rid death of much of its horror and enable physicians to care for persons approaching death. A "yet more powerful motive" for lifting the veil that separates doctors from care for dying persons pertains to physicians' eliminating the suffering caused by "the prejudices and indiscretion" of non-medical "attendants" at the deathbed. "To soothe the last moments of existence" when "all hopes of revival are lost" is a professional duty for doctors.[20]

These are historically powerful criticisms. They link physicians' emotional and moral escapism to medical escapism, a reliance on the common use of "heroic treatments" rather than putting the emphasis on mastering the art of symptom-easing medical and personal care. Ferriar's criticisms forecast the voices of palliative care advocates in later centuries when the capabilities of curative medicine became far more powerful. They also usher us into the world of the cure-oriented therapies in Ferriar's time, therapies being used on persons who were dying.

The only hint that Ferriar provides about what ignorant practitioners were using to prolong "the flutter of the pulse for a few more vibrations" is found in the phrase that they were seeking "to stimulate the dissolving system."[21] What stimulants were used as therapies in the late 18th century? Their use constituted one side of medical theory and practice. Two broad medical approaches were being employed—first, medicines and procedures that would calm down or relieve the tension of the system such as rapid heart rate and fevers; second, medicines that would stimulate or increase the body's tension and vitality.

These therapeutic approaches were based on the assumption that if the symptoms of medical conditions were altered, the diseases themselves would be controlled and hopefully cured. The three therapeutic methods of the time were bleeding by opening veins and using live leeches to suck out blood; purging "impurities" by using emetics that caused vomiting, profuse diarrhea, and copious levels of salivation; and using opium as both a calming and a stimulating agent.[22] Soluble in alcohol, opium was developed into a drug tincture by the renowned English physician Thomas Sydenham (1626–1689). Sydenham promoted his drug under the name laudanum, which became widely used as both a stimulant and a sedative for numerous ailments from the time of Thomas Browne in the 17th century to the end of the 19th century.[23] None of these treatments were scientifically tested or proven. They were instead predicated on personal observation with respect to drugs, concoctions, and bleeding that would remove worrisome symptoms and presumably restore health.

Ferriar's reference to stimulants indicates how dying persons who were manifesting signs of lost vitality—weakness, abnormally low pulse, lessened or lost communication—were being treated. To reverse their symptoms and thereby keep them from dying, physicians could use popular stimulants to restore the body's vitality—in particular, alcohol, opium, arsenic, and quinine. Some physicians who used these and other remedies on dying persons were, in fact, not ignorant about the effects of the therapies they were using. For example, the Scottish physician Alexander Gordan (1752–1799), who was greatly influenced by John Gregory, wrote about the treatment of patients—especially elderly patients—who appeared to be dying. When these persons were beset with conditions that appeared to be hastening toward certain death, "any Remedy, however desperate, that may have a chance of saving the Patient's life, ought to be tried."[24] Gordan's approach was similar to the recommendations in the often-revised 18th-century medical manual titled *The London Practice of Physic*. The manual recommended two types of stimulants for persons in "great danger, where the respiration is much affected": physicians should induce the patient to breathe in a vaporous stream of hot vinegar, or they should use a huge dose of white vitriol (zinc sulphate) to shrink mucous and other secretions, and thus stem further outflows of energy.[25]

With respect to the treatment of dying persons, Ferriar emphasizes that he is talking about the normal course of dying, not about threats of death that occur due to unexpected accidents and circumstances in which "it is certainly proper to employ [various] means of recovery," even though "the efficacy of those means has been over-rated." But when the approach of death is clearly ascertained "either from the symptoms of the disease, or the patient's own feelings," the physician should turn to palliative care, which will be welcomed no less by the dying person than by surrounding family members.[26]

Ferriar outlines what he considers the essential guidelines for expert palliative care by physicians. Physicians must first accurately ascertain whether death is approaching. That requires expert knowledge about how different diseases have a variety of effects on the quickness or slowness of the patient's loss of speech, loss of breathing ability, and final loss of sensibility and awareness of her or his surroundings. Ferriar also speaks of the differences between these losses in patients beset with different types of illnesses—fevers, peripneumony (pneumonia), heart failure, chronic diseases including consumption, and difficulty in breathing (apnea). Physicians must realize that the process of dying varies depending on particular disease conditions. A patient who is suffering from depleted blood circulation, for example, can experience a lucid interval that should not be confused with recovery.[27]

All of these disease conditions cause patients whose senses are intact to sink into inaction and languidness, to breathe less normally, and finally to become insensitive to their surroundings. To respect and value a patient during this dying process, Ferriar asserts that as long as the senses remain intact, "the patient ought to direct his own conduct, both in his devotional exercises, and in the last interchanges of affection with his friends."[28] As patients become weaker and incapable of speaking, they should not be disturbed. "I have always been impressed with an idea," Ferriar says,

> that the approach of actual death, produces a sensation similar to that of falling asleep. The disturbance of respiration is the only apparent source of uneasiness to the dying, and sensibility seems to be impaired, in exact proportion to the decrease of that function. Besides, both the impressions of present objects, and those recalled by memory, are influenced by the extreme debility of the patient, whose wish is for absolute rest. I could never see the close of life, under these circumstances, without recollecting these beautiful lines of Spenser[29]:
>
> > Sleep after toil, port after stormy seas,
> > Ease after war, death after life doth great please.[30]

Ferriar backs up what he says about the painlessness of death with his own palliative care experience, with a quotation from an eminent anatomist of his time, and with references to refutations of "the general opinion" that death is painful. His sources include the French essayist Michel de Montaigne (1533–1592) and the French natural scientist Georges Louis Leclerc de Buffon (1707–1788).[31]

He then instructs his readers regarding how patients should be treated from the time of their becoming insensible to the "the absolute cessation of existence." Like Francis Bacon and Thomas Browne, Ferriar refers to Hippocrates' signs of death as "the surest indications of the nearness of death." Here are Ferriar's bottom lines for physicians and family members:

> When the tossing of the arms ... the rattling noise in respiration, and difficulty of swallowing have come on, all unnecessary noise and bustle about the dying person should be prohibited. The bed curtains should be drawn nearly close, and unless the patient should place himself in a posture evidently uneasy, he should be left undisturbed. Exclamations of grief, and the crowding of the family round the bed, only serve to harass him.
>
> The common practice of plying him with liquors of different kinds, and of forcing them into his mouth, when he cannot swallow, should be totally abstained from.
>
> Everything should be conducted as if he were in a tranquil sleep.[32]

This association of death with sleep means that a physician or some other responsible person should keep family members from harassing dying persons when they are becoming insensitive to their surroundings and desire absolute rest. Ferriar is not saying that because he wants physicians to display power. He wants, instead, to protect dying persons from harmful and disturbing interruptions when they begin to enter into the phase of insensitivity. He knew about that harm from personal experience—how persons with consumption expressed their "great uneasiness" when the cries of their friends at the bedside "recalled" them from the beginning of insensitive peacefulness, and how those who could no longer speak expressed their opposition by looks and gestures.[33]

In keeping with his many roles as a social reformer, John Ferriar turns his attention to the correction of two common cultural practices in his time: the practice of crudely removing insensible, dying patients from their warm and pillowed beds[34] and the practice of rushing the bodies of patients thought to be dead off to their final rites and ultimate burial. Beyond cultural fascination, these sections of Ferriar's essay show that, unlike former authors, Ferrier is addressing both physicians and the public, whom he also enlists as a "means of prevention" of such practices. These sections likewise point to the ritual- and ethically-laden features of dying in all cultural settings, including past and present medical cultures.[35] And they highlight the importance of physicians who should employ their knowledge and experience at the bedsides of dying persons for the purpose of enabling them to die peacefully.

Concerning the first of these cultural practices, Ferriar says that over the last two centuries,

> it was very common to strip the dying, to drag them out of bed, and place them on mattresses of straw or hair, in the middle of the room.... It is a prevalent opinion among nurses[36] and servants, that a patient, whose death is lingering, cannot quit life while he remains on a common bed, and that it is necessary to drag the bed away, and place him on the mattress. This piece of cruelty is often practiced when the attendants are left to themselves. A still more hazardous practice has been very prevalent in France and Germany, and, I am afraid, is not unknown in this country. When the patient is supposed by the nurses to be nearly in a dying state, they withdraw the pillows and bolster from beneath his head; sometimes with such violence, as to throw the head back, and to add greatly to the difficulty of respiration.[37]

He refers to an essay by a German lawyer to prove that this practice was still occurring in his time, which the lawyer said was being done for the purpose of putting the patient out of pain. Ferrier counters that the practice suffocates dying persons because they can no longer breathe without the aid of pillows propping up their heads. Those who perform these practices are called "executioners" by Ferriar, who adds that it is the responsibility of the patient's family members and friends to stop "this barbarity." Ferriar assumes that physicians will join him in ending these practices.[38]

Almost 50 years later, the English physician James Mackness confirmed the accuracy of Ferriar's concern over these cruelties. Referring to Ferriar's essay, Mackness says,

> It is well known to everyone who has had much experience, that this is actually the case, and therefore it is the duty of a medical man to look carefully into the cases that come under his observation, and to take care that the dying patient shall not be abandoned to the care of those whose officious folly or unfeeling indifference are likely to distress the last moments.[39]

Physicians should seek out "affectionate and intelligent relatives" to attend to the patient when the physician cannot be present, or, if such relatives are not available, the practitioner should endeavor to find others who can "protect the patient against every species of suffering but that which is inevitable."[40]

Ferriar opposes two other folk customs, both of which relate to persons who were incorrectly thought to be dead. The first involved taking presumably dead persons out of their beds, placing them on a table, and covering them with a sheet. Ferriar refers to a story told by Thomas Sydenham, who described how a young man with smallpox revived when his body cooled, going on to live for several more years. Ferriar adds that in some instances that practice would extinguish "the feeble remains of life." The second custom involved laying out the bodies of persons presumed to be dead and hurrying to bury them. In France persons were at times buried within twelve hours, which admits to "the dreadful possibility of their being buried in a state not destitute of consciousness." He observes that keeping bodies unburied for several days is a "firmly established" practice in England. The greatest horror is that a helpless dying person "feels all these cruelties, after he has become unable to express his sensations directly."[41]

Ferriar's criticisms of these customs are predictive of laws that would eventually require physician certification of death. They also foreshadow present-day concerns with respect to the ways that the practice of medicine inescapably involves negotiations between physicians' medical knowledge and patients' cultural backgrounds—presently termed "cultural competency" of the part of healthcare professionals.[42]

Fully agreeing with John Gregory, Ferriar holds that it is the duty of physicians to soothe the last moments of existence and to comfort surrounding relatives. But Ferriar is far more detailed than Gregory. Ferriar displays the interconnections between specialized medical knowledge and palliative care. He describes the natural process of dying—awareness, increasing weakness, loss of speech, indications of not wanting to be disturbed, insensibility, and final cessation. This process becomes the foundation for what all persons—physicians, family members, friends, and nursing attendants—should do or not do with respect to the care of persons who are dying. He attends to particular things that should be done regarding posture in bed, opened windows for air, regulation of light, and abstinence from forced drinking.

Ferriar deeply respected persons as they entered the dying process. As long as they are able to do so, he believed, patients ought to direct their devotional exercises and interchanges of affection with family and friends. Like Bacon, Gregory, and Rush, Ferriar recognized the value of spiritual concerns. For apparently the first time in Anglo-American history, Ferriar roundly criticized ignorant practitioners who tormented their patients with vain attempts to extend signs of life—a critique that would become all the more notable in ensuing centuries. And like Francis Bacon and Thomas Browne, Ferriar associated death with sleep, which deeply informed his approach to palliative care: "Disturb him not—let him pass peaceably."

Thomas Gisborne on the Necessity of Truthfulness: 1794

The Reverend Thomas Gisborne (1758–1846), an Anglican priest, poet, and widely published author, displayed his brilliance in mathematics and classic languages and literature as a student in St. John's College at Cambridge. Expected to have a brilliant career, Gisborne was offered a seat in Parliament, which he turned down to enter the priesthood in 1783. Like Benjamin Rush and John Ferriar, he became a staunch campaigner for the abolition of slavery. In 1794 he published his 900-page *Enquiry into the Duties of Men in the Higher and Middle Classes of Society in Great Britain. Enquiry* was reprinted six times by 1811. The twelfth chapter of this work continued to be published as a separate book titled *On the Duties of Physicians, Resulting from Their Profession* as late as 1847.[43]

Not one to neglect attention to women, the Reverend Gisborne also published *An Enquiry into the Duties of the Female Sex* in 1797, which even Jane Austen said she was pleased to have read.[44] Gisborne maintained that women should remain in domestic roles, but he believed they should not conceal their intellectual abilities and never be forced into marriage. In search of harmonizing new geological discoveries with scripture, he wrote extensively about the relationships between geology, the Bible, and Christian tradition.

Gisborne's position on truth telling with fatally ill persons opposed the position Thomas Percival would take and defend in his profoundly influential *Code of Medical Ethics*[45] (the discussion of which will follow). Like John Gregory, Percival advanced physician paternalism with respect to what should or should not be communicated to dangerously sick patients. Gisborne's disagreements with Percival are recounted below.

Before Gisborne completed his chapter *On the Duties of Physicians* in his *Enquiry*, he received a considerable portion of the manuscript copy of the work Percival was compiling on medical ethics.[46] Due to tragic losses of members of his family, Percival did not resume work on his book for a number of years; nevertheless, he received a great deal of correspondence from the physicians (including John Ferriar), lawyers, and clergy to whom he had sent his manuscript and from whom he received support and assistance.[47] Gisborne decided to write to Percival about one issue in his manuscript. He advised Percival to add the words "as far as truth and sincerity will admit" to the sentence, "A physician should be the minister of hope and comfort to the sick." Gisborne's recommendation accords with the duty specified by Benjamin Rush that physicians should "inspire as much hope of recovery as you can, consistent with truth."[48]

Gisborne wrote to Percival,

> I know very well that [your] sentence, as it now stands, conveys to you, and was meant by you to convey to others, the same sentiment which it would express after [my] proposed addition. But if I am not mistaken in my idea, there are few professional temptations to which medical men are more liable, and frequently from the very best principles, than that of unintentionally using language to the patient and his friends, more encouraging than sincerity would vindicate, on cool reflection. It may be right scrupulously to guard the avenues against such an error.[49]

That's about as verbose, nice, and indirect as a clergy friend could ever sound. We will soon see what Percival did with Gisborne's counsel.

In the meantime, nine years before Percival published his *Code of Ethics*, Thomas Gisborne published *On the Duties of Physicians*, in which he is far more pointed about what he so mildly suggested to Percival.

> Humanity ... and the welfare of the sick man, commonly require that his drooping spirits should be revived by every encouragement and hope which can honestly be suggested to him. But truth and conscience forbid the Physician to cheer him by giving promises, or raising expectations, which are known or intended to be delusive. The Physician ... is invariably bound never to represent the uncertainty or danger as less than he actually believes it to be, to the patient or to his family, any impression to that effect. Though he may be misled by mistaken tenderness, he is guilty of positive falsehood. He is at liberty to say little; but let that little be true.[50]

This paragraph puts teeth into the phrase "as far as truth and sincerity will admit," which Gisboune had previously recommended to Percival. Humanity and the well-being of dispirited sick persons call for encouragements from physicians. But those encouragements must conform with truthfulness, not deception. Nor should doctors misrepresent the severity of patients' conditions. Mistaken tenderness can lead to lying. Whatever the physician says must be true.

To support his positions, Gisborne appeals to both Christian scripture and consequence-based ethical reasoning. Concerning scripture, "Saint Paul's direction, not to do evil that good may come,[51] is clear, positive, and universal." That the Apostle Paul's imperative is universal means, for Gisborne, that it is grounded in natural reasoning. So he adds that even if scripture contained no such injunction, a consideration of the moral consequences of deception proves that it is immoral.[52] Consider the consequences. First, expectations of good results from false statements are, at best, temporary. Second, patients will learn—indeed, they will undoubtedly discover—that the physician's words are often "vain encouragements and delusive assurances." When that happens, physician assurances will "cease to cheer the sick man and his friends." And third, patients and their friends may well begin to believe that anxiety lurks underneath the physician's comforting words. They may think that the doctor actually views the patient's disease as "highly formidable," which will foster distressing apprehensions in the hearts and minds of patients even if these apprehensions eventually prove to be groundless. The physician should not slide "into deceit, either expressly or implied."[53]

It logically follows that

> the state of the malady, when critical or hazardous, ought to be plainly declared without delay to some at least of the patient's near relations.... On many occasions it may be the duty of the Physician spontaneously to reveal it to the patient himself. It may sometimes also be incumbent on him to suggest to the sick man, or to his friends, the propriety of adjusting all unfinished temporal concerns; and conscience will frequently prompt him discreetly to turn the thoughts of the former towards Religion. Not that the Physician is officiously to intrude into the department of the Minister of the Gospel. But he may often smooth the way for the Clergyman's approach.[54]

Having previously set forth his position on the necessity of veracity, these statements by Gisborne are full of latitude. They speak of what the physician may do, may reveal, or may sometimes suggest. Gisborne recognizes that physicians can and should use a variety of approaches to fulfill their duties to dying persons and their relatives, but he holds that whatever they decide to do should be truthful and that terminal care involves jointly fulfilled roles by both physicians and clergy.

In addition to these concerns, Gisborne speaks briefly about two additional guidelines with respect to care for dying persons: physicians should never abandon patients who are beyond hope of recovery, and they should be moderate in their fees for palliative care services. He remarks that even though life cannot be retained, pain may be mitigated, and the presence of the physician "will compose the minds and alleviate the sorrow of friends and relations." Then he appeals to the virtues of generosity and compassion as motives behind physicians' modest fees for palliative care.[55]

Gisborne emerges as an impressive medical ethicist within the setting of his time. Percival recognizes this when he refers to Gisborne's chapter on physicians in his *Enquiry Into the Duties of Men* as the work of an "excellent moralist."[56] Gisborne's thinking and contributions are also occasionally recognized as historically important by 21st-century authors.[57]

Thomas Percival and the Codification of Palliative Care: 1803

Thomas Percival (1740–1804) studied in Edinburgh's college of medicine as that college was being recognized as the leading medical school in Great Britain and at the center of the Scottish Enlightenment.[58] After receiving his MD from Lyden in Holland in 1765, he settled in Manchester, England. From Manchester, Percival increased his influence through numerous publications, became deeply involved with the Manchester Literary and Philosophical Society, and cultivated friendships with the medical, philosophical, political, and religious figures of his time, including Benjamin Franklin, Voltaire, and the great surgeon and anatomist, John Hunter (1728–1793). Along with John Ferriar, who also practiced in Manchester, Percival made outstanding contributions to public health—limiting the labor time of children in factories to 12 hours, requiring clean and ventilated lodging for the rural poor who came to work in Manchester's factories, mandating cleaner water supplies, and establishing "The House of Recovery," a fever infirmary for the control of infectious disease.[59]

The physicians and surgeons of the Manchester Infirmary urged Percival to "frame a general system of Medical Ethics" for the purpose of governing the conduct and interactions of physicians both in hospitals and in private practice.[60] Between 1792 and 1794 he composed the first draft of the work he eventually published in 1803 under the title of *Medical Ethics; or, A Code of Institutes and Precepts, Adapted to the Professional Conduct of Physicians and Surgeons.* As previously indicated, Percival circulated his draft to numerous acquaintances, including Thomas Gisborne, who made "valuable suggestions for its improvement."[61]

Holding with Bacon that doctors are debtors to their profession, and thereby are duty-bound to strengthen its foundations, contribute to its dignity and protect it from abuses, Percival shouldered the task of constructing an exceedingly comprehensive code of professional conduct for physicians and surgeons.[62] Its first chapter deals with professional conduct in hospitals and other charitable institutions, such as infirmaries for women, for persons with syphilis, and for mentally ill persons. Its second chapter specifies rules of professional conduct for physicians in private and general practice. This chapter covers rules of consultation, the care of dying persons, gratuitous services to one's fellow physicians and to apothecaries and members of the clergy, and physicians' obligation to upbraid patients who manifest "vicious conduct." Its third and fourth chapters address the relationships between physicians and apothecaries, as well as guidelines for physicians in relation to laws and testimonies in courts. The fourth chapter also covers a fascinating array of topics, ranging from manslaughter, abortions, and dueling to physicians' duties to protect the public from the smoke of factories, fumes from smelting houses, and the stench of hog farms.[63]

Percival says that his code of *Medical Ethics* sets forth his own opinions, but also reflects a consensus of medical and moral opinion. He secured "the aid and support" of an impressive number of "judicious and learned friends, in different stations of life"— physicians (including John Ferriar), clergy-scholars (including the Reverend Thomas Gisborne), philosophers, and barristers. He circulated copies of a later draft to infirmaries "in different parts of the kingdom."[64] He also profited from "the excellent lectures of Dr. [John] Gregory."[65] Composed as a code of ethics, Percival notes that his style is aphoristic, which "precludes the discussion of many interesting points."[66] Percival also discusses a number of the most important of these points in the extensive "Notes and Illustrations" attached to his code.[67]

Percival sets forth guidelines for the care of dangerously ill and dying persons in three places in his code of medical ethics. In the seventh section of his first chapter, he holds that at times hospitalized patients "on the bed of sickness and death should be reminded, by some friendly monitor, of the importance of a *last will and testament* to his wife, children, or relatives, who otherwise might be deprived of his ... future ... legacy." Percival views this as a duty that should be performed by the house surgeon, who regularly attends hospitalized persons and thereby secures their confidence.[68]

His far more explicit directives regarding the care of dying persons are given in the third and thirteenth sections of his second chapter on the professional conduct of physicians in private and general practice. These widely adopted sections are fully quoted below.

In the third section he says,

> A physician should not be forward to make gloomy prognostications.... But he should not fail, on proper occasions, to give to the friends of the patient, timely notice of danger, when it occurs, and even to the patient himself, if absolutely necessary. This office, however, is so peculiarly alarming, when executed by him, that it ought to be declined, whenever it can be assigned to any other person of sufficient judgment and delicacy. For the physician should be the minister of hope and comfort to the sick; that by such cordials to the drooping spirit, he may sooth the bed of death, revive expiring life, and counteract the depressing influence of those maladies which rob the philosopher of fortitude,[69] and the Christian of consolation.[70]

This section of Percival's code raises critical issues about the ethics of truth concealing versus truth revealing to fatally ill persons, the details of which are discussed later in this chapter.

Percival's last section on terminal care appears in the thirteenth section of the second chapter. Logically, this last section should have come first, because it sets forth Percival's fundamental convictions concerning the duty of physicians to attend to fatally ill patients. Here is the wording of that thirteenth section:

> Sir William Temple has asserted that "an honest physician is excused for leaving his patient, when he finds the disease growing desperate, and can, by his attendance,

expect only to receive his fees, without any hopes or appearance of deserving them." But this allegation is not well founded. For the offices of a physician may continue to be highly useful to the patient and comforting to the relatives around him, even in the last period of a fatal malady; by obviating despair, by alleviating pain, and by soothing mental anguish. To decline attendance, under such circumstances, would be sacrificing, to fanciful delicacy and mistaken liberality, that moral duty which is independent of, and far superior to, all pecuniary appreciation.[71]

With these words Thomas Percival elevates the palliative care proclamations of Francis Bacon to the status of widely endorsed medical policy. Like Theophile Bonet, John Gregory, Benjamin Rush, and Thomas Gisborne, Percival holds that it is morally unacceptable for physicians to abandon desperately ill and dying patients.

Percival begins section thirteen by refuting the position of the English statesmen and essayist Sir William Temple.[72] Temple was not a physician, but he nevertheless advocated that physicians were not obligated to attend to dying patients because they did not deserve to be paid for noncurative interventions. Percival labeled Temple's position "mistaken liberality" because it appears to manifest a noble lack of greed at the cost of leaving the bedsides of fatally ill persons who might greatly benefit from physicians' continued ministrations.

Versus Temple, Percival's code holds that physicians' attendance at the bedsides of dying persons is a "moral duty" far superior to monetary gain. Physicians should accompany persons even in the last period of their fatal conditions, and they should do so for the purposes of reviving their drooping spirits, preventing despair, alleviating their pain and other depressing symptoms, and, if possible, reviving expiring life.

To return to the third section of the second chapter of Percival's code, Percival's position on truth concealing and truth telling mirrors the paternalism of John Gregory. First, physicians should decide whom to tell when the patient's life is in danger. They should not fail to find a proper occasion to tell the friends of the patient about that danger. Without further comment, he adds that, "if absolutely necessary," the patient can be told. He then quickly says that if telling the patient "is so peculiarly alarming," this office should be avoided by the physician and assigned to "any other person of sufficient judgment and delicacy," which probably refers to a member of the clergy.[73] In short, doctors at the deathbed should seek to avoid becoming the bearers of bad news.

Second, in the extensive "Notes and Illustrations" that he appended to the four chapters of his code, Percival discusses at great length the sentence in section three that the physician "should be the minister of hope and comfort to the sick." That was the phrase Thomas Gisborne had found wanting. As previously discussed, upon receiving a copy of the code Percival was developing, Gisborne wrote to Percival suggesting that he should add the words "so far as truth and sincerity will admit." Gisborne held that the truth is compatible with silence: the physician "is at liberty to say little, but let that little be true."[74]

Gisborne's arguments seized Percival's attention and laid bare their conflicting viewpoints about truth telling. In "Notes and Illustrations" Percival wrote ten pages pertaining to the duty of physicians to be ministers of hope and comfort to the sick. He begins with a full review of Gisborne's letter to him, as well as the stronger positions Gisborne took in his book *Enquiry Into the Duties of Men*, first published in 1794. Percival says that the moral differences between them are "of high importance," and they have given rise to opposing opinions. He surveys the opinions of ancient and modern authors, one of whom argued that the maxim from the Apostle Paul—"We must not do evil that good may come of it"—is "of no use in morals, as it is quite vague and undetermined."[75]

At stake for Percival are questions regarding the morality of concealing the truth from patients, on the one hand, and deceiving patients, on the other. Moral truth, Percival argues, has two references—the first to the person or persons to whom it is delivered and the second to the person who is speaking. Concerning the second, the physician who is doing the speaking should "generously relinquish every consideration, referable only to himself," such that he is willing on occasion to "sacrifice [his] delicate sense of veracity." The physician's truthfulness or lack of truthfulness should be determined by the situations of the patients to whom he is speaking. The physician's personal sense of veracity is morally secondary to his professional and social duties centered on the good of his patients.[76]

Percival argues that concealing the truth is justified when it protects persons from harm. Consider, for example, the father of a large family and a leader in the community who asks about the danger of his illness. In this case, "it would be a gross and unfeeling wrong to reveal the truth." The truth might cause his death, such that its conceivable benefits would be reversed: "It would be deeply injurious to him, his family, and to the public."[77]

What about overt deception, a direct violation of truthfulness? Deception presents the practitioner with "a painful conflict of obligations" between upholding or sacrificing veracity. For Percival, deception is morally justifiable, but only "in cases of real emergency, which happily seldom occur."[78] To illustrate cases of morally permissible outright deception, Percival concludes his discussion with two biographical stories that warrant deception, to the point of overt lying.

> The husband of the celebrated Arria, Caecissa Paetus, was very dangerously ill. Her son was also sick at the same time, and died. He was a youth of uncommon accomplishments; and fondly beloved by his parents. Arria prepared and conducted his funeral in such a manner, that her husband remained entirely ignorant of the mournful event.... Paetus often inquired with anxiety, about his son; to whom she cheerfully replied, that he had slept well, and was better. But if her tears, too long restrained, were bursting forth, she instantly retired, to give vent to her grief; and when again composed, returned to Paetus with dry eyes.

> Lady Russel's only son, Wriothesley, Duke of Bedford, died of the small pox in May 1711, [followed by] the loss of her daughter, the Duchess of Rutland, who died in child-bed.[79] Lady Russell, after seeing her in the coffin, went to her other daughter ... from whom it was necessary to conceal her grief, she being at the time in child-bed[80] also. Therefore she assumed a cheerful air, and with astonishing resolution ... answered he anxious daughter's inquiries with these words: "I have seen your sister out of bed today."[81]

Percival's examples raise questions worthy of discussion. Do they convincingly justify concealing the truth or overt deception? What might happen if these persons discover that they are gravely or terminally ill? Like John Ferriar, Percival believed that physicians should very rarely inform extremely ill patients about the gravity of their conditions even if asked. One of Percival's just-quoted cases also illustrates why patients should not be told about the recent deaths of their children: the patient might die from the shock of such news.

Lurking in the shadows of Ferriar's and Percival's moral paternalism is death as the king of terrors. To them it is truly alarming for the physician to speak about the gravity of the patient's condition. Learning that death is approaching, or even hearing about the death of a loved one, may prove fatal to the dangerously sick patient. Due to the placebo and nocebo effects of the physician's interactions with his patients, physicians should benevolently shield patients from those horrifying realities.[82] Similar to John Ferriar, Percival also justifies the physician's presence at the deathbed as a source of comfort for surrounding relatives. That comfort would become another dimension of palliative care.

Percival's *Medical Ethics* became exceedingly influential, serving as the foundation for the codes of ethics adopted by medical societies and fraternities in Philadelphia, Pennsylvania, and Lexington, Kentucky, in 1821 and 1823, and by the New York State Medical Society in 1823. His code was also republished in 1807 and 1827. These were forecasts of its increasing influence in years to come.[83]

Concluding Perspectives

Francis Bacon demystified death as natural for all of nature's creatures, including human beings. Less a philosopher, but experienced as a physician, John Ferriar held that "the physical process of death loses much of its horror, on a near view." Based on his close observations of dying persons, he held that "the approach of actual death produces a sensation similar to that of falling asleep," a metaphor dear to the heart of Thomas Browne.[84]

Percival thought differently. Motivated by beneficence, physicians should protect patients and families from humankind's mortal enemy—death.[85] With rare and unspecified exceptions, Percival wanted physicians to protect patients from knowledge of impending death even if it meant sacrificing personal duties of truthfulness. Percival thereby relegated Thomas Gisborne's defense of truthfulness to his "Notes and Illustrations," which silenced the concerns of Gisborne for a time. That season of silence would be shattered in 46 years. Nevertheless, the wording and duties in Percival's code would resonate in the minds of numerous practitioners for centuries.

Apart from these diverse understandings of death and differing assessments of truth telling, John Ferriar made a momentous contribution. He took his readers to the besides of dying persons and innovatively explored details about the process of dying and the care of dying persons. His observations and recommendations are still informative. To this day, family members and caregivers can profit from his description of the process of dying—for example, how persons at the end of life often desire absolute rest and are no longer interested in food and drink, to say nothing of stimulants that will jolt them into a level of consciousness. Some family members become worried and alarmed when their dying relatives do not want to eat. Some are haunted by the idea that Mom or Dad may be committing suicide. Crafted well over 200 years ago, Ferriar's insights still resonate with meaning.

Momentously, Samuel Bard, Ferriar, Gisborne, and Percival shared the conviction declared to be imperative by Francis Bacon and put into practice by a generation of physicians who followed Bacon: physicians should attend to patients in the last periods of their fatal maladies in order to alleviate pain and soothe mental anguish. To his great credit, Percival carved that conviction into the stone of his historic code of medical ethics. Palliative treatment and care had progressed from proclamation to recognition, and now to codified establishment.

3

That Science Called Euthanasia

1826–1854

The bookends to the story of the quest for a good death between 1826 and 1854 are richly detailed essays on the care of dying patients. The first was given as a lecture by Carl Friedrich Heinrich Marx (1796–1877) in 1826 and published that same year. The second is a handwritten essay by Hugh Noble, which he crafted as a requirement for his medical degree from the University of Edinburgh in 1854. Both essays merit recognition as classics in the literature on palliative care. Both likewise expand upon and add to the themes of the groundbreaking essay by John Ferriar in 1798 discussed in Chapter 2.

Marx titled his lecture "Medical Euthanasia," and Noble titled his dissertation "Euthanasia." Both affirm that *euthanasia* refers to good or peaceful dying—the meaning inherent in the term coined by Francis Bacon in 1605. Both strongly oppose what euthanasia now denotes—physician-induced death, which neither author would have ever called euthanasia.

Between these bookends are important developments within the expanding palliative care tradition. These include the import of findings from physiology, the influential career and publications of Christoph Wilhelm Hufeland, and the officially adopted Code of Ethics of the newly founded American Medical Association (AMA) in 1847, which includes texts on end-of-life care from Thomas Percival's code of medical ethics.

These developments also include increasing controversy over the ethics of telling the truth to terminally ill patients. In his cogently written book, *Physician and Patient*, published in 1849, Worthington Hooker (1806–1867) directly and publicly confronted Thomas Percival's defense of the morality of lying to patients about the seriousness of their conditions. To register the intensity of his opposition to Percival, Hooker first gives a word-for-word account of Percival's two graphic stories used to justify deceptive lying.[1] Hooker then asserts, "The falsehood in the two cases ... is of the most egregious character, and yet they are fair representations of that kind of deception" that many physicians "feel authorized to use in the sick room." Hooker marshals a powerful critique against such deception in full knowledge that by so doing he is publicly opposing how sections of the newly approved AMA Code of Ethics were being interpreted.[2]

Carl F. H. Marx on the Science and Art of Enabling Persons to Die Peacefully: 1826

Marx (1796–1877) received his MD from the medical school in Jena, Germany. At the time of his installation as an assistant professor of medicine at the University of Gottingen in 1826, he delivered an oration titled in English "Medical Euthanasia," which was published in Latin that same year. His numerous publications thereafter included studies of famous physicians and a seminal study on the anatomical sophistication of Leonardo da Vinci.[3]

In his oration before the medical faculty of the University of Gottingen, Marx displays how the palliative care legacy of Francis Bacon had reached the European continent. He asserts that the physician is expected to offer "skillful alleviation of suffering" when life is ending. "This," he says, "is that science, called euthanasia, which checks oppressing features of illness, relieves pain, and renders the supreme and inescapable hour a most peaceful one." Marx further claims that "our greatest efforts should be devoted" to those ends, as "urged by that great Englishman" Francis Bacon. Marx then supplies his listeners and readers with Bacon's entire text on "outward euthanasia" from *Advancement of Learning*.[4]

Marx quickly turns to how physicians possess the means to ensure peaceful dying, beyond the abilities of philosophers and clergy, who remove fear of death by strengthening hope in immortality. Physicians can be present when continued life becomes perilous. They can skillfully alleviate suffering. They can best judge when illness turns for the worse. They can remove "everything that might increase the patient's pain and suffering." They can cheer the patient's mind and soul with gracious and convincing comfort.[5] End-of-life care is both a science and an art.[6]

Most physicians, Marx says, are not thoroughly acquainted with the essential components of good dying. They start to lose interest when the patient's case appears to be hopeless. They think that their duties are discharged when they have exhausted their use of curative therapies. They assume that they are treating diseases, not human beings. In contrast, some physicians have nobler hearts. They "consider it their more lofty duty to lay to peaceful rest a life they can no longer save." They carefully follow the patient's changing circumstances and know how to use "palliatives" whenever possible.[7]

The body of Marx's essay covers four subject areas: ways to alleviate patients' symptoms and discomforts; what must be avoided; how to give "gracious and convincing comfort" to the patient's mind and soul; and a series of special topics.[8] Because the subject is so vast in its particulars, he focuses on points of general interest, the great importance of which leads him to exclaim, "May the reading of this paper fall on fertile ground."[9]

Ways to Alleviate Patients' Symptoms and Discomforts: Nursing, Palliative Medicines, and Palliative Care

Marx begins by telling his hearers and readers something new and remarkable: "Whatever can possibly be done through the doctor's foresight is best of all carried out by attendants and by properly trained nurses" who are considerate and free of prejudice, and who adhere to the doctor's orders. He praises a nurse training program in Heidelberg, Germany. Nurses, physicians, friends, and relatives should all enable persons facing death to feel that they are receiving affectionate attention and the best of care.[10]

His reference to "properly trained nurses" foreshadows a new era that would give birth to the historic activities of Florence Nightingale in the 1850s and thereafter. Programs to train nurses apparently began in 1780, when Dr. Franz May in Mannheim, Germany, provided nurses with levels of formal education and practice under physician supervision. May's efforts were furthered by the Protestant minister Theodore Fliedner, who established a program of nurse training in Kaiserswerth, Germany, in 1836. Intrigued by nursing, Florence Nightingale traveled to visit Kaiserswerth in 1850, and then returned to complete training in 1851 and receive certification as a "trained nurse."[11]

Concerning palliative remedies, Marx says,

> The entire plan of treatment will here confine itself within symptomatic and palliative indication. The doctor will indeed keep only in mind, not by what means he may restore to normal the whole organism, but in what way he may eliminate or curb any particularly harassing episodes and attacks of the disease and the stern signs of nature in battle, such as anxiety, pain, torment, spasm, convulsion, restlessness, long-drawn-out sleepless nights as well as excessive secretions and excretions. Soothing, soporific, sedative, analgesic, and antispasmodic medicines will answer such a purpose.... Their choice and composition depend on the type of illness and on the type of patients.[12]

He knows the medicines of his age. Narcotics are enormously useful for all types of diseases, but especially for enabling patients to experience peacefulness at the end of life. They temporarily remove bodily pain and anguish, enable patients to sleep, and ease mental fretfulness. Drugs containing cyanide and opium can be used for cancerous ulcers of the uterus and breasts, extractions of the plant belladonna for hardened areas and cancers, and the milky fluid from the lettuce-like plant lactucarium for restful sleep. Juice from the flowering plant hyoscyamus should be used as a replacement for opium when opium harms bowel function and when patients are coughing up bloody sputum. Marx adds a modern note about persons who can no longer swallow and who become so short of breath that they endure torturous and labored breathing: opium can be used to deprive persons of conscious awareness and "make life's end a lenient one."[13]

In addition to palliative medicines, Marx expands upon practical measures, many of which would later become hallmarks for Florence Nightingale. He says persons facing the end of life should be cared for in secluded rooms with pure and freshly renewed air. Cleanliness is especially imperative because of bowel and urine incontinence, diarrhea, and pus secretions. Special beds should be used, the heads and foots of which can be raised and lowered to offer greater relief. The often "vicious and almost unbearable affliction" of bedsores should be tended to by keeping patients clean and using thin sheets of buckskin to keep sores from occurring. As a matter of routine, the patient's dry tongue and pharynx should be moistened.[14]

What Must Be Avoided: Cure-directed Remedies, Surgery, and Dangerous News

Marx opposes all "that might increase the patent's pain and suffering," such as plying them with curative remedies, attempting "cruel surgical exploits," and revealing any news about dangers and death. Beyond John Ferriar, who opposed the use of stimulants for dying persons, Marx asserts that use of all the standard "heroic" treatments used at the time should cease.[15] He does not mince words:

> [The physician] must see to it that no medicines are senselessly given from which all human nature, and not the least the sick, shrinks back in horror, like the harsh, the bitter, the sickening ones, or the external irritants or those causing blisters, the caustics, and other tortures for a nearly disintegrating body.[16]

These "so-called remedies ... never are of any help," he says. Worse still, they cause dying persons' last breaths to be "choked with pain and sorrow." Marx asks, "What good will it do the incurable patient to apply dangerous and dubious therapeutic measures?"[17]

As a background to his words,[18] the therapeutic remedies Marx is referring to include purging sick persons' systems with emetics that would cause them to vomit and with cathartics or purgatives that act as extremely powerful laxatives. Furthermore, calomel (mercuric chloride) given in large doses became a favored cathartic and a medical panacea. Its side effects included profuse salivation as an additional means of removing impurities, at the cost of painful mouth sores and sometimes rotting and lost teeth.[19] External irritants that caused blisters on the skin would be drained to remove harmful liquids.[20] For many physicians, "the lancet [for letting out blood through the veins], mercury, [and] antimony or opium, are the great guns that they always fire on all occasions.... Whoever sends for a physician ... expects to be bled, blistered, or vomited, or submitted to some other painful or nauseous medication."[21]

One may well ask why these therapeutically intended measures were ever used on sick persons. The best answer seems to be that patients could *feel* them and thus assume that these methods would counteract their painful conditions. Nothing of value could be achieved without suffering.[22] Partly due to the popularization of far more mild and natural remedies by medical "sectarians,"[23] U.S. physicians proceeded with greater caution and moderation in the use of medical heroics after the 1850s.

Marx reveals that the drive to extend the lives of dying patients was so great that questionable surgical operations were also being used if "a slight chance to save a life" was thought to exist. He notes that surgery was being performed on patients with abdominal cavities swollen with fluid,[24] with gallstones, and with life-threatening hernias.[25] The most common surgical procedures were limb amputations.[26]

The early decades of the 19th century in England and on the Continent witnessed bold operative feats inspired by new and detailed anatomical studies, the rising status of surgeons, and close connections between surgeons across the Western world.[27] Because anesthesia had not yet been discovered, surgical operations were exceedingly painful, such that the skills of surgeons performing amputations were measured in part by the brevity of their procedures. Perhaps the fastest knife in the first half of the 19th century was held by Robert Liston (1794–1847), who would call out to those in the galleries witnessing one of his amputations, "Time me, gentlemen."[28]

Marx mentions that surgery sometimes saves or extends life. "But on the other hand, just as many, who with equanimity and with greatest patience submitted to the surgeon's incision, died under excruciating pain either right under [the surgeon's] eyes or a few days later." He responds that anyone with a sense of mercy would recoil when "the most cruel operation is performed" on persons whom knowledgeable physicians recognize as approaching the end of life. With passion, he concludes that "the experienced physician should apply himself much rather to euthanasia than to surgery."[29]

To enable persons to pass from life peacefully, Marx adds a third prohibition. Similar to Thomas Percival, he asserts that dying patients should not be told about "any misfortune, danger, or death." Concealing the truth about the patient's condition, according to Marx, becomes all the more imperative as hopes for maintaining health and life recede.[30]

Comforting Dying Patients' Minds and Souls

While recognizing that clergy soothe longings of the soul, Marx also believed them to be "quasi-harbingers of death."[31] In contrast, physicians can be sources of less compromised comforting, as patients are accustomed to their presence and know that physicians are relieving their physical miseries. So physicians should extend their comforting roles:

> With encouragement and with promise [the physician] will bring spirit to the dejected, hope to the fearful, confidence to the despairing. Likewise he may tell [persons approaching death] how often other people have recovered from more serious illness, and how many effective medicines for aid and support are still available, or he may cheer up his patient's mind … [by] holding out the prospect … of fairer weather, and even a trip to hot and medicinal springs.[32]

The practitioner will also remind dying patients to make out their last wills if they have not done so. That will enable physicians to confer confidence about "the safe and secure future of those to be left behind, his wife, his children, his dearest stakes in life." Taking on the role of a priest, the doctor will also relieve fears of complete extinction by giving patients hope of immortality.[33]

Parallel to the imperatives of John Ferriar, Marx holds that when dying persons approach the end of life, quietness must be maintained. Loved ones should conceal their grief. Since hearing is the last sense lost, lamentations and mournful funeral songs should not be voiced. However, as opposed to the views of some physicians who claim that the presence of loved ones makes death more difficult, "dearest ones" should be welcomed: "Where there is love, life is sweet and death is not bitter. Thus it is related that Caesar Augustus passed away calmly under Livia's kisses."[34] Predictive of a feature of Cicely Saunders' hospice care beginning in the 1960s, Marx adds that unless silence is preferred, dying persons can be soothed and lulled to sleep with sweet chords from harps and flutes.[35]

Special Topics: Culturally Inclusive Care, Ending Life, Psychology and Death, Age and Death

In his final remarks Marx displays his great sense of fairness and inclusiveness by emphasizing that some groups of patients deserve especially gentle and supportive care as they "go to meet death"—those who are poverty stricken, those from a foreign country, and adherents of different religions.[36]

He also contends that it is never moral, even when prompted by requests or by his own sense of mercy, for the physician "to end the patient's pitiful condition by purposely and deliberately hastening death." Directly shortening or ending life is illegal and goes against the goals of medicine, against religious teaching, and against the utterances of the wisest of persons, such as the Greek mathematician, philosopher, and mystic Pythagoras.[37]

Marx's discussion of the ways patients with differing psychological temperaments face death would be called, centuries later, the psychology of death and dying. He divides patients into groups of four temperaments, which reflect ancient medical concepts known as the four humors (blood, yellow bile, black bile, and phlegm). These humors were thought to give rise to four personality traits and behaviors: sanguine (outgoing and personally impressionable), choleric (passionate, energetic, and ambitious), melancholic (sensitive and contemplative), and phlegmatic (quiet, relaxed, and passive).[38] Marx associates these temperaments with differing responses toward death. Persons with sanguine temperaments become "extremely stirred up" by the specter of death. Choleric personalities will reluctantly realize that they are bound to die and will "spend [their] last moments in struggle and violence." Melancholic persons will bear the dread of death with a balanced and serene mind. And phlegmatics will manifest little response, such that death is concealed in solitude.[39]

Finally, and also innovatively, Marx summarizes how the care of persons in different age groups requires a "separate study of the treatment appropriate to each." He speaks of babies, children, adolescents, mature adults and aged persons. For the mature adult, for example, dying is bitter:

> He realizes that medical resources have reached an end, he realizes the affection of his family, the kindness of his friends, and he goes over his earthly possessions, often acquired by hard labor and toil. To bid farewell for all this fills him with sorrow and grief, and the mind of the dying is greatly shaken with worry about those he is about to leave behind.[40]

In old age death "takes place much easier." Rather than presenting itself as hostile, death is often regarded as a "beckoning" whereby "the bonds with life are loosed one by one." Nature often ushers aged persons with a peaceful passage out of life.[41]

Indebted to Francis Bacon, whose *Advancement of Learning* was available in Latin, Marx adopted the term *euthanasia* and viewed it as a "lofty and sacred duty."[42] Far beyond Bacon and even beyond Ferriar's historic essay, however, Marx presents his audience with an overarching and expansive description of palliative care as a distinct area of medical knowledge and practice.

Marx's medical paternalism rivaled that of Thomas Percival: physicians should conceal bad news about misfortunes, dangers, and the patient's own failing conditions; and they can instill false hopes when the clouds over the patient's conditions are darkening. Unlike Percival, however, Marx urged practitioners to "speak out freely" if patients have failed to complete their last wills and testaments. As stated earlier, they should also assume priestly roles, rather than work closely with members of the clergy.[43]

Like John Ferriar, Carl F. H. Marx was a visionary. His innovativeness with respect to palliative care included the use of trained nurses as caregivers; unvarnished opposition to the use of heroic cure-directed concoctions and surgeries for dying persons; inclusiveness of palliative care for poor persons, foreigners, and persons of different faiths; ardent opposition to a physician ever purposefully ending the life of a suffering and dying patient; and attention to the temperaments and ages of dying persons.

Robley Dunglison on Physiological Proof About the Painlessness of Death: 1837

The remarkable career of Robley Dunglison (1798–1869) epitomizes the interconnections between outstanding physicians in the 19th century. Dunglison's career spanned continents: he was born in England; studied medicine in London, Edinburgh, and Paris; obtained his MD from the University of Erlangen in Germany; accepted a professorship in anatomy and medicine at the University of Virginia in 1824; and then moved to the University of Maryland in 1832, where he spent the remainder of his career.

In 1837, Dunglison presented an *Address to the Medical Graduates of the Jefferson Medical College,* in which he asserts that it is the unfailing duty of physicians to enable patients to experience "euthanasia, or easy death." He thereby upheld the wording and tradition advanced by Bacon, Gregory, Percival, Ferriar, and Marx.

> The most trying cases ... are those in which all earthly hope is lost; where every resource of art has been found unavailing. Even here, the attention of the physician is most consolatory. It is indeed his duty to persevere unremittingly in his cares, however distressing to his feeling this may be; and until the very last, to smooth the pillow of suffering.
>
> A euthanasia, or easy death ... may be facilitated by his agency, and hence his aid is often invoked until the very period of dissolution.[44]

Dunglison then employs his knowledge of physiology to demystify terrors associated with death. By so doing, he voiced the findings of numerous other physiologists.[45]

> The idea of intense torment immediately preceding death is so general, that the term <u>agony</u> has been applied to it in many languages. In its origin, the word means nothing more than a violent contest or strife; but it has been extended so as to embrace the pangs of death, and any violent pain.
>
> The agony of death, however—physiologically speaking—instead of being a state of mental and corporeal turmoil and anguish, is one of insensibility. The hurried and labored breathing, the peculiar sound on inspiration, and the turned up eyeball, instead of being evidences of suffering, are now admitted to be signs that the brain has lost all, or almost all, sensibility to impressions.[46]

As the "Father of American Physiology," Dunglison knew that he was talking about.[47] Beyond his and others' findings about the physiology and painlessness of expiring, Dunglison urged his medical audience and readers to convey to family members

> how consolatory ... for the affected attendants on the last scene of all, to be informed, that all these indications of painful strife are such in appearance only. Even the convulsive agitations, occasionally perceived, are the nature of epileptic spasms, which we <u>know</u> to be produced in total insensibility, and to afford no ... evidence of corporeal suffering.... This kind of euthanasia is what all must desire, and fortunately, whatever may have been the previous pangs, the closing scene, in most ailments, is generally of this character.[48]

The centuries-old worries and alarms about the agonies or painful struggles at the end of life were thus being put to rest by physicians schooled in physiology. These findings were used to soothe the minds of persons surrounding the deathbeds of friends and loved ones.

Christoph Wilhelm Hufeland on Terminal Care and Euthanasia Induced by Opium: 1836–1855

While he chronologically belongs in an earlier era, Christoph Wilhelm Hufeland (1762–1836) did not send his famed *Enchiridion Medicum* to his publisher until just days before his death in 1836. Based on 50 years of medical teaching and practice, *Enchiridion* received immediate attention in Germany and was soon published in France. Six German editions were published before it was first translated and published into English in 1842, then again as a second edition in 1844 and a fourth edition in 1855. *Enchiridion* voices Hufeland's convictions about palliative care.

In English editions, *Enchiridion Medicum* (double-titled as *The Practice of Medicine)* greatly advanced Hufeland's fame. The U.S. editions began with testimonials from well-known American physicians. James R. Manley, formerly president of the Medical Society of the State of New York, spoke of the book's unparalleled popularity in Germany and its concise, comprehensive, and rational contents, which justified its being "in the hands of every medical man, whether pupil or practitioner." Others spoke of its close observations, soundness of judgment, usefulness, and overall excellence. One physician referred to the "the great Hufeland" as a well-established medical authority who did not need anyone's recommendation.[49]

Hufeland's medical career manifested profound dedication to the sacrificial nobility, moral duties, and workable therapies of medical practice. After receiving his MD from Gottingen in 1783, he inherited his father's medical practice in Weimar, became a professor in Jena in 1793, and transferred to a professorship in the new University of Berlin in 1801. Like Francis Bacon, he published a book on ways to prolong human life through healthy living. He actively participated in a transformative period of German medicine by pressing for clinical training as an essential component of medical education. While he believed that training in hospital settings was helpful, he favored training in medical dispensaries or polyclinics, from which students would attend patients in their homes apart from the strictly controlled environments of hospitals. Hufeland wanted medical trainees to experience firsthand the way medicine was practiced at the time.[50]

Written as a clinical guide for junior practitioners, *Enchiridion* begins with an essay on the physician's duties regarding sick and dying patients, as well as physicians' relationships with the public and with colleagues. Appended to its 630 pages are 70 pages on "The Three Cardinal Means of the Art of Healing": the "heroic" remedies of venesection (bleeding), opium, and emetics (or "vomits").[51] Hufeland considered himself a therapeutic eclectic opposed to narrow systems of medical theory. He adjusted all of his prescriptions to the particular circumstances, body builds, occupations, ages, living conditions, and emotional temperaments of each patient. That, he believed and taught, was the "science" of medicine.[52]

Hufeland asserts that physicians' highest ends are saving life, restoring health, and relieving the suffering of humanity, including the suffering of dying persons. These are divine and sublime callings. He tells his physician readers, "You are employed by God as a priest of the holy flame of life," so they should exercise their tasks "purely, not to your advantage, nor to your fame, but to the glory of the Lord, and to the salvation of your fellow man."[53]

Hufeland speaks authoritatively about essential aspects of palliative care, even though (unlike John Ferriar and Carl F. H. Marx) he does not systematically outline its details. Yet, similar to Samuel Bard, John Gregory, Benjamin Rush, Ferriar, and Marx, he holds that end-of-life care is an essential professional duty: "Even in the stage of dying the physician ought not to forsake the sick; even then he may become a benefactor, and if he cannot save, may at least relieve departing life."[54]

He narrowly navigates through the options of using curative therapies on mortally ill patients or ceasing to use them. Because he believes that preserving, and perhaps prolonging, life is the highest end of the medical art, Hufeland censures physicians who do nothing when the patient might possibly be cured.[55] When the physician believes that even a dubious and dangerous cure might save a patient's life, he should "not hesitate to use ... this last resort." In such cases, he will "either enjoy the triumph of seeing his honest attempt crowned with success, or the still greater triumph" of knowing that he has been faithful to his highest, life-saving calling. The physician must be prepared to bear the unjust judgment of the public when his honest intention to save life has directed his actions.[56]

Hufeland augments these therapeutic attempts to cure with the psychosomatic power of hope, which forbids speaking truthfully to patients in danger of dying. The hopes of severely ill persons should be raised because hope elevates the mind to the possibility of new endeavors and can render impossibility possible. "I consider it as one of the most important rules of practice," Hufeland asserts, "never to give up hope." Without hope, apathy will follow and the sick will die.[57]

In like manner, the physician must "avoid all things which have a tendency to discourage the patient and lower his spirits."[58] Every word, every look, all his glances, and all his conduct must conceal the dangers the physician feels about the patient's condition. Why? Because anxiety and fear of death "are pernicious poisons" that directly paralyze the vital power of life within the patient. As if taking pages from Thomas Percival, Hufeland holds that physicians should give "a true description of the patient's situation to the relatives"—all the more darkly if the relatives seem to be fickle and negligent. And doctors should never announce danger of death to the sick person even if she or he desires to know the truth: "To announce death is to give death, which is never the business of him, who is employed to save life." Hufeland then refers to two cases in which the patients committed suicide when their expert physicians, induced by their patients' entreaties, revealed the incurability of their conditions.[59]

Far more reprehensible are physicians who put an early end to the lives of patients suffering from disease and praying for death. Physicians who acquiesce to patients' pleadings are annihilating their life-saving vocations. Actions to shorten life are criminal. The doctor who performs them "becomes the most dangerous person of the community."[60] Everything that approaches the modern meaning of euthanasia is totally forbidden by Hufeland.

Even though Christoph Hufeland urges physicians to do everything possible to save a patient's life, he also believes they should know when patients' conditions are incurable and when "the act of dying" begins. In a section subtitled "Palliation," he discusses opium as "the highest gift of God" for easing physical and mental suffering in the last stages of life.

> No other remedy can alleviate pain and anxiety equally with opium, even act like a charm.... Not a hundred, but a thousand times I have seen my patients quite changed in physiognomy, speech, and whole external expression in the morning, after taking opium the preceding evening.[61]

He maintains that "the palliative virtue and effect of opium" has generally been considered insignificant, whereas in his experience opium "surpasses every other narcotic." Its soothing virtue "manifests itself in the most splendid manner, in relieving death in severe cases, to effect the *euthanasia*, which is a sacred duty and the highest triumph of the physician, when it is not in his power to retain the ties of life."[62] Opium is not only capable "of taking away the pangs of death, but it imparts even courage and energy" to dying persons, and it elevates their minds to "heavenly regions."[63]

Hufeland ends his discussion of the palliative effects of opium by telling the story of a man who was experiencing anguish and despair due to a constant sense of suffocation. Even those around him were experiencing unrelieved torment. Upon being given large amounts of opium, the man slept quietly for several hours, and then awakened quite cheerful and free from pain and anxiety. Strengthened and emotionally appeased, "He bade farewell with the greatest composure and satisfaction to his relatives; and after he had given them his blessings and many a good admonition, fell again asleep and ceased to live while sleeping."[64]

Numerous practitioners who relied on Hufeland's *Enchiridion* to aid their medical practice and teach physicians-in-training were surely influenced by his enthusiastic and unconditional recommendations of the use of opium for palliative care. They were also instructed by this famous physician to try to cure exceedingly ill patients if at all possible; to never, ever reveal by word or demeanor the seriousness of the patient's condition to the patient; and to honestly and forthrightly convey that seriousness to relatives. The framers of the American Medical Association's Code of Ethics would rely on the palliative care teachings of Thomas Percival to create their guidelines. In what ways were they also indebted to Christoph Hufeland?

The Code of Ethics of the American Medical Association (AMA): 1847

The first Code of Ethics of the AMA was adopted in 1847 and remained as the official statement of professional ethics by AMA members until it was revised in 1903. Before 1847, medical societies in a number of American states set forth codes of professional conduct. With the founding of the American Medical Association, a common code of duties would regulate that conduct. Sections regarding terminal care were taken by and large from Thomas Percival's *Medical Ethics* of 1803. Percival's recognition of palliative care as a moral imperative, his views of medical paternalism, and his assumptions regarding death's terrors were thereby officially promulgated for decades to come in the United States.

Because of their great influence, the words of AMA's Code of Medical Ethics that pertain to terminal care are given here (the additions to Percival's text are underlined):

ARTICLE I, Paragraph 4. A physician should not be forward to make gloomy prognostications, because they savor of empiricism,[65] by magnifying the importance of his services in the treatment or cure of the disease. But he should not fail, on proper occasions, to give the friends of the patient timely notice of danger when it really occurs; and even to the patient himself, if absolutely necessary. This office, however, is so peculiarly alarming when executed by him, that it ought to be declined whenever it can be assigned to any other person of sufficient judgment and delicacy. For, the physician should be the minister of hope and comfort to the sick—that, by such cordials to the drooping spirit, he may soothe the bed of death, revive expiring life, and counteract the depressing influence of those maladies <u>which often disturb the tranquility of the most resigned, in their last moments. The life of a sick person can be shortened not only by the acts, but also by the words or the manner of a physician. It is, therefore, a sacred duty to guard himself carefully in this respect, and to avoid all things which have a tendency to discourage the patient and to depress his spirits.</u>

ARTICLE I, Paragraph 5. <u>A physician ought not to abandon a patient because the case is deemed incurable</u>; for his attendance may continue to be highly useful to the patient, and comforting to the relatives around him, even in the last period of a fatal malady, by alleviating pain and other symptoms, and by soothing mental anguish. To decline attendance, under such circumstances, would be sacrificing to fanciful delicacy and mistaken liberality, that moral duty which is independent of, and far superior to, all pecuniary consideration.[66]

The words in Article I, Paragraph 5, are historically momentous because they officially oppose physicians' abandonment of incurably ill patients, and they set forth the care and treatment of terminally ill persons as a nationally established imperative.[67] This official endorsement of terminal care as a duty constitutes a milestone in the quest for a good death.

With respect to truth revealing and truth concealing, Article 1, Paragraph 4, of the 1847 code keeps most of the words of Percival's code. In particular, the AMA code holds that the physician should not "make gloomy prognostications" and "should be the minister of hope and comfort to the sick." But the last part of Paragraph 4 favors concealing the truth about patients' dire conditions even more strongly than Percival had done. Percival had focused primarily on what physicians should or should not say, as well as the duty to supply fatally ill persons with medical "cordials."[68] Beyond Percival's imperatives, the AMA code stresses that the doctor's role as a minister of hope and comfort includes the manner of the physician—his behavior, bearing, and everything he says. The physician should "*avoid all things* which have *a tendency* to discourage the patient and to depress his spirits"[69] because these, too, can shorten the lives of dangerously and fatally ill persons. This addition to Percival precisely accords with the directives of Christoph Wilhelm Hufeland.

Worthington Hooker on Hope and Truthfulness with Dangerously Ill Patients: 1849

Two years after the adoption of a Code of Ethics by the AMA, Worthington Hooker (1806–1867) published *Physician and Patient*, which he wrote for both the medical profession and "the community at large."[70] Hooker's purposes for writing were wide ranging, including an exposé of quackery and false advertisements, descriptions and critiques of medical sects such as Thompsonism and Homeopathy,[71] and a lengthy discussion of insanity. His book includes two chapters on medical ethics, the second of which directly confronts Thomas Percival's defense of occasionally lying to severely ill patients.

Hooker graduated from Yale College in 1825 and obtained his MD from Harvard Medical School in 1829. After practicing medicine in Norwich, Connecticut, from 1829 to 1852, he became professor of the theory and practice of medicine at Yale Medical School from 1852 to 1857.[72]

Hope and Medical Treatment

Chapter 16 of Hooker's *Physician and Patient* is titled "The Influence of Hope in the Treatment of Disease." Hooker explores what it should mean or not mean for physicians to be "ministers of hope" to sick and dying persons as set forth in the AMA Code of Medical Ethics. He, too, believes that hope, not despondency, should "characterize the prevailing cast of the physician's mind.... For hope stimulates to action—steady, clear-minded action—while despondency is prone to inaction," fitfulness, and confusion.[73] So Hooker, the AMA code, and most physicians of the time agreed that hope is a physical-emotional stimulant, "a curative agent" similar to alcoholic beverages for body and mind.[74]

Not one to leave the meaning of "ministers of hope" unexamined, Hooker seeks to specify what roles hope requires or forbids. Here are his conceptual guidelines: "The hope of the physician should be an intelligent hope ... based upon just and definite conclusions. It should be discriminating, and should be varied in its degree according to the character of each individual case."[75]

Hooker's position is daunting because he believes in both the therapeutic effects of hope and the harmful effects of revealing a prognosis of death. Therefore, Hooker opposes practitioners who, upon thinking that a patient is very likely to die, believe that they "ought frankly to tell him so."[76] He objects to such frankness for three reasons: First, it is extremely difficult to be "absolutely certain that the patient will die," and even when certainty exists, hope may extend life.[77] Second, physicians who prognosticate death are siding with "the grim visage of death," the "king of terrors," that depresses vital forces of life.[78] And, third, hope is sometimes life-saving.[79]

Concerning the first reason, Hooker appears to deviate from truthtelling. He recognizes that sometimes physicians know death is imminent, but he thinks they should not reveal that prognosis to patients because hope can prolong meaningful life and also alleviate suffering. He illustrates these ideas with a story from his practice:

> In reply to the inquiry of [a patient's] friends [as to] whether I had any hope of his recovery, I frankly said that I had not, and that from all I could see I supposed that the relief which he experienced was to last but a short time, and that he must die very soon. They urged me to tell him so, but I declined.... The condition of comfort and relief lasted in this case, contrary to my expectations, for several weeks; and they were weeks of delightful intercourse, of affectionate counsel, and of triumphant faith and

joy. And I have not a doubt that his life was thus happily prolonged in part by the cordial influence of hope, that the remedies which relieved his distress might effect a cure.[80]

The last line in this story shows that Hooker allowed this patient to falsely believe the remedies Hooker was prescribing might reverse his terminal disease. He adds that "the hope of recovery should occasionally light up ... cases which are certain to end fatally, especially when the patient is the subject of protracted chronic disease. It breaks in upon that painful monotony of mind."[81] These cases exemplify beneficence-based deception.

Concerning Hooker's second objection to a frank disclosure regarding approaching death, he views acquaintanceship with the so-called king of terrors as productive of despair, cheerlessness, physical debilitation, a sense of fatalism, loss of a love for life, and loss of the beneficence of hope.[82] The historic duty of the physician to do no harm thereby justifies truth concealing, which Hooker distinguishes from overt lying.

Concerning his third objection, Hooker tells the story of a patient who was expected to die, but recovered thanks to the administration of a medical remedy accompanied by hope:

> A physician was called in great haste to a patient upon whom he had been attending with deep anxiety. He found the family and the friends assembled around the bed of the patient weeping over him as a dying man.... [H]e prepared a [medical] cordial at once, and with the look of hope and uttering the words of hope, he administered it. The patient not only revived but recovered. In his convalescence he told the physician that as he lay there dimly seeing with his glazed eyes the sad countenances of his friends, and feeling the oppressive languor of death, as he supposed, upon him, and panting for some cordial and for the pure air of heaven, and yet unable to speak or even to raise the hand, no words could express the relief which he at once felt, spreading a genial glow over his benumbed body, when he heard his cheerful voice speak of hope, and it seemed to him that this had more influence in reviving him than the cordial.[83]

Up to this point Hooker has fundamentally agreed with the entire second half of Article I, Paragraph 4, of the AMA code, which calls for physicians to be ministers of hope for grievously sick and dying patients. His contribution consists of infusing the words of the code with an ethical analysis based on bedside experience.

However, believing that hope should be morally limited, Hooker opposes an apparently common practice of his time. He argues that discriminating hope forbids a "wide departure from truth" in the form of falsely assuring patients that they will recover. To Hooker, this is clearly dishonest (and even worse when it is fueled by greed). Physicians and "quacks" alike are guilty when they excite "unwarrantably the hopes of the sick for their own selfish ends."[84] It follows that Hooker believed his deceptive silence was moral insofar as it instilled life-prolonging hope without uttering false assurances.

He concludes this chapter precisely in accordance with the advice that the Reverend Thomas Gisborne gave to Thomas Percival: "A physician should be the minister of hope and comfort to the sick *as far as truth and sincerity will admit.*" Benjamin Rush also voiced that view.[85] Hooker says that "the obvious rule in regard to the use to be made of hope as a curative agent is this—that its cordial influence should always be employed, as far as it can be done consistently with truth, and no farther."[86]

Truth Telling

So what more does "consistent with the truth" mean in medical practice? That is the topic of Hooker's 17th chapter, an innovative chapter that is far more tough-minded than his chapter on hope. Theophile Bonet had favored telling the truth about the patient's terminal condition to patients who ask. Thomas Gisborne's arguments in favor of truth telling, however, were rejected by Thomas Percival. Hooker published his book two years after Percival's paternalistic truth concealing had been inscribed into the code of the American Medical Association. Insofar as Hooker opposed Percival, he also opposed how the AMA's code was being interpreted.

While Hooker titled Chapter 17 "Truth in Our Intercourse with the Sick," his chapter focuses almost entirely on opposing outright and verbalized deception of sick and dying patients with respect to the seriousness of their medical conditions. He begins by noting the great differences of opinion among both medical practitioners and members of the community regarding the permissibility of such dishonesty. Some scrupulously oppose it. Others are generally scrupulous, but make occasional exceptions in "cases of great emergency," while "others still (and I regret to say that they are very numerous) give themselves great latitude in their practice, if they do not in their avowed opinions."[87]

As indicated in his chapter on hope, Hooker opposes overtly verbalized deception. He begins his critique of those who occasionally or regularly deceive patients by forcefully refuting Percival, whom Hooker rightly interprets as occasionally endorsing outright deception. He quotes extensively from Percival's "Notes and Illustrations" in his 1803 Code of Ethics, which included two examples of permissible dishonesty.[88] Hooker exclaims that "the falsehood" of the two cases Percival used to illustrate permissible lying "is of the most egregious character, and yet they are fair representations of that kind of deception which many [physicians] feel authorized to use in the sickroom." Sometimes, he admits, that deception is not as gross as in Percival's examples, but it is real. The question at stake is not whether truth can be *withheld*, but whether "falsehood is justifiable, in any form, whether direct or indirect."[89]

"The preciousness of the principle of truth" is ever-present and right-making in the moral order. It is "the soul of all order, and confidence, and happiness, in the wide universe." Its preciousness is underlined by attending to consequences of deception even in exceptional cases.[90]

First, those who practice outright deception erroneously assume that the knowledge concealed from the patient would, if communicated, be injurious. Hooker claims that such knowledge is not harmful (even though, ironically, he discussed its harmful effects in his chapter on hope). Second, it is erroneously assumed that deception can be successfully carried out. In contrast, Hooker asserts that unguarded expressions or acts by physicians, or even statements by children, "very often either reveals the truth, or awakens suspicion and prompts inquiry with the most skillful equivocation may not be able to elude." And, third, if the deception is discovered or suspected, "the effect upon the patient is much worse than a frank and full statement of the truth can produce."[91]

To illustrate the power of his second and third arguments, Hooker tells about a case that occurred during an epidemic. The death of a woman from the epidemic was "studiously concealed" from her friend beset by the same disease. She was doing well until a neighborhood child alluded to her friend's death, the shock of which was "almost overwhelming." The woman concluded that those who had been deceiving her were doing so because she was "exceedingly in danger of dying from the disease." She soon followed her friend to the grave.[92]

Fourth, the moment physicians are revealed as lying to patients, their veracity is impaired or destroyed. All that they do afterward will be questioned.[93] Hooker drives home this point with seven pages of discussion about the injurious effects of deception on children and insane persons—including their loss of trust and confidence in those who deceived them.[94]

His fifth point analyzes the general effects of deception, which are so injurious to the medical profession that "the momentary good which occasionally results to *individual* cases" pales in comparison to "the vast and permanent evils of a *general* character."[95] Lying to patients affects the profession of medicine as a whole. Among other things, it undermines physicians who adhere to veracity: "Every day we see evidence of the fact ... that the profession, as a whole, has to a greater or less degree the imputation [of deception] fastened upon it."[96]

Sixth, Hooker uses an intriguing philosophical argument that frequent deception destroys the usefulness of deceiving in rare instances. Why, he asks, is deception successful in rare and urgent cases? "It is because the patient supposes that all who have intercourse with him deal with him truthfully."[97]

And finally, he sets forth the cogent rational argument that the actual short-term and long-term consequences of deception are unknowable, such that appeals to consequences cannot serve as the foundation of moral conduct.

> In order to make out a justification of deception, on the ground of expediency in any case, all the possible results, direct and indirect, must be taken into account. But this is impossible except to omniscience itself. Even in those cases which appear the most clear to us, there may be consequences of the most grave character utterly hidden from our view.[98]

It follows that "when the truth is sacrificed for what is deemed to be a greater good, it is in fact the sacrifice of a greater good." It also sacrifices "the eternal principle, which binds together the moral universe in harmony, for a mere temporary good, which after all may prove to be a shadow instead a reality."[99]

Hooker ends his chapter by emphasizing that he is not speaking about withholding information from sick persons when the physician fears the knowledge might be injurious to them. "All that I claim," he asserts, is "that in withholding the truth no deception should be practiced." The physician has the moral right—indeed, the moral duty—to withhold his opinion about the severity of a patient's condition "if he can do so without falsehood or equivocation." If the incurably ill patient asks, "Do you think on the whole that I shall recover?" the doctor can say something like this: "It is difficult to decide that question.... You are very sick, and the issue of your sickness is known only to God."[100]

Worthington Hooker's Chapter 17 has been assessed as "the most original contribution to medical ethics by an American author in the nineteenth century."[101] Notably, debates over truth telling in the doctor-patient relationship were primarily exemplified by cases of patients who were seriously ill and threatened with death.

The lengthy review of *Physician and Patient* by Hooker's medical peers testifies to the cogency of his reasoning against the background of persisting resistance to that reasoning. His reviewers agreed with Hooker that "absolute truth" should rule medical discourse with patients, but then they hedged, suggesting that "deviation from truth" is permissible in "rare and altogether exceptional cases."[102] Their hedging agreed with Thomas Percival, and betrayed Worthington Hooker's objections to the permissibility of lying in urgent cases.

Hugh Noble: Continuity and Change in the Care of Dying Persons: 1854

In England, Scotland, Ireland, Australia, Israel, and elsewhere, the MD is regarded as an advanced degree that requires the writing and defense of a thesis that displays original research.[103] Hugh Noble wrote and defended his articulate, beautifully handwritten, and unpublished MD thesis on palliative care in 1854, which he titled "Euthanasia"— good death by means of skilled palliative care.[104] In Edinburgh, advocacy of palliative care as a fourth dimension of medical practice had been initiated by Gregory in the 1760s.

Hugh Noble's thesis for his MD differs from the innovativeness and authoritative power of the address by Carl C. H. Marx 28 years earlier. Nevertheless, it embodies the thoughtful study of a medical graduate whose work, without scholarly references, reflects how terminally ill persons were being treated and the degrees to which end-of-life care was (or was not) being valued. Noble sometimes thinks independently, and he regards medically aided euthanasia as a normal part of medical practice.[105]

Noble first states that euthanasia is being neglected and sometimes abandoned. "It is true," he says, "that the grand object of the physician is to cure disease." But isn't he also obligated to do all that he can

> to mitigate suffering wherever he may meet it, and surely not less in cases beyond all hope of recovery? ... This part of practice is ... undeniably too much neglected. No sooner does the patient show indications of approaching dissolution than he is apt to be abandoned by his medical attendant as one for whom medical art can do no more, and often little is done or thought worth attempting to render the last painful struggle easier or more endurable ... surely this should not be.[106]

Because dying is often painful and protracted, Noble argues that it is the physician's duty to alleviate the pangs of death. All persons are entitled to all means of medical comfort, and physicians are able to ease much of the misery that many dying persons experience. It is true that efforts to relieve the suffering of persons who cannot recover are not always successful. But, appealing to the intrinsic worth of all living human beings, Noble asserts that the patient "does not forfeit all claim to attention merely because his disease is mortal." It is "criminal" to think and act otherwise.[107]

Like palliative care advocates beginning with John Ferriar in 1794, Hugh Noble holds that when hope of recovery has vanished, the practitioner must re-envision the case from a different point of view. Blistering, bleeding, and purging "may well be dispensed with as soon as it becomes apparent that the patient's fate is sealed." He believes that "great relief may often be afforded by this step alone."[108]

Note, however, that Noble says that these remedies "may well be dispensed with." In fact, his thesis reveals that many cure-directed practices of the time were being employed for palliative purposes. Consider, for example, bleeding, which Noble says might have the effect of giving degrees of comfort without shortening life. He mentions that bleeding patients with acute inflammations and lung diseases will likely ease their symptoms. Noble then discloses an apparently new development: surgery may also palliate symptoms. Patients with difficult, labored breathing or with an aneurism at the arch of the aortic artery can be made more comfortable by means of a tracheotomy or through chest surgery, which, thanks to the discovery of anesthetics, could be performed painlessly. However, he does not mention how these patients might die from infection.[109]

All things considered, Noble does not want to "be held as condemning the use of such measures in proper cases," even though he wants dying persons to be saved from any additional afflictions that will not be beneficial. Through his equivocations Noble is revealing what was being done in the mid–1850s in Edinburgh to patients nearing the very end of life. As a medical student, he is reluctant to oppose those practices forcefully.[110]

Similar to Carl F. H. Marx, Noble emphasizes that the art and science of enabling persons to pass from life peacefully requires expert prognostic knowledge of fatal diseases. Sometimes the approach of death is gradual and painless, such that nature, not palliative measures, effects the transition between life and death. But in other cases the mode of dying proves to be tedious and severe—mortal wounds, the bursting of aneurisms, weakness and disability, apnea, poisoning, starvation, chronic vomiting, and obstruction of the bowels. Apnea may involve horrible anguish, including distended nostrils, heaving of the chest, exhaustion and wakefulness. Additionally, diabetes, "that mysterious error of nutrition," is intractable and ends in extreme emaciation.[111]

He then turns to the ways pain and other symptoms can be relieved. Pain often points directly to the cause of the disease and thus demands attention. Pain, sleeplessness, and anxiety can be mollified by an array of soothing, calming and hypnotic remedies. Historically innovative, Noble writes at some length about chloroform, which was being used as an anesthetic during surgery, but which, he feels persuaded to say, "might be made available far more than it is in the closing scenes of many unhappy victims of disease."[112] He has in mind the same practice recommended by Marx—namely, that persons who are suffering interminably can be "kept in a state of imperfect anesthesia (unconsciousness)" during their last days of life. Chloroform has the advantage of being easily controlled, and its effectiveness is independent from the ability to swallow.[113]

The two modes of emotional comfort Noble discusses are highly important and emotionally laden moral issues. The first, still-haunting issue involves whether the truth about the patient's condition should be concealed or revealed. Noble notes that the truth about a patient's mortal illness is "usually ... studiously concealed" from the patient out of fear that that news will accelerate his death. "Is this always right?" he asks. Except for extremely difficult cases, his answer is "No."

> I have heard a patient ... bitterly complaining that he had never been made aware that his sickness was to terminate fatally.... [D]oes not some responsibility rest upon those who are best qualified to tell beforehand that a patient is to die, and who nevertheless neglect to do so?[114]

Noble claims that in many cases the true state of matters might well be communicated to the patient, thereby giving him the opportunity to prepare for death. At the same time, there are cases of great delicacy in which a slender chance of recovery will be "destroyed entirely by the fear of death."[115]

Noble's second moral-emotional concern is astonishing for his time. He argues that the practitioner should respect the wishes of dying persons: "A judicious acquiescence in the dying man's expressed wishes must often have a great effect in augmenting his comfort ... conducing to his tranquility of mind."[116]

In step with notable advocates of palliative care who preceded him, Hugh Noble opposes ever actively ending the lives of suffering persons. He is deeply acquainted with the extent of suffering that some dying persons are experiencing:

> There are diseases so horrible a character and accompanied by so great an amount of distress that the arrival of death comes to be very desirable, and when the severity of suffering becomes very acute, one is constrained to wish that nature were less capable of resisting and that death would triumph more easily.[117]

But because human life is sacred, "no combination of circumstances can be imagined in which it would be in the least degree warrantable to seek to abridge the sufferings of the dying by means having any tendency to hasten the close of even a fast-ebbing existence."[118] His words are painfully graphic, yet morally determined and conclusive:

> However painful the mode of dissolution—however loathsome the disease—however vehemently the wretched patient may cry for the merciful arrival of death, yet no one **dare dream** of using means to shorten the period of his misery, we are only at liberty to endeavor to lessen its <u>degree</u>. The patient must wait for deliverance at the hand of nature however protracted the process may prove.... [T]he only relief he is to expect from human hands is the application of such means as may be calculated to mitigate the intensity.[119]

Hugh Noble ends his dissertation by returning to the morality of truth telling—not to the question of whether the truth should be revealed, but to whether outright deception is ever permissible. In the last sentence of his thesis, he asks whether "it is ever right to prevaricate or deny the existence of manifest danger" to the patient. He quickly responds, "I shall not here attempt to discuss" that question.[120] He surely knew that his question would seize the attention of his thesis examination committee. Under the pressures of a dissertation defense, he was smart to decline getting involved in the debate.

Noble's dissertation reflects continuities with former proponents of the art and science of peaceful dying: the great value of palliative care, its reliance on updated medical knowledge, its commitment to soothing suffering, its steadfast opposition to physician-induced death, and its recognition of ethical concerns embedded in palliative care. His essay also reflects discontinuities and change—namely, his remarkable points about listening to and acting in accordance with patients' wishes and the increasing use of heroic remedies and even surgeries as palliative measures for dying patients.

Concluding Perspectives

Advocacy of palliative care for dying persons continued in Britain and Scotland and on the European continent between the 1820s and the mid–1850s. Thomas Percival's inclusion of palliative care as a prescribed duty in medical practice became officially promulgated in the United States by the newly formed American Medical Association in 1847.

Between 1826 and 1854 ever more attention was being given to the specific and manifold diseases and types of suffering endured by many dying patients—in particular, diseases that cause terrible suffering. Carl F. H. Marx talked about the necessity of giving one's utmost attention to persons dying of chronic arthritis, yellow fever, leprosy, lung diseases, and cancer. And Hugh Noble described the exceedingly various degrees of suffering with respect to a long list of tedious and severe conditions.

The science and art of enabling dying persons to experience good and peaceful deaths rested on the essential preconditions of suspending, greatly curtailing, or wisely using life-prolonging medical treatments and surgeries. Increased attention was also given to effective pain-relieving medicines, particularly the uses of opium and chloroform.

The care that was being advanced proved to be filled with ethical issues: why dying persons should not be abandoned, why and when the curative treatments of the time should be suspended (or sometimes used), what levels of hope should be offered, what information should be concealed from or revealed to persons thought to be dying, whether outright deception was ever warranted, and why dying persons should be asked about their wishes.

Truth telling or concealing emerged as an especially contentious ethical issue because doctors were of several minds on the matter. Worthington Hooker indicated that some physicians believed patients should be told forthrightly when they were dying. Others, in the tradition of Percival, Marx, and Christoph Hufeland, believed that patients in the throes of life-endangering illness should not be informed about their conditions and could at times be overtly deceived. Hooker marshaled cogent rational arguments against such deception, which he believed was morally compatible with withholding judgments about the likelihood of death.

In contrast to Thomas Percival and a moral continent removed from Carl F. H. Marx and Christoph Hufeland, Hugh Noble sided with truth revealing in most instances. He based his judgment on the comforts dying patients derived when physicians respectfully acquiesced to their expressed wishes and also on the case of a patient's bitter disappointment over never being informed about his fatal illness.

In one voice these proponents held that palliative care is antithetical to deliberately hastening death. Vividly, and with greater force and detail than all others, Noble exclaimed that no one should dream of intentionally shortening the period of a patient's misery. There is no little irony that the word "euthanasia" in the titles discussed in this chapter would within decades become identified with actions these authors ardently opposed.

Within the literature on comfort-directed care during these years, however, a worrisome problem was registered by Marx and Noble—care for dying persons was too much neglected. Noble credited the lack of attention to physicians becoming enamored with the great art of curing disease. But that art, he declared, should not eclipse the duty of the physician "to do his utmost to mitigate suffering wherever he may meet it, and surely not less in cases beyond all hope of recovery."[121]

4

Polarities Between Attention and Disregard

1859–1894

Before 1859 women remained behind the curtains of the stage where the quest for good dying was being enacted. In 1826 Carl F. H. Marx spoke of their taking an acting role when none had yet taken center stage. Marx uttered something bordering on the scandalous: attendants and "properly trained nurses" could best carry out everything that "can possibly be done through the doctor's foresight."[1] He envisioned nurses becoming pivotal with respect to care for terminally ill patients.

Florence Nightingale (1820–1910) took center stage in 1859, which inspired generations of nurses to play leading roles in the care of sick and fatally ill persons. Another heroine performed anonymously. In 1890 "a Hospital Nurse" commended the study by William Munk (1816–1898) to her reading audience. Published in 1887, Munk's book was a systematic, scholarly treatise about the care of dying persons. The hospital nurse found the book enormously helpful for her duties with the terminally ill, and she quoted from it extensively as she informed her nurse sisters about her discovery.[2]

Between 1859 and 1894 several other physicians besides William Munk spoke about their commitment to palliative care. The most notable of these physicians, D. W. Cathell, takes us into the common culture venues of his times. Yet worries had become alarming over both the neglect of detailed attention to persons in their last stages of life and the academic study of their physical and emotional suffering. Reasons for neglect were not given, but they were reflective of an increasing equation of medicine with diagnosing and curing disease.

A brief summary of medical theory, knowledge, and practice during this time of transition between traditional and modern medicine provides background for what follows. In an oration before the Royal College of Physicians in London in 1862, C. J. B. Williams equated the diagnosis of specific diseases as "the object of the scientific physician."[3] He speaks of the necessity that physicians keep records of the cases they treat and says his analysis is based on notes of some 23,000 cases. Williams dwells at length on the causes and cures of pneumonia. It is caused by poisons, but especially "that great cause" of becoming chilled. For example, soccer-playing school boys become chilled and catch pneumonia when, at the end of play, they "throw themselves carelessly and exhausted on the wet grass." The great cure of pneumonia is bloodletting, which arrests the symptoms of hot skin and strong and rapid heartbeats. Coolness of the skin and lowered pulse rates should be sustained through further depletions of blood by means of leeches, blistering, and using the powerful mercury compound, calomel, and other stimulants if circulation flags.[4]

Traditional use of bloodletting, calomel, and other caustic remedies was receding at the time of Williams' oration.[5] The demise of heroic therapeutics was due in part to studies in Europe that showed, for example, that calomel produced gangrene and obstructed the flow of bile from the liver. More judicious uses of bloodletting were still defended in the 1870s, but by then therapeutic thinking had shifted away from getting rid of fevers and toxins to building up strength.[6] Some physicians questioned and castigated the heroic remedies of the past and replaced them with dietary aids, fresh air, and other comforting practices. That required courage in the face of patient and family questions: "Aren't you going to do something, Doctor?"[7]

Medical rigor was maintained by stimulants and turning to agents to decrease fever. Fever reduction and physical ease were accomplished through such agents as aconite and quinine, the first a poisonous vegetable compound with harsh side effects. Quinine became a panacea in the 1870s and 1880s as both a fever reducer and a stimulant.[8] Opium was widely used as a pain reliever and as a treatment for diarrhea for sick and dying persons alike. Alcohol as a stimulant was invested with a host of beneficial effects for acute diseases such as typhoid fever and pneumonia, as well as chronic diseases such as tuberculosis. In keeping with Christoph Hufeland's instructions, alcohol also served as an anchor in terminal care.[9]

Important changes on the horizon would greatly enhance the status of curative medicine. Joining the recently established Johns Hopkins Medical School, William Henry Welch (1850–1934), for example, established a laboratory in pathology and bacteriology. Among many other studies, Welch explored the effects of an anti-diphtheria serum, which, he announced in 1895, all physicians should be obliged to use.[10]

Surgery changed remarkably after the 1850s, and within decades it became the most prestigious of all medical specialties. In addition to having a far greater knowledge of human anatomy, surgeons could deaden pain with anesthesia—nitrous oxide, ether, and chloroform. This greatly increased numbers of amputations and, as discussed in the previous chapter, also increased other types of surgery. But without asepsis or antiseptics, these amputations resulted in death rates of 15–20 percent even when performed in hospitals.[11] The 1880s were transitional years in surgery. Modern surgery based on anesthesia, antisepsis, and asepsis that made abdominal, chest, throat, eye and other surgeries possible began on the European continent in the 1870s and in the United States a few years later.[12] Chloroform and ether continued to be used as agents to ease conditions of patients with painful conditions.

Florence Nightingale and Trained Nurses: 1859

When Florence Nightingale published *Notes on Nursing* in 1859, she was already world-famous and revered.[13] She and the nurses she trained saved the lives of thousands of wounded and sick solders during the Crimean War[14] by radically altering unsanitary conditions and erratic care in military hospitals. Her book became a cornerstone of the curriculum at Nightingale's training school for nursing established in 1860 at King's College in London. *Notes on Nursing* became required reading in numerous other newly established nursing schools across the Western world and was widely read by the general public. Nightingale pivotally influenced the professionalization of nursing throughout her long life.[15] When Queen Victoria awarded her the Royal Red Cross in 1883, it symbolized her ever-increasing acclaim.

The training of nurses as caregivers for wounded, sick, and dying persons, particularly patients in hospitals, increased after 1836 in Kaiserswerth, Germany, where Florence Nightingale received her training. Programs similar to Nightingale's school were developed for children and women in New York in 1859 and Philadelphia in 1865. By the 1870s other training programs that followed "Nightingale's Plan" were established in New York, New Haven, and Boston. Fifteen such programs were in existence by 1880, 35 by 1883, and 432 training programs (with some 3,456 graduates) in 1900.[16] Trained nurses contributed to the popularity of hospitals by making them clean and less productive of disease transmission. They would become registered nurses—RNs—starting in 1914.

Physicians also recognized Nightingale's life-saving contributions. Before London's Royal College of Physicians, C. J. B. Williams said that the great saving of the lives of injured soldiers "has been primarily due to.... Miss Nightingale."[17] Kindness was no longer enough. Knowledge and skill were also essential.[18]

Florence Nightingale's *Notes on Nursing* discusses the care of hospitalized sick persons, including persons who are dying or in danger of death. Concerning dying patients, she says:

> Patients are frequently lost in the latter stages of disease from want of attention to ... simple precautions. The nurse may be trusting to the patient's diet, or to his medicine, or to the occasional dose of stimulant which she is directed to give him, while the patient is all the while sinking from want of a little external warmth. Such cases happen at all times, even during the height of summer.
>
> A careful nurse will keep a constant watch over her sick, especially weak, protracted, and collapsed cases, to guard against the effects of the loss of vital heat.... In certain diseased states much less heat is produced than in health; and there is a constant tendency to the decline and ultimate extinction of the vital powers by the call made upon them to sustain the heat of the body. Cases where this occurs should be watched with the greatest of care from hour to hour.... [W]henever a tendency to chilling is discovered, hot bottles, hot bricks, and warm flannels, with some warm drink, should be made until the temperature is restored.[19]

Nightingale's precautions are not always simple. They include many factors that she discusses at great length under separate headings: ventilation and warming, light and darkness, hygiene, noise and conversation, and beds and bedding. She speaks about ventilation and air almost to the point of preoccupation[20]:

> The very first canon of nursing, the first and the last thing upon which a nurse's attention must be fixed ... is this: TO KEEP THE AIR HE BREATHES AS PURE AS THE EXTERNAL AIR, WITHOUT CHILLING Him.... [W]here it is thought of at all, the most extraordinary misconceptions reign about it. Even in admitting air into the patient's room or ward, few people ever think, where that air comes from.[21]

As she explains, the air in hospitals may come from the rooms of other sick persons. In hospitals and homes it may come from sinks, washrooms, toilets, or open sewers loaded with filth, such that the air is poisoned. Windows and chimneys must be open to let in fresh air. Chimneys should be swept. Night air must be let in. The noxious smells of excreta from bedpans must be stopped. Nightingale asserts that hospital pus-exuding abscesses and consumptive coughing are "the *immediate* products of foul air."[22]

Writing at a time before the discovery of germs and before the germ theory of disease created the discipline of bacteriology (one of the foundation stones for modern medicine and preventive health),[23] Florence Nightingale believed that infection and disease were caused by contagions and miasmas. Contagions are the poisonous emanations arising from the bodies of affected persons, while miasmas are the poisonous emanations and smells of musty rooms, hospital wards, rotting garbage, sewage, decomposing flesh and bodies, and swampy, low-lying land. These convictions led to extensive and effective "scientific sanitation" reforms, and they account for Nightingale's steadfast interest in sanitation and hygiene, to the point of her saying that "*sanitary* nursing is the subject of these notes."[24] At one point in her *Notes*, she even directly opposes the notion that diseases result from "separate entities, which *must* exist, like cats and dogs.... I have seen with my eyes and smelt with my nose small-pox growing up ... either in close rooms, or in overcrowded wards."[25] These separate entities would soon be called germs.

In keeping with the sanitary reforms of her time, Nightingale also sets forth nursing rules regarding rinsing utensils and bedpans; cleaning musty carpets and curtains; and shaking, drying out, and airing the bedding of sick and dying persons with sunlight. Mattresses, sheets, and blankets, she says, should be aired out every twelve hours. Second to fresh air, sick and dying patients need light. "Who," she asks, "has not observed the purifying effect of light, and specifically of direct sunlight, upon the air of the room?" For Nightingale, "A dark house is always an unhealthy house, always an ill-aired house, always a dirty house.... People lose their health in a dark house."[26] For dying patients, special attention should be given to the use and placement of pillows. They should not be used merely to raise the head, but also spread out to support the lower back for breathing. Correcting the "almost universal error among nurses," the right amounts and digestibility of food and drink should also be carefully considered.[27]

Florence Nightingale likewise displays concern for the emotional well-being of patients. Similar to the counsel of physicians beginning with John Ferriar, she says loud and sharp noises that jar patients awake and disturb their sleep must be muffled. Spoken and whispered conversations can be cruel if overheard by grievously ill persons. (She relates the story of the death of a patient who overheard a discussion of her impending surgical operation.) The value of and respect for each person must also be upheld by sitting down directly within the patient's sight when talking. No patient should be spoken to at a distance or from behind a door. Patients should always be told beforehand when the nurse will be leaving and when she will return.[28]

To fulfill these duties, nurses must be "in charge" to ensure that a system of caring exists:

> To be "in charge" is certainly not only to carry out the proper measures yourself but to see that everyone else does so too; to see that no one either willfully or ignorantly

thwarts or prevents such measures. It is neither to do everything yourself nor to appoint a number of people to each duty, but to ensure that each does that duty to which he is appointed.[29]

Nightingale's *Notes on Nursing* do not dwell on palliative care, but they include information on this topic. Her reference to nurses being "in charge" likely means that nurses were in charge of medical wards, which was clearly true by 1890 (as discussion that follows will show). John Ferriar in 1792 and Carl F. H. Marx in 1826 talked about the need to open windows to purify and renew the air and to pull back the curtains for light, but Nightingale addressed these and other matters with greater detail and passion, and she deemed them utterly necessary.

S. D. Williams Initiates the Modern Definition of Euthanasia: 1870

Little is known about S. D. Williams, an English schoolmaster, apart from the speech he gave to members of Birmingham, England's Speculative Club in 1870. Titled "Euthanasia," his speech, printed in *The Spectator* (and then reprinted several times as a book of essays by the Speculative Club), became pivotal in reversing the meaning of the term *euthanasia*.[30] Previous chapters have shown that, beginning with Francis Bacon in 1605, euthanasia denoted easing the symptoms and sufferings of mortally ill patients without ever putting them to death. Euthanasia would continue to convey that meaning well after Williams gave his speech. But over time the term increasingly denoted its modern meaning: doctors putting suffering, dying patients to a quick and painless death. They could accomplish this with large doses of sedatives and, for Williams and many others, by administering chloroform or some other anesthetic until life was extinguished.[31]

Unlike other scholarly works, this 400-year history of palliative care does not intertwine palliative end-of-life care with other major types of euthanasia—topics in their own right.[32] Yet Williams' lecture merits attention here because it eventually reversed the historic meaning of euthanasia and thereby broke the history of medically assisted palliative care into two eras: first, the era from 1605 to the last decades of the 19th century, during which it was termed euthanasia; and, second, the era thereafter, when, shunning the term *euthanasia*, this care was designated as medically managed dying, death with dignity, care for dying patients, and, of course, palliative care.

Here is Williams's proposal:

[I]n all cases of hopeless and painful illness, it should be the recognized duty of the medical attendant, whenever so desired by the patient, to administer chloroform—or such other anesthetic as may by-and-by supersede chloroform—so as to destroy consciousness at once, and put the sufferer to a quick and painless death.[33]

He calls this medical duty a "boon conferred on mankind" because it relieves patients from "the hideous tortures of a lingering disease"—horror that abounds everywhere.[34] He amplifies his case with copious rhetoric: these tortures are protracted, fiercely painful, often lengthy, fruitless, pitiless, writhing, victimizing, cruel, terrible, ever-present, appalling, and agonizing, but "happily, often remediable."[35] He asks, "Why should not the [chloroform] inhaler not be seen as unfailingly by the bed of death, as it is by the operating table?"[36]

Williams relies on his Darwinian worldview to secure the validity of his thesis. Nature is "red in tooth and claw," a dreadful and blind force that is anything but a kindly mother. Instead, nature is a "scene of carnage" in which the strong prey upon the weak in a never-ending struggle.[37] Pain to all living creatures "is the one great reality amid a crown of appearances and illusions."[38] Nature knows nothing of the sacredness of life to which those opposed to physician-induced death constantly appeal but which, upon reflection, should be dismissed as irrational.[39] He argues, instead, that human life is not intrinsically valuable, and it becomes useless when persons are no longer useful to themselves and others.[40] Physicians, therefore, should align themselves with modern progress that opposes all forms of cruelty, including the cruelty of protracted dying and the cruelty in slaughterhouses.[41]

Within a year, editors of *The Spectator* revisited Williams's essay with their own article titled "Euthanasia." They confessed that his proposition created "a terrible perplexity," but then they set forth counter-arguments that would typify physicians' opposition to Williams's proposal in decades to come. The arguments included a concern that the type of euthanasia Williams proposes would be sorely abused. Also, the actions he urges are irrevocable. His position degrades physicians' noblest aspirations by turning healers into executioners. And, finally, Williams fails to address the "far reaching wisdom" of belief in an overruling Divine Order.[42]

D. W. Cathell: Palliative Care by Physicians in the Trenches of American Culture: 1882

D. W. (Daniel Webster) Cathell (1839–1925) takes us into the worlds of patients outside hospitals. His *Book on the Physician Himself*, first published in 1882, was written as a no-nonsense guide on how physicians in private practice can get on in the world where diverse populations of patients live.[43] For more than thirty years, Cathell revised and republished his book,[44] which continued—and continues—to be praised for its savvy advice on becoming a successful and respected practitioner.[45] He widely influenced common medical practitioners of his time and generations of physicians in private practice thereafter. His advice is straightforward and full of practical suggestions. His targeted readers are doctors in search of a decent, lower-middle-class living in competition with numerous independent general practitioners, many of whom were poorly educated.[46]

Beyond his book's fame, little is known about D. W. Cathell's life and career. He received an MD from the New York Downstate College of Medicine in 1865 and practiced in Baltimore, Maryland, for the rest of his life.

The term "trenches of American culture" does not exaggerate the sort of patients Cathell has in mind:

> The white and the black, the rich and the poor, the courtesan, the outlaw, the swaggering rowdy and the reprobate, will all be represented in your practice.... Remember always that such people respect no doctor who does not respect himself.[47]

Cathell also refers to hard drinkers and drunkards, fine ladies, hod carriers (laborers carrying heavy loads of coal, bricks, and plaster), broken-hearted wretches, lawyers, sailors, and persons with differing temperaments and religious persuasions, especially Roman Catholics.[48]

The range of persons the doctor treats day and night[49] calls for a mixture of open-ended education and caution. Consider drunken patients with accidents and injuries. For these patients, practitioners should

> have the presence of mind to give a provisional opinion only, till they return to a sober state. It is better to say, "He is certainly drunk; whether his drunkenness obscures other and more important features it is at this time impossible for anyone to say."[50]

Consider patients who are terminally ill:

> The truth is that life is a **different** quantity in different people, and you will usually have no other way to judge a patient's prospect of recovery than by the **average** human standard. You will sometimes have cases which will surprise you by their having a great deal **less** than the **average** tenacity of life, and others by having a great deal **more** than average; and no matter how careful you are, you cannot with our present aids accurately prognosticate the endurance power of every patient.[51]

Cathell's counsel to his readers is ever guarded—indeed, at times it is indicative of defensive medicine. Practitioners are commonly assumed "to foreknow all conceivable things related to disease ... and its terminations." So when death occurs unexpectedly, "do not let your manner indicate that you were entirely ignorant of its possibility." When the danger of rapid or sudden death exists, readers are told to be wary of ordering opiates or other potent drugs that might "create a belief that they caused or hastened" death. It is wise at times to order such drugs under names that make them appear to be harmless. That will keep physicians from being "unjustly charged with doing harm." And when called to make a determination of the cause of sudden death, "the utmost composure of mind and manner is of great importance." In order to keep from being censured, never express "any opinion of the cause ... until you have calmly and coolly collected and weighed all the circumstance."[52]

He combines caution with an emphasis on life-long learning, or, in his words, the "full use of all the teachings of experience, and of ... every aid offered to you by medical science."[53] Physicians attending patients in their homes should know how to perform surgery, know the natural histories of numerous diseases, understand how the varying temperaments of patients (stoical, apathetic, nervous, hysterical) affect how they respond in sickness and in death, know the basic signs of death, and know how to determine the causes of death. Physicians should use the findings of physiology to comfort families and friends and to assure them that "the dying struggle" is painless even though it may appear painful and harrowing.[54] They should also bravely perform autopsies on patients who died unexpectedly or mysteriously in order to learn about death and, if censured by relatives, to meet their criticisms as squarely as possible.[55]

With respect to truth telling, truth concealing, lying, and hope, D. W. Cathell sides, knowingly or not, with Theophile Bonet, Thomas Gisborne, Worthington Hooker, and Hugh Noble. However, he also adds his own notes of propriety: It is permissible to conceal the truth about the danger of death from patients who might give up all hope or be overcome by apprehension and terror. But in all cases, family members and friends should be told. If an extremely ill and mentally composed patient asks his physician plainly about his condition, "answer him frankly and truthfully, but if possible in bland terms." Give him "all the encouragement you honestly can" and "if you know anything favorable either in his physical or spiritual condition," mention those as a solace.[56] Maintain hope as much as possible, but, reflecting the language of Hooker, he says, "Of course you must not, you cannot, put falsehood in the place of truth, even when talking to the sick and dying, for you cannot sacrifice principle or truth for expediency under any circumstances. But tell it in a proper manner.... Veracity should ever be your golden shield."[57] Quoting, perhaps unknowingly, from Francis Bacon, he says, "It is just as natural to die as it is to be born." Everyone's time must come. Physicians and their patients "can neither see what is written in the book of life, nor detain the sick soul when the Angel of Death summons."[58] It is better to be prepared for death than to allow terrors of death to undermine one's devotion to truth.

In addition to its unique purpose, Cathell's book breaks new ground regarding the roles of religion in the care of sick and dying persons. Ministering to these persons day and night in their homes, he would have had to put blinders on to dismiss the interconnections between sickness, dying, and religious faith and practice.

Like hope—indeed, as the ultimate source of hope for most of his patients—Cathell believes that faith is medically therapeutic and that it is ignorant to think otherwise.

> The great prospect of Eternity certainly overshadows all temporal things. Be ever ready, not only to allow, but to advise patients to have spiritual comfort. Religion does good, not only hereafter but here. Indeed, the presence of religious faith is a wonderful power, and if any physician does not recognize it he lacks the a b c of philosophy and the rudiments of observation.
>   The ministrations of a cheerful, sensible and pious clergyman are sometimes more useful to a worn and irritated patient than medicine; and even where death is near and inevitable, resignation often takes the place of fear when the sick one is skillfully informed of the probability of death. In fact, when cheered by religion, many show as little regret upon learning that they will probably die as a traveler does when about to start on a pleasant journey.[59]

Furthermore, doctors should never thrust their personal religious beliefs on patients, nor should they voice political opinions. Physicians should confine their ministrations to the worldly welfare of their patients and "never suggest anything in religious matters that involves a creed different from that of the sick one."[60]

Because they were so widely prevalent in the northeastern United States at the time and constituted a large percentage of the working-class patients, Roman Catholics are discussed at length by Cathell. By 1880 the Catholic population had risen to 12.5 percent of the entire U.S. population and outnumbered all other religious groups. At this time, most American Catholics were overcoming former levels of poverty and becoming policemen, firemen, and active members in the labor movement.[61] Cathell describes Catholic beliefs and rituals to his readers, explaining that the family of the dying patient should be told of the danger of the patient's becoming unconscious so that a priest can be called to take the patient's confession, give the Holy Eucharist, and administer the last rites. If you err at all in these matters, he tells his readers, "let it be on the safe side."[62] Cathell gave special attention to the relationships between religion and medicine a century before their interconnections would be far more thoroughly explored.[63]

William Munk's Historic Contributions to Terminal Care: 1887

William Munk (1816–1898) began his study of medicine at University College, London, in 1835 and received his MD from the University of Leiden in 1837. He secured five honorary appointments in medical institutions, including the Royal Hospital for Incurables,[64] and became a fellow in the Royal College of Physicians in London in 1854. His service as the Royal College's Harveian Librarian for almost 30 years expanded his social connections and fostered several publications in the history of medicine. Paying no attention to the definition of euthanasia set forth by S. D. Williams, Munk published his own book titled *Euthanasia or, Medical Treatment in Aid of an Easy Death* in 1887 at the age of 71. The stellar review of *Euthanasia* in *The Lancet* praised Munk's "large store of erudition ... experience ... [and] calm reflection"—all "worthy of the attainments and character of the Harveian Librarian of the Royal College of Physicians."[65]

Munk's *Euthanasia* is substantive, systematic, impressively researched, and informed by 50 years of medical experience—a scholarly classic in the literature. Beyond all previous writers, he researched and referenced the writings of prior and contemporary authors and practitioners.[66] Both his preface and later chapters recognize the "short but valuable essay ... by Dr. [John] Ferriar of Manchester in 1798" and the publications of many others, including Florence Nightingale.[67]

He frames his study within the unbroken sweep of the palliative care narrative and identifies that care with the term *euthanasia*. His first chapter begins with the recognition that "one of the wisest of our countrymen, Lord Verulam [Francis Bacon], saw reason to censure the physicians of his own time for not making the Euthanasia a part of their studies."[68]

> Lord Verulam held it to be as much the duty of the physician to smooth the bed of death, and render the departure from this life easy and gentle, as it is to cure diseases and restore health. And this doctrine ... is commended to us by that most estimable and judicious of modern physician, Dr. Heberden[69]; as it was also by the example and counsel of one of the most popular and successful physicians of the present century—the late Sir Henry Halford.[70]

In his preface Munk says that Halford "was confessedly a master in all that concerns the management of the Dying." Munk adds that Halford's remarks on terminal treatment and care occur incidentally in the course of his various essays and are "now but little known," but they manifest "an experience so large, and so carefully thought out" that he (that is, Munk) will harvest them in his book.[71] Munk also incorporates the insights of many others, including the prominent surgeons Benjamin Collins Brodie (1783–1862) and William Scovell Savory (1826–1895).[72] He completely agrees with Christoph Hufeland's passionate belief in the value of opium, and he extensively quotes from Hufeland's instructions.[73]

Munk wrote with the conviction that the medical treatment and aid of an easy death needed and deserved special study, especially for the purpose of enabling young physicians to know "what to do, and what not to do, in the most solemn and delicate position in which [they] can be placed."[74] Published as a small book, his treatise inspired and informed physicians, nurses, and several of the founders and caregivers of the hospice movement. He outlines his study under the three headings that follow.

Some of the Phenomena of Dying

William Munk begins this chapter by lamenting the lack of attention given to the medical management of dying persons:

> The subject is not specially taught in any of our medical schools; and the young physician entering on the active duties of his office has to learn for himself, as best he may, what to do, and what not to do ... in attendance on the dying, and administering the resources of the medical art, in aid of an easy, gentle, and placid death. The whole subject of the Euthanasia, or of a calm and easy death, insofar as it respects the physician is in need of special study; and of a systematic treatment that has not hitherto been accorded to it.[75]

However, he will only trace the outlines of this subject and leave more extensive studies to others.

The disregard he highlights is all the more deplorable because modern science has thrown great light on the diverse modes of dying and death.[76] Quoting from John Ferriar's 1798 essay and predicated on his personal experience, Munk says that "the physical process of death loses much of its horror on a near view."[77] This horror is also eased because the process of death does not usually involve severe bodily suffering.

> Physicians, the clergy, and intelligent nurses—all, indeed, who are practically conversant with the dying—testify to the truth of this statement.... Sir Benjamin Brodie, whose experience of death from surgical disease was second to none, states that, according to his observation, the mere act of dying is seldom, in any sense of the word, a very painful process.[78]

Convulsions that dying persons manifest, and which are viewed as evidence of suffering, for example, are the reverse of suffering. Voicing the findings of Robley Dunglison and other physiologists, he says these convulsions usually signal a loss of conscious sensibility and, therefore, an incapacity to feel pain.[79] (Brodie and Dunglison published their views years before S.D. Williams built his case for doctor-induced death by equating death with ever-present tortures.)

Nevertheless, Munk describes several conditions that cause grievous suffering for dying persons—namely, diseases of the heart and great vessels of the chest, angina pectoris, obstruction of the bowels, and diseases such as tetanus and spasmodic cholera, which create spasms in external muscles. These cases are rare, "but they are so terrible that they fix themselves in the memory, exert an undue influence on the judgment, and ... come to be ... assumed [as] the universal and inevitable lot of the dying. Happily for mankind it is not so."[80]

Furthermore, Munk believes that concern for the emotions of patients is critical. Suffering can be eased by the great solace of hope—hopes voiced by physicians, the hope of religious faith, and the patient's retrospective reflection on a well-spent life. At times these are infinitely more efficacious than "all the resources of the medical art." Concerning the solace of religion, he says that

> a firm belief in the mercy of God, and in the promises of salvation will do more than anything in aid of an easy, calm, and collected death. To those who are skeptical on this point, and such there are, I would remark, that unless a man has himself felt the influence of religion on his own mind, he is unable fully and accurately to understand its influence on others.[81]

In Munk's experience, atheists and agnostics are more often beset with anxiety that makes dying peacefully impossible.[82] Munk himself converted to Catholicism in 1842, after which he became the medical advisor to Cardinal Nicholas Wiseman from 1857 until the cardinal's death in 1865.[83]

Munk writes at length about the fear of death—the hush-hush topic that Thomas Percival and others hardly mentioned except to say that talking about it with patients may well kill them. Having researched the topic and based on his own experience, Munk found that "an urgent fear of death" usually does not occur "when death is actually impending." When death is near, the desire to live eases and finally ends. The fear of death takes place in "that earlier period when the individual realizes for the first time that he is about to die." The shock at that moment may be great, but it is usually transient, such that later contemplation of approaching death will make it seem far less terrible.[84]

Notably, Monk contends that postponing the intimation of death until the last moment does not give the patient time to get over the shock and regain serenity. The alarm over imminent death in such cases disturbs peaceful dying and explains why some persons manifest harrowing responses that occasionally mark deathbeds. Therefore, "An earlier intimation to the dying person of the great change he is about to undergo is in all respects desirable, and if the communication be made tenderly and with prudence, nothing but good is likely to result from it."[85] The good that follows includes the patient's making arrangements for worldly affairs, engaging in spiritual contemplation, carefully reviewing her/his past life, and expressing sorrow and contrition that will secure pardons from family members and acceptance into the life to come. Urged by the physician, it is best for the patient's friends to suggest the danger of the patient's dying, but no single rule can be followed, because each case requires its own considerations.[86] Munk then observes something unique, something that would become widely known in the 20th century: "In some instances the patient himself is the first to discover, and this from his own internal feelings, that he is about to die, and he announces the fact calmly, and for the most part without alarm, to those about him."[87]

Munk concludes this chapter with a lengthy discussion of the different mental processes associated with dying and with cases illustrative of those processes. Some die fully conscious and intellectually alert. Some form of delirium is often present—usually talkativeness that later becomes low muttering and preoccupation with events in childhood. Delirium is sometimes interrupted by keen visual sensations, or else ends with comas and death during sleep. The interval between insensibility and death varies from a few seconds to several hours, and even to days. The senses of smell, taste, and touch generally fail first, along with sight; hearing is usually the last sense that is lost. All who attend to dying persons should, therefore, be careful not to say "anything in the presence of the patient which they would wish him not to hear" even if he appears to be insensible.[88]

The Symptoms and Modes of Dying

Munk's second chapter is based on the "modern science" of its time.[89] It covers two topics—symptoms and signs that indicate when death is near and updated knowledge about the modes of death in relation to its physiological causes. He gives a late 19th-century version of the late 20th-century bestselling book by Sherwin B. Nuland. Nuland believed that "everyone wants to know the details of dying, though few are willing to say so." Like Munk, but with the aid of a century of medical research, Nuland also argued that how persons die largely depends on what they die from.[90]

Munk says that it is often difficult to determine when the final stage of dying begins, but in keeping with centuries of medical tradition, he states that

> the Father of Physic [Hippocrates] is perhaps still our best guide. A sharp and pinched nose, the eyes sunk in the orbits and hollow, the ears pale, cold, shrunk, with their lobes inverted, and the face pallid, livid, or black; these together make up the celebrated **facies Hippocratica**, and show that the work of dying has commenced, and has already made some progress.[91]

Other signs include glazed, half-closed eyes, cold clammy sweats on the head and neck, slow and labored breathing, and an irregular, weak, and rapid pulse.[92]

Munk traces the beginnings of dying to three sources—the heart, the lungs, and the brain. Much that he says is based on the convictions and findings of Thomas Watson.[93]

> "Although," says Sir Thomas Watson, "all men must die, all do not die in the same manner. In one instance the thread of existence is suddenly snapped ... in another the process of dissolution is slow and tedious, and we scarcely know the precise instant in which the solemn change is complete. One man retains possession of his intellect up to his latest breath; another lies unconscious and insensible to all outward impressions for hours or days before the struggle is over."[94]

Munk discusses at length dying that begins in the heart, in the lungs, and in the brain, including descriptions of comas and strokes.[95] He concludes with pointers about the interplay between these modes of dying and their sometimes increasing and sometimes lessening effects on suffering:

> The several modes of dying described above are often combined in the same person, complicating the process and confusing our views of it; with the effect too, in some cases, of increasing the sufferings of the dying, but in others of lessening them. Thus coma ... first lessens the perception of the distress and anguish that attend them, and then extinguishes it.[96]

The General and Medical Treatment of the Dying

William Munk impressively and thoroughly discusses essential features of palliative medicine and care in his final chapter. When the process of dying begins, physicians should dismiss all thought of cure and do all they can in aid of euthanasia or easy dying.

Munk quotes approvingly from John Ferriar: the physician "will not torment his patient with unavailing attempts to stimulate the dissolving system."[97]

In lieu of attempts to cure patients, a host of medical and practical measures should be employed to comfort dying patients, depending, of course, upon their conditions. Patients with the "urgent conditions" will greatly benefit from palliative medical treatments as well as practical measures, with the proviso that "no medicine should be given without a distinct—I had almost written urgent—need for it."[98]

For example, patients suffering from a lack of oxygen that causes interrupted breathing can be relieved by placing them on one side, as well as by supporting them with well-arranged pillows. "The suffering of dying patients, says Miss Nightingale, is immensely increased by neglect of these points."[99] Since difficulty of breathing to the point of gasping is increased by heat and closeness of air, the patient's room should be supplied with fresh and cooler air. Sometimes medical treatments are also essential. "Paroxysms of great suffering" should be treated by ether or opium as the best possible palliative treatments.[100]

In numerous cases in which patients are not beset with symptoms of dangerous diseases, there is no need of medicines of any kind, although stimulants and light nourishment *cautiously* administered are useful.[101] Good nursing and due administration of light food and stimulants are all that is needed for many persons, including aged persons.

> Death from old age—the natural termination of life, and the simplest form of death that can occur, creeps on by slow and almost imperceptible degrees. It is characterized by a gradual and proportionate decay of all the functions and organs of the body, and as a rule presents no symptoms that call for special treatment.... The approaches to death are so gentle, and the act of dying so easy, that nature herself provides a perfect euthanasia.[102]

Much that Munk discusses about comfort-directed care is still timely and perhaps, at points, worthy of greater attention. Consider his discussion of food and drink: "There is nothing of greater importance in the treatment of the dying than the right administration of nutriment."

> Errors in feeding are the cause of much of the disquietude and of many of the sufferings that attend the dying. The sinking and exhaustion that are in progress throughout the system, are assumed by the attendants to demand a free administration of food and stimulants [and who] forget that the stomach shares in the exhaustion, and has lost its tone, and in great part, if not wholly, its power of digesting. Food is given too frequently, and in quantities too large. The dying person is induced by the wearisome importunity of his attendants to take food or stimulants, against which nature and his stomach revolt.[103]

It is an "act of cruelty" to force food and drink on these individuals. The best way to determine what to feed patients is to ascertain what they want, and great discretion is required in clarifying what kinds and qualities of food should be given.[104]

Munk greatly values alcoholic beverages as medicinal and pleasurable stimulants. They readily pass into the bloodstream, stimulate the failing heart, and thereby promote circulation through the lungs.

> The quantity of wine or spirit which is needed varies exceedingly, and no definite rule can be laid down on this point. They should be given in small quantities at a time and

repeated at short intervals.... Of wines, sherry is perhaps the most useful. Port, if preferred by the patient, may be substituted.... Champagne is most refreshing and is often eagerly taken; but its effects are evanescent and it needs repeating at shorter intervals than other wines. A teaspoonful of brandy, or some liqueur may sometimes be advantageously added to it.[105]

Wines, sherry, and champagne for terminally ill persons? William Munk does not render the last stage of life as morose and pleasure-drained as it might otherwise be.

Next to the value of these stimulants, opium, as Hufeland asserted, is "worth all the rest of the material medica" as long as its purpose and actions are clearly understood. Its benefits are numerous—it serves as an anodyne to relieve pain, a cordial to allay "that sinking and anguish" which frequently occurs, a drug that will induce sleep, and the frequent relief from distress and anxiety.[106] Munk quotes Hufeland on how opium also imparts courage and energy for dying patients. The amount given—preferably large doses—should be governed solely by the relief afforded, and it should always be given in liquid forms.[107] Ether is especially indicated when difficulty of breathing becomes gasping or spasmodic, or when the bloating of the stomach cannot be relieved by belching.[108] The judicious use of all the above—liquors, opium, and ether—"are equal to the emergencies we are called upon to meet."[109]

Munk also speaks at length about the practical measures that should be put in place for all dying patients. Restless agitation and cold extremities can be relieved by bed coverings that, in accordance with the counsel of Florence Nightingale, are not excessively weighty.[110] Parched lips, tongues, and mouths need constant attention and can be alleviated by spoonfuls of cold water, bits of ice, or small amounts of lemonade or weak black tea. Patients who cannot swallow should never be forced to drink even small amounts of liquid.[111] Distended bladders cause restlessness that should be relieved by catheters. Attention should also be given to the temperature, ventilation, light, and noise within the person's room.[112]

Excessive noise, on the one hand, and whispering, on the other, should be controlled. Agreeing with Nightingale, Munk asserts that talking around the deathbed should be clear, distinct, and ordinary. Agreeing with Ferriar, he believes that exclamations of grief and the crowding of the family around the bed only harass persons approaching death. Physicians should manage the social dynamics of the patient's room.

Nurses are first on Munk's list of those who should be caring for dying persons. "Good nursing" with respect to administering the right amounts and kinds of food and stimulating drinks, as well as putting in place the practical measures Munk discusses, often "comprise all that is needed." He draws extensively from Florence Nightingale's *Notes on Nursing*.[113]

Upon praising William Munk as a thoughtful and experienced practitioner and his treatise as a compelling call for physicians to return to "their office as *ministers at the bedside*," the reviewers of his book in *The Lancet* announced, "We have not a fault to find with this treatise." In agreement with Munk, *Lancet*'s reviewers observe that terminal care "is not discussed ... in clinical treatises on medicine," nor covered in medical schools or hospital lectures. "The truth would appear," they hold, "that it is almost ignored."[114] A year after Munk's book was published, William Osler praised Munk's book as full of valuable suggestions and sound advice.[115]

These accolades were well deserved. Munk based his book on his own extensive experience, as well as the work of his predecessors and contemporaries. Similar to John Ferriar, Carl F. H. Marx and Hugh Noble in their own times, he utilized updated physiological findings to show how various causes of death inextricably relate to how persons die in differing ways. Against that background, Munk comprehensively discussed palliative medical treatments and practical measures that were useful and effective. He believed that dying persons should conduct their own affairs as much as possible. As opposed to many advocates of palliative care, he believed that these persons should become aware of the danger of their fatal conditions. Innovatively, he also pointed out that some dying patients know they are dying, thus enabling them to review their lives, attend to spiritual concerns, and, if needed, make amends with family members. Munk's work is filled with still-valid insight and counsel.

The importance of Munk's *Euthanasia* was not lost on physician authors who continued to regard expert and sensitive care for dying patients as a physician's "sacred duty."[116] In 1894 Charles B. Williams, a dispensary surgeon in the Methodist-Episcopal Hospital in Philadelphia, succinctly summarized Munk's treatise.[117] At the end of his essay, Williams acknowledged the controversy initiated in 1870 by S. D. Williams, who argued that doctors should use chloroform or some newly discovered anesthetic to put sufferers to a quick and painless death. Williams replied that it would be "better, by far, that chloroform had never been discovered" if it were "put to so base and awful a use as to willfully take away the life of a fellow creature."[118] Munk gave no attention to that debate. Like his palliative care predecessors, he ardently opposed any physician actions that "might hasten death."[119]

With Munk's Assistance, Nurses Fill the Breach: 1890 and 1894

During and after the time William Munk's book was published, nurses in hospitals were being told by doctors that there was nothing more to do for hopelessly ill patients than to make them comfortable. "Make him as easy as you can, sister," physicians were saying. "Make him as easy as we can?" a nurse asked. "That is just what we wish we knew how to do."[120]

These points are made in the insightful and lucidly written article by an anonymous nurse author (known only as "A Hospital Nurse") in 1890.[121] Distressingly, she adds that lectures and training about palliative care for nurses seldom occur. "When I first took charge of wards there was nothing I so much dreaded as attending death-beds and nursing the dying." To ease her dread, she began searching: "I in vain enquired for any book to help me and, with the exception of a few sentences in various medical works, found nothing; until a short time ago I read a most interesting and suggestive book called 'Euthanasia,' by Dr. Munk."[122]

Because Munk's book eased her past troubles, she decided to make parts of it available to her fellow nurses. His last chapter, "On the General and Medical Management of the Dying," is especially valuable, so she greatly abbreviates selections from that chapter in her article to her nursing sisters. She comments that the title of Munk's work—*Euthanasia*—has almost become synonymous in the public mind with "putting people quietly out of the way when for one reason or another their demise seemed desirable to themselves or their friends." She immediately points out that the word really means "a good death," and enabling good death to occur is the topic of Dr. Munk's book.[123]

Her nurse readers will agree "that our one duty, in every way, is to make the patient as comfortable as is possible. The great question is how to do this." They know only too well about the "often long hours of painful waiting and watching, with weeping friends around, either entreating you to do something to ease the last hours, or officiously making all sorts of horrible suggestions, that you have in the interest of the dying patient gently but decidedly to negate."[124] They also know that visits of clergy are often greatly soothing to dying persons and their families. Concerning spiritual needs, she adds a modern touch for "the inexperienced sister":

> You may be suddenly asked to pray, and if there is no one else more suitable, you will have to do so or disappoint a dying patient. Unless you happen to have the extremely uncommon gift of extemporary prayer, don't trust to your memory, but have a prayer book where you can get at it.[125]

The anonymous nurse also discusses the difficult question concerning the extent to which dying persons should not be disturbed by the usual routines. Those in danger of immediate death should be left in peace, but those expected to live longer should be given comfort care: "I must say I have so often seen wonderful temporary relief given to dying persons by their hands and face being gently sponged with hot water, perhaps the hair smoothed, and clean, warm sheet[s] and nightgown[s] exchanged for clammy soiled ones."[126]

On all other subjects respecting nursing care, she gives substantive, abbreviated and, for the most part, uninterrupted quotations from William Munk's book. The topics she covers include lightening bed coverings, allowing cool and fresh air to circulate, using pillows to change the patient's posture, feeding and using alcoholic stimulants, and relieving dryness of mouth and tongue. She knows nurses cannot administer any form of opium, but she wants her sisters to know how valuable it is so they can request sedatives from doctors. Recognizing the importance of opium and other pain-relieving drugs, she quotes from Munk about opiates, ammonia, and ether. She also quotes from Munk about limiting noise and bustle around the bedside, as well as dealing with labored breathing and other matters.[127]

This nurse author concludes her essay by saying that it was difficult to decide what to quote because Munk's book is so excellent: "I can only recommend the perusal of Dr. Munk's book to those nurses who find the efficient nursing of the dying one of their most anxious and difficult duties."[128] That she is writing anonymously suggests that what she is writing may be personally perilous. What lines might she fear she may be crossing?

Some physicians also recognized the great value of William Munk's book for nurse professionals. This is evident in the lectures the English physician Oswald Browne gave to nurses in 1892 and 1894. Browne published his remarks as a small book titled *On the Care of the Dying: A Lecture to Nurses* in 1894. In his preface he writes, "Those who are familiar with Dr. Munk's charming little book on 'Euthanasia' will appreciate how full a measure of acknowledgment is due from me to him."[129] He assesses Munk's book "as a short compass" on "most of what is specially know upon the subject," and he surveys all the topics discussed by Munk.[130]

The most innovative topic in Browne's lecture dwells on the ethics of truth telling. Should patients learn that they are going to die? He answers "yes." In his opinion, the harmfulness of knowing the truth has been overplayed. Knowing that one is going to die does not shorten life. That knowledge can even have beneficial effects. Beyond these consequences, "an adult has a right to know the state of his own body and its prospects," such that physicians "have no right to mystify or deceive" their patients, including "under the specious pretext of doing what is best" for them.[131] Then Browne puts nurses in a moral bind: "I hold that it is no part of a nurse's duty to foretell the issues of disease." If patients ask nurses about the seriousness of their conditions, nurses should respond, "Don't you think that you had best ask the doctor that, or if you would like it I will ask him for you?" Tightening the bind, Browne recognizes that most doctors shrink from "prophesying evil" to their patients.[132]

Oswald Browne fervently believes that no medical duty "touches or approaches" the privilege of caring for dying persons, which "amply repays most careful study." Yet he knows that the treatment and personalized care of dying "are far too little studied." He asks why do "we hear nothing of this [topic] in lectures [and] we read little of it in books?"[133] As he discusses Munk's recommendations about the practical measures, Browne makes a fascinating and humorous observation. He quips to his audience of nurses,

> I shall tell you perhaps little that is not already known to you. Indeed, I feel that here our positions should be reversed, and that my own proper place would be somewhere at the back of my audience [as the] "Chief amang ye takin' notes."[134]

Browne thus realizes that nurses were responsible for most of the palliative care available in hospitals.

Concluding Perspectives

With respect to the quest for good death, the years encompassing 1859–1894 vacillated between the polarities of impressive attention and festering disregard. The attention came from nurses, from the popularized advancement of palliative care and treatment by D. W. Cathell, and from the scholarly, updated, and comprehensive book by William Munk.

At the same time, doctors and nurses were noting how these subjects were being neglected and ignored in medical and nursing teaching and training. As he introduced his groundbreaking study, William Munk noted that the subject "is not especially taught in any of our medical schools."[135] The British reviewers of his book agreed the subject was almost ignored. Worries over the attention given to palliative medicine had previously been registered by Carl F. H. Marx in 1829 and Hugh Noble in 1854. Concerns over the lack of attention in the literature were also voiced by the anonymous nurse author in 1890 and by Oswald Browne in 1892 and 1894.

The disregard became virtually enshrined in updated textbooks on the practice of medicine. By the 1860s textbooks on the principles and practice of medicine were no longer listing end-of-life care as one of the major dimensions of medical practice. In 1862, the British pioneer in pulmonary medicine, C. J. B. Williams, outlined the ultimate goals of medicine as the cure, mitigation, and retardation of disease; the prolongation of life; and the relief of suffering.[136] In the first sentence of his 1868 medical textbook, the renowned clinician and researcher Austin Flint narrowly equated the goals of medicine with the knowledge and cure of disease.[137]

Yet interest in the treatment and care of dying persons remained. D. W. Cathell brought its relevance and basic features to practitioners in the trenches of American culture. In addition, attention was profoundly advanced by William Munk, who showed how differing forms of palliative treatment must be given to patients with differing medical conditions, and he comprehensively outlined the numerous components of palliative care for all persons. It was also advanced by nurses, beginning with the remarkable, passionate, and lasting contributions of Florence Nightingale. It continued in the duties assigned to and shouldered by nurses who were becoming responsible for the care of dying persons in hospitals as that care was being abandoned by doctors. The torches carried by palliative caregivers were thus far from extinguished.

5

Challenging the Overreach
of Modern Medicine

1895–1935

By 1910 modern medicine became robed with an aura of salvation. That year Sir William Osler (1849–1919), a renowned figure in the development of scientific medicine, gave a layperson's Sunday sermon at the University of Edinburgh titled "Man's Redemption of Man."[1] He equated modern medicine with the "the glad tidings of a conquest *beside which all others sink into insignificance … the final conquest of nature.*"[2] Medicine's contributions to humankind's "physical redemption" include "The Death of Pain" via anesthesia and the "glory of the science of medicine" in the prevention of surgical infections and waves of infectious disease, including smallpox, typhoid fever, yellow fever, and tuberculosis—all predictive of a "vast dominion of greater peace, pleasure, and happiness."[3]

> Measure as we may the progress of the world—intellectually in the growth and spread of education, materially in the application to life of all mechanical appliances, and morally in a higher standard of ethics between nation and nation … there is no one measure which can compare with the decrease of disease and suffering in man, woman, and child.[4]

Four years later, a brief article titled "The Doctor" depicted a physician with a mighty sword preparing to sever the rope that the skeleton of death on a gaunt horse was using to drag humanity toward "the dark abyss." The article announces, "While eventually Death will claim his own, the worthy doctor will retard his progress and safeguard humanity from too early a visitation of Death."[5] Death had always been fought by the profession of medicine, but scientific practitioners were winning battles against their historic adversary. As early as 1892, George E. Ranney proclaimed that death, the king of terrors and dread destroyer, was being confronted by physicians "panoplied with science."[6]

Medical Science, Surgery, Modern Hospitals, and Professional Authority

"Panoplied with science" symbolizes the remarkable progress in scientific medicine from the last decades of the 19th century into the 1930s. Medicine—distinguished for a moment from surgery—relied on scientific experiments to overturn centuries of medical tradition. By rendering the past antiquated, the profession became all the more equated with progress. Momentous discoveries in physiology, pathology, bacteriology, and correlations between pathological findings and the symptoms of disease vastly expanded the numbers and types of identifiable diseases and radically revised disease diagnoses. These changes were mirrored in the regularly updated comprehensive medical texts by Austin Flint and William Osler between 1866 and 1947.[7] In addition to pathological anatomy, diagnosis was greatly improved by medical technology—X-rays after the 1890s and bronchoscopes, ophthalmoscopes, proctoscopes, and electrocardiograms in the 1920s.[8]

Scientific physicians focused on diagnosing, and then following, the courses of particular diseases until the time of death. Deaths from common diseases were widely regarded as uninteresting.[9] The practice of the renowned doctor Richard Cabot (1868–1939) reflects his preoccupation with scientifically accurate diagnosis and the effects of the diseases diagnosed. Cabot authored a 600-page text that outlined classifications of heart disease. He also established the famed clinic-pathological conferences in the Massachusetts General Hospital beginning in 1909.[10] He relegated most of the personal, social, and spiritual dimensions of care to social workers and the clergy. Except for his intense focus on the course of his wife's terminal cancer and his own failing heart condition, he rarely gave attention to patients nearing death.[11]

In addition to advances in diagnosis, medicine's progress discredited traditional therapies and focused on innovative therapies proven to be effective. Abandoning the heroic remedies of the past, Osler and his generation adopted a "diagnose-and-wait" perspective, which emphasized sophisticated diagnoses and far fewer medical prescriptions.[12] More targeted and effective therapies began to emerge—antitoxins for diphtheria in 1891 and for tetanus in 1894, salvarsan for syphilis in 1907, insulin for diabetes in 1921, and so on.[13] Modern medicine became linked to "sanitary science," which rendered the older theories of contagion and miasmas passé. Via historic discoveries in bacteriology, public hygiene campaigns prevailed over the scourges of cholera, tuberculosis, typhoid fever, hookworm disease, and yellow fever.[14]

Beyond internal medicine, surgery enormously enhanced modern medicine's ability to rescue thousands of patients from dreadful conditions and the jaws of death.[15] The fundamental components of modern surgery included anesthesia, a thorough knowledge of pathophysiology, and antiseptic (later aseptic) prevention of infection. Excitement became virtually overwhelming. The cascade of progress between the late 1870s and the 1920s included painless repairs of fractured bones, abdominal injuries, hernias, and appendectomies; remedies for patients with gallbladder disease; excisions that prolonged the lives of persons with breast, brain, and rectal cancers; surgeries on the pituitary gland; and initial efforts to perform vascular surgery on arteries of the heart.[16]

These historical changes in medicine and surgery became institutionalized in modern hospitals, the expansion and sophistication of which were remarkable. In the United States there were 187 hospitals with 35,453 beds in 1873, 5,000 hospitals by 1920, and 6,655 hospitals with 1,649,254 beds in 1943.[17] Hospitals also multiplied in the United Kingdom and Continental Europe during these years, including specialty hospitals for skin and urological disorders. The opening of the Johns Hopkins Hospital in 1889 symbolized the adoption of the German medical-science model of medical education and training in the United States. Johns Hopkins served as an ideal for other medical schools.[18] The model included linkages between universities and hospitals, joining science and research with clinical hospital practice—medical diagnosis, the treatment of diseases, and surgery. The new university hospitals contained pathology laboratories for postmortem examinations and theaters for modern surgery. They were also the training grounds for nursing professionals, who played invaluable roles in carrying out the complex work hospitals were taking on.[19]

Hugh Cabot called the growth of hospitals where diseases were "scientifically managed" the "most characteristic development of modern medicine" between 1871 and 1921.[20] Beyond their inner dynamics, modern hospitals changed the landscape of medical and surgical practice. Visually, they displayed the power and promise of modern medicine.

Recognizing that hospitals were the safest place to go, patients entered them in ever-increasing numbers, and those who were seriously ill were often kept there for weeks, even months.[21] The revolution occurring in public transportation accompanied that growth. Naturally, larger and larger numbers of patients died in hospitals—21 percent in New York City by 1926.[22] More often than not, trained nurses became the main caregivers of persons who were dying.[23] Some nurses, such as the anonymous nurse writer whose words are recorded in the previous chapter, became superb caregivers.[24] Other nurses manifested no knowledge of the palliative care tradition, lied to patients who asked them about the seriousness of their conditions, and related to terminally ill patients so matter-of-factly that the patients' relatives thought their services were insensitive.[25]

All the just-discussed topics contributed to the ever-advancing cultural authority of the medical profession.[26] Medicine's association with science and technology directly and vastly improved its therapeutic capabilities. Its soaring scientific status occurred in an era transfixed by scientific advances in education, transportation, communication, and architectural wonders. Its newfound and amazing abilities to cure and free human beings from the former scourges of disease both stunned the imagination and created far greater levels of patient dependency on doctors. The dependence was all the greater due to the gulf between patient knowledge and physician erudition. Medicine's institutionalization within modern hospitals and medical schools gave doctors new levels of sophistication, occupational independence, peer loyalty, wealth, public acclaim, and authority over patients.

Palliative Care Besieged by
Battles Against Disease and Death

The lack of physician attention to palliative treatment and care depicted in Chapter 4 continued after 1894. Textbooks on medicine equated the practice of medicine with scientific sophistication in the cure of disease. The rewriting of the American Medical Association's (AMA) original, 1847 Code of Ethics in 1903, and again in 1912, reflected and perpetrated flagging interest in the care of dying patients. The revised 1903 principles abbreviated, partly changed, and partly preserved essential points of the AMA's 1847 Code of Ethics pertaining to palliative care. Far less detailed than the 1847 code, the 1903 principles say that patients with incurable illnesses should not be abandoned, that *ordinarily* patients should not be told about their fatal conditions, and that by alleviating pain and soothing mental anguish, the physician should be "a minister of hope and comfort to the sick."[27]

In 1912 the principles of the AMA were revised again—radically. Under the title PROGNOSIS, the 1912 principles say,

> A physician should give timely notice of dangerous manifestations of the disease to the friends of the patient. He should neither exaggerate nor minimize the gravity of the patient's condition. He should assure himself that the patient or his friends have such knowledge of the patient's condition as will serve the best interests of the patient and the family.

Under the heading PATIENT MUST NOT BE NEGLECTED, the 1912 principles talk about the physician's right to choose his patients and his duty to respond to emergencies. In the middle of that section, only one sentence pertains to palliative care: "Once having undertaken a case, a physician should not abandon or neglect the patient because the disease is deemed incurable."[28] Non-abandonment remained intact, but all the details about what physicians should do at the bedsides of patients—and why they should do them—were deleted. The new 1912 AMA "Principles of Medical Ethics" thus allowed modern practitioners to decide how they would treat dying patients. This created a vacuum that was filled by at least four approaches to dying persons on the part of physicians.

The first approach reflected the historic legacy of Francis Bacon—making dying and death easy through palliative treatment and care. This included Thomas Percival's emphasis on the physician's providing hope and comfort to soothe the drooping spirits of dying persons, a tenet voiced in the AMA Code of Ethics of 1847. William Osler and an unknown number of practitioners in Europe, Canada, and the United States held to this first approach. Osler credited William Munk with giving "valuable suggestions" and "sound advice" on the medical management of dying persons.[29] In 1909 he said that "careful clinical observations have taught us to recognize our limitations, and to accept the fact that a disease itself may be incurable, and that the best we can do is to relieve symptoms and to make the patient comfortable."[30]

The second approach was described by the anonymous nurse in 1890, who noted how physicians were directing nurses to assume the duties of palliative care when patients were thought to be hopelessly ill.[31] The discussion below will indicate how this practice continued in decades to follow.

The third approach is strange and raises questions about its frequency and influence. It involves the notion that death does not merit professional attention because dying is natural and gentle. Why give attention to the details of terminal care when dying can be so peaceful? In 1875 a physician described how nature tenderly, "like a mother with her foot on the cradle," will "rock us all gently out of the world."[32] With no mention of palliative care, E. P. Buffett in 1891 compared the process of dying to education and training that leads to a tranquil retiring from life for the vast majority of dying persons. An acute disease can "complete the training in a few days, an accident in a few hours."[33]

The fourth approach is, and for decades would remain, alarming. Increasing numbers of modern scientific practitioners would undertake so-called heroic attempts to extend the lives of dying persons in order to postpone medicine's and humankind's greatest enemy—death. Toward that end, they would employ their new skills and vested professional authority. They would also overturn a bottom-line principle of proponents of palliative medicine and care first voiced by John Ferrier in 1798, and then reaffirmed by Carl F. H. Marx in 1826, Hugh Noble in 1834, and William Munk in 1887. To recall Ferriar's words, when some physicians discover that their patient is dying, they attempt "to stimulate the dissolving system, from the idle vanity of prolonging the flutter of the pulse for a few more vibrations."[34]

New efforts to prolong the lives of patients in extremity were predicated on scientific findings about how dying can be manipulated and death postponed. Experiments on animals proved they could be kept alive in spite of severe disruptions to their organ systems. Extensive vivisections on animals, followed by reparative procedures, proved that animals and humans were "physical-chemical and mechanical entities," whose survival could be extended in ways that were formerly considered unimaginable.[35] Human life could and should be prolonged as long as possible, many doctors came to believe, and death began to symbolize treatment failure.[36]

Cardiopulmonary resuscitation of persons apparently drowned or struck by lightning began in the eighteenth century and included electric shocks, chest compressions, and doses of stimulants. Attempted life prolongation was utilized on new populations of patients after the 1870s—endotracheal intubation and tracheotomies beginning in 1900, epinephrine (adrenaline) as a stimulant by 1906, open-chest CPR in experimental animals in 1882, and electric defibrillation of laboratory animals around 1900.[37]

Graphic reports of heroic attempts—occasionally successful—to prolong life were described in the medical literature. In 1889 A. H. P. Leuf told how a Brooklyn doctor sought to save the life of a child with diphtheria. After the child lost consciousness and appeared to be only a corpse, the doctor went to his office and returned twenty minutes later with an electric battery. He shocked the child's nerves and chest muscles until he witnessed gasps of air and a flicker of the heart, but ignorant relatives compelled the doctor to desist, such that the child died. Leuf also told the story of a wealthy man who was treated with bottles of hot water applied to his limbs, red pepper and whiskey injected into his bowels, and nearly four hours of attempts at artificial respiration. After still more injections and efforts at respiration, the man eventually recovered consciousness and lived for another twenty years. Leuf asserted that it is "our duty as physicians to attempt to return life until there is undoubted evidence of cellular death" that ends with rigor mortis. He ended by listing different modes of exciting the heart's action, including cardiac punctures, intra-cardiac injections, and flagellations.[38]

In 1895 L. Pierce Clark described the use of stimulants to revive heartbeat. First, to restore the loss of heart function on the part of three persons with delirium tremens, various stimulants were injected into muscle tissue. But these shots of digitalis, nitroglycerin and other drugs "failed to ward off ... cardiac paralysis." So Clark decided to use a long needle syringe to inject sulphate of strychnine directly into the heart muscle of a patient. The pulse was restored, and the patient eventually recovered and was discharged after five days. Clark concluded that this case, as well as a second one mentioned briefly, showed that injections of stimulants into the heart can save lives. He indicated that ammonia was being similarly used, but without success in two cases.[39] By 1922, Julius Gottesman wrote about emergency measures being used to restore cardiac activity either by massaging the cardiac muscle through the abdomen or by the action of drugs on the myocardium tissue. He praised the injection of epinephrine directly into the heart because the injection mechanically stimulated neuromuscular connections.[40]

These stories about medical struggles—and successes—in the saving of human life overshadow palliative care insofar as it enables patients to die peacefully and accepts death as natural and inevitable. Telling of her experiences as a trained nurse responsible for the care of dying persons in hospitals, Hermine Kane asserts, "No adult wants to die"—neither those who say they're willing to die nor the rich and the poor, suicidal patients, non-religious persons, truly religious persons, she herself, and, above all, doctors. When patients learn that they will die, they become hysterical. As a result, she tells her dying patients that they will soon get better. That makes them more comfortable, and it makes her work easier because once they know that they're on their deathbeds, patients "usually break down completely." Then she speaks of doctors who hate for patients to die:

> The death of a patient hurts a doctor. He has done all that he can to prevent it, and he can do no more; he feels defeated, and he wants to avoid all reminders of his defeat. It is necessary for him to avoid them if he is to remain confident and effective.[41]

Simeon E. Baldwin's "No!" to the Excesses of Modern Medical Practitioners: 1899

In 1899 Simeon E. Baldwin (1840–1927) articulated a powerful, perhaps first-ever resounding critique of the excessive ways in which modern medical practitioners were seeking to prolong the lives of fatally ill persons. In the annual president's address of the American Social Science Association, he publicly condemned modern medicine's overreaching and vain attempts to save patients from the clutches of certain death. Baldwin was a jurist and Yale law professor who was elected governor of Connecticut in 1912. His critique, "The Natural Right to a Natural Death," was quickly published in a medical journal.[42]

Baldwin was no enemy of modern scientific medicine: "If recovery is possible, all means of recovery should be exhausted." Nor is he sanguine about death. He contends that human beings instinctively shrink from death as that which is mysterious and unknown, and that which takes us away from friends, from the work we want to do, from familiar scenes, from "yielding to an overmastering force," and from being "beaten down and conquered against our will."[43]

Nevertheless, there is a time to die. "Birth, marriage, death: these are the landmarks of normal human life, and each one of them is as natural as the other."[44]

> A time comes to every man when the dominance of the mortal is attacked by a force which he cannot long resist. The physician can recognize the coming and predict the end. We call it a fatal disease. Fatal! Rather let us say, kindly, divine. One by one nature reclaims ... the forces that have stirred this transitory being, to energize

in new forms some other of her manifold creation. Medical art cannot stop this process.[45]

Therefore, "Let us not fight, when there is no fighting chance."[46]

The "us" in that last sentence refers to modern scientific practitioners who, according to Baldwin, have lost their moorings with respect to forcing patients to endure unnatural deaths when, in plain English, the patient's "time [to die] has come."

> In civilized nations, and particularly of late years, it has become the pride of many in the medical profession to prolong such lives at any cost of discomfort or pain to the sufferer, or of suspense and exhaustion to his family.
>
> The patient has come to a point where he cannot bear the thought of eating. The throat declines to swallow what the stomach is no longer able to digest. He craves nothing but to be let alone. A few hours, and nature will come to his release.... The vital forces have been spent. The main spring is broken and the watch has run down. It can be made to tick feebly for a minute or two by shaking it hard enough; but **cui bono?** [To whose benefit?][47]

Yet many practitioners keep persisting in fruitless attempts to prolong the lives of patients whose physiological watches are broken and rundown:

> The family asks the doctor if there is not hope, and he responds with some sharp stimulant; some hypodermic injection; some transfusion or infusion to fill out for a few hours the bloodless veins; some device for bringing oxygen into the congested lungs that cannot breathe the vital air; some cunning way of stimulating another organ to do the stomach's work or perhaps, with strychnine to poison the fountains of life [actions of the heart] into spasmodic activity, as they struggle to reject it. The sufferer wakes to pain, and gasps back to a few more days or weeks of life.[48]

For Baldwin, these attempts at life prolongation are contrary to nature and to human morality. That they are contrary to nature is, in his view, inseparable from their immorality. Heroic efforts to prolong life force pain, suffering, emotional misery, and weakness on often unwilling patients. They evince cruelty, rather than mercy. Baldwin describes the case of an elderly widow—one of several cases communicated to him— to illustrate his moral reprehension:

> X, a widow in advanced years, was seized by a cancer in the stomach. She suffered acutely for nine weeks, at the end of which time her stomach refused to retain anything but a little water, and even that caused great pain. For several days she was kept alive and in agony by injections of mutton broth. She had no living descendants. A relative who had been sent for arrived from a distant State to find her in this condition. [The widow] was a person of great strength of character, and full in possession of all her senses. "They will not let me die; I want to die," was her complaint to the new-comer. The latter took the place of the friends who ... had urged in vain that a different treatment should be pursued. The attending physician was asked, "Is it not a hopeless case?" "Yes." "Is she not suffering?" "Yes." "Is she not a Christian, and longing to die?" "Yes." "And do you think it merciful to keep her living by these artificial means?" "I can do nothing else," was the reply. "It is my duty to keep her alive as long as possible. I will leave the case in your hands. You can stop the injections, or continue them, as you think right. I can do nothing about it." They were stopped, and the poor sufferer allowed to sink away as nature meant; but had the physician had his way, there might have been days more of useless agony.[49]

Horrifyingly, this woman's physician dismissed her wishes to be allowed to die. He dismissed them in the name of what he regarded as his higher duty—"to keep her alive as long as possible." So, in addition to adding to her suffering, the doctor overruled her rights, or, in Baldwin's words, her "right to reject such aids to the continuance a little longer of a life that has no remaining value."[50] If the patient does not wish for her suffering to be prolonged, why should this unnatural pain be forced upon her?[51] Concerning patients like this woman who will be treated by authoritarian doctors, Baldwin claims, "Happy [is] he, if nature calls him quietly away, before the doctor can be sent for."[52]

In contrast to the widow's case, Baldwin tells about another that illustrates the care he thinks dying persons deserved:

> Y, an elderly man, had fatty degeneration of the heart. Acute symptoms were suddenly developed. He asked his family physician what was the matter with him, and was frankly told. "Is my cure possible?" "No." "How long have I to live?" "A very short time; perhaps a few hours; perhaps a few days." "Can you keep me alive long enough to let Z get here to see me once more?" "Probably, by the use of champagne." "Then, I will take it, till he comes." A telegram brought Z from a distant State. After their interview, the patient said: "Now, no more champagne"; and in a few hours the end came, with no further attempt by the physician or family to protract his suffering.[53]

Champagne! That was what William Munk recommended in 1887 as the "most refreshing ... and often eagerly taken" palliative stimulant for many fatally ill persons.[54] Baldwin does not talk at length about palliative treatment, although he does mention that fatally ill patients should have the violence of their conditions mitigated by palliative changes of diet and air and by the use of medicines. But no food or stimulants should be forced on these persons.[55]

Simeon Baldwin believes that modern scientific medicine reflects a spirit of altruism, but its zealous attempts to prolong life often only prolong an inhuman parody of life. He challenges modern medical practitioners to accept their limitations and cease cruel and unwanted patient suffering. "Why is it now, in these days of larger hope," he asks, "do we ever engage in this contest at the finish, in this struggle for a little more time, when we know that it must be a brief and losing one?"[56]

> No code of medical ethics of any school of practice countenances that which I denounce. The physician is enjoined in cases of fatal disease to continue in attendance for the purpose of alleviating pain, but not to protract or produce it.
> I ... say that it is not right that ... a life should be prolonged in hopeless misery, by medical art, against the sufferer's will, when nature has plainly called him away.[57]

As if he were drawing from a page of modern surgery, Baldwin's language cuts like a deftly used scalpel—the "pride" of many medical professionals, the "cunning" means they use, the irony of unnatural prolongation of life as "the highest medical art," life prolongation as a "contest" at the finish line of life, the impressive power of medicine "to hold us back from the grave"—in a state "of long-drawn agony."[58] He asks, "*cui bono?*"[59] To whose benefit? Or, in our words, "What's the point?"

Like Francis Bacon and palliative caregivers of the past, Baldwin views death as natural and inevitable. He uses the naturalness of death to critique the excesses of medical practices in his time. He also confronts the disturbing development that some doctors view aggressive and sometimes unproven life-extending medical measures as a medical duty that trumps the wishes and rights of patients and family members. That turns the historic legacy of medical paternalism into paternalistic authoritarianism for the presumed good of humanity.

The innovativeness and eloquence of Baldwin's lecture are remarkable. He argues that allowing patients to die is a moral imperative, preceding the momentous pronouncement of Pope Pius XII on the rights of patients by 50 years, not to speak of defenses of that imperative during and after the 1970s.[60]

Harrington Sainsbury on Patients' and Families' Rights to Make End-Of-Life Decisions: 1906

Similarly concerned about the issues raised by Baldwin, the London physician Harrington Sainsbury, in his widely acclaimed *Principia Therapeutica* (1906), asked, "To what end then this formidable array of remedies?"[61] Sainsbury replied that the aims of medicine include relieving pain, mitigating disease, and prolonging life. He then adds, "Singly or jointly these aims will call for our utmost endeavors until that time, which will come, which must come, when the **cui bono** can receive no satisfactory answer." The endeavors are unsatisfactory when the expectation of life is too short and when physicians' efforts "to eke out existence" only lengthen a hopeless struggle marked by fretfulness rather than comfort. At that point, "we physicians should remember that the obligation to protract life at any cost is not laid upon us."[62]

Sainsbury knows that modern medicine and surgery challenge physicians to face difficult decisions. If futility of further treatment is apparent, physicians should put aside attempts to cure in order to ease the suffering of the patient. But decisions in some cases are dauntingly difficult. According to Sainsbury, when a skillful surgeon informs an internist that surgery to remove a tumor is warranted, the internist's rejection of surgery is equivalent to a passive acceptance of defeat. But exceedingly careful deliberation and debate must be used to determine the best course of action. If such reasoning leads physicians to expect a prolongation of life, the surgery can be advocated, but if a rational balancing of probabilities indicates otherwise, the surgery must be "unhesitatingly rejected."[63]

The above process of decision making may well end, however, with conflicting and confusing hopes and fears. When this occurs, the physician must dispassionately determine what the reasonable probabilities are. How, then, should a decision be made? It should be made according to the data the doctor has gathered, but by whom? Primarily, Sainsbury affirms,

> by the patient, if we judge that he or she is capable of bringing a sound mind to bear upon these data [and], secondarily, by the relatives and friends, and preferably by these in council with the patient.... The one thing that is obligatory is that we bring before the patient and his circle all the facts which we deem to have an essential bearing upon the case. Finally, should the decision be left to us, as in many, perhaps in most, cases it will be, and we conclude that all things considered, it is wiser to stay the hand than to be active with it, then we must have the courage to let it be idle, and to abide the issue.[64]

Sainsbury's affirmation is momentous. His conviction that end-of-life treatment decisions should be made by the patient and/or the family would have greatly pleased

Simeon Baldwin, who objected to the authoritarianism of doctors who believed that they, and they alone, should dictate treatment decisions. Sainsbury gave two corrective answers to that behavior. First, the physician should provide patients and/or a circle of loved ones with all the medical facts and ask them what they prefer. Second, if the decision is left in the doctor's hands, the doctor should carefully weigh what to do, not automatically opt for aggressive treatment. All things considered, it may well be best to suspend life-prolonging treatments. In opposition to the spirit of the times, doctors must have the courage to cease active treatments and stick with that decision.

Remarkably, Sainsbury is opposing the physician authoritarianism of his time, which uncritically sanctioned aggressive treatments. He voices a moral principle that would not become normative in medical ethics for at least another 65 years—the principle of respecting the patient's own choices (via relatives and friends if necessary) regarding whether further life-prolonging treatments should be attempted.

After Baldwin and Sainsbury

Apart from occasional journal articles, few authors discussed palliative care between 1903 and 1928. Little mention was made of the bearing of scientific diagnosis and prognosis, of new discoveries of pain management, of insights from psychiatry, and of other matters regarding the care of terminally ill persons. Medical attention lay elsewhere.

In 1921, Arthur MacDonald, an anthropologist from Washington, D.C., published a long article titled "Death in Man," which he expanded and republished in 1928.[65] The thirtieth of his thirty-three sub-sections was called "Euthanasia," the entire contents of which summarized William Munk's book on palliative euthanasia. MacDonald's only contribution involved his keeping Munk's ideas before readers of the *Medical Times* thirty-four years after Munk's book was published. However, he does so in a backhanded fashion by giving an overview of Munk's work without directly referencing Munk as his source of information.[66]

J. Norman Glaister's Remarkable Use of Psychiatry in Terminal Care: 1921

J. Norman Glaister, a psychiatrist in the Royal Free Hospital of London, should be brought out from the shadows of medical and psychiatric history.[67] One of the few who wrote about palliative care between 1895 and 1929, Glaister published a brief and groundbreaking article on "Phantasies of the Dying: Some Remarks on the Management of Death" in 1921. His article was published in one of *The Lancet*'s miscellaneous sections—its minor section on "Notes, Short Comments, and Answers to Correspondents" that appeared after "Birth, Marriages, and Deaths."[68] Glaister deserved better press than that.

Glaister begins by affirming the theme boldly set forth by Francis Bacon, reaffirmed by palliative caregivers after Bacon, and powerfully defended by Simeon Baldwin: "The suggestion here brought forward is that we should regard death as being, like birth, a natural process."[69] When death is regarded as natural, "we shall escape the futile struggle, well known to every general practitioner, against a death known to be both inevitable and desirable."[70]

He focuses on "the typical case of a patient dying from inoperable cancer." These persons are trapped in a terrible emotional bind. Glaister describes this bind impressively:

> The illness of the patient is steadily progressing; his friends know that he is dying, but he is supposed not to know—or at least, not to know how advanced it is. He is perfectly sane, presumably capable of drawing inferences from his own observation of facts, and growing steadily worse; the efforts of those about him to dissuade him from taking his illness seriously are in marked contrast with their earlier attitude of urging him to seek ... treatment. The atmosphere of unreality soon shuts him off completely from the world of common-sense and normal conversation; the word "cancer" is never mentioned, and the friends avoid any remarks which might encourage him to ask a direct question as to the verdict.
>
> The patient's mind is therefore in a condition of continual conflict. He knows that he is dying of cancer, and this for him is very likely the most important fact in the world; it appears constantly in his dreams, but in the waking world there is not a living soul with whom he can discuss it.... The one thing which he craves—human companionship up to death as in normal life—is denied him. As the end approaches, the effort of those around him to encourage him becomes such a mockery that it is abandoned; but there is nothing to put in its place.

Doctors, Glaister observes, are not easing this emotional conflict and loneliness because they view their roles as treating symptoms, prolonging life as much as possible, and relieving physical pain by morphine or other medications. These are important, but hardly sufficient. "For all human purposes the patient is ... thrust out from the company of living minds and buried away from contact ... weeks or even months before his death."[71]

Glaister advocates a radically different approach. Through the case he presents, he shows how honesty-based psychotherapy with patients beset by inoperable cancers will relieve their fears, ease the terrors of their dreams and fantasies, and enable psychotherapists and others to truly "accompany him as far as possible on his road" to the end of life.[72]

He provides his readers with the case of Miss A, a woman past middle age with inoperable cancer in both breasts. In the boarding house where she lived, he initially found her very depressed, cheerless, unable to concentrate, and incapable of displaying her emotions.

He describes his care and treatment of Miss A as follows: On his first visit he asked her to face the realities of having the type of cancer she admitted she had—the facts being that most people with her type of cancer will die, and that she probably would die similarly. She refused to see Glaister on his second visit, which Glaister interpreted as her attempt to "avoid this brutally truthful doctor," as well as a desire on her part to feel as if she was getting well.[73] But over the next three weeks Glaister counseled her seven times, and they became friends as she described her dreams and fantasies. During that time she expressed her extreme dislike of the matron of the house and the special nurse who was attending to her physical needs. The "cheery conventionalities" of her nurse became "thoroughly unreal to her, even as her dreams and fantasies became all the more real." Glaister entered into her world of dreams, and based on his relationship with Miss A, she began to overcome her emotional difficulties. Learning of her great affection for a niece in a convent school in France, Glaister convinced the niece to come take care of her. The niece agreed with Glaister's instructions that she should talk freely in her aunt's presence on the assumption that she knew of her aunt's approaching death and welcomed it.[74]

Continuing with his psychotherapy, Glaister enabled Miss A to experience a transformation. She not only ceased being a painfully difficult patient with her nurse but also "took a great liking to the nurse and made friends with her old enemy the matron." She sent for a priest and was received into the Roman Catholic Church. She gave up denial and pretenses. She regained strength and began to sleep peacefully. She ceased needing sedatives altogether. She said that she was quite ready to die. "She was fully conscious half an hour before her death, and died apparently without any discomfort."[75] "There is no doubt," Glaister said, "that the last week of this patient's life was quite exceptionally pleasant and satisfactory both to herself and those around her, and it seems not unreasonable to attribute the fact to the special attention devoted to the solution of her mental difficulties."[76]

Glaister concludes with a brief and eloquent plea for "The Necessity for Plain Speaking." He recognizes that "an immense amount of skilled effort" is being directed toward the surgical excisions of malignant disease, "to the great advantage of those patients who are cured as a result." But he notes that most patients with cancer cannot be cured, and for them little help is being offered. He asks, "Has not the time arrived for a broad re-survey of the whole treatment of the inoperable cancer case?"

> When cancer has been diagnosed, the facts in their least painful guise ought to be laid before the patient, and this may be a mental operation of considerable difficulty. The patient and his medical attendant can then discuss adequately their plans for extirpating [surgically removing] the disease, or failing that, for making the best possible use of the remainder of life.[77]

Nothing in the literature of palliative care up to this time matches this astonishing essay by J. Norman Glaister. He is modeling how to provide psychological care for patients with end-stage diseases—care according to the psychotherapy of his time. He advances truth telling as a prerequisite for that care. That was all the more pioneering during the years when telling patients they had cancer was taboo. The tradition of concealing the truth about cancer continued during the 75 years between 1890 and 1965, when cancer-phobia reigned. The treatment of the famed Babe Ruth, baseball's "Sultan of Swat," manifests the power of that phobia: with pride, the writer of Ruth's obituary in 1948 said that his having cancer was "one of the best kept secrets in modern times."[78] In contrast, learning the truth via his persistent counseling became the foundation for the mental stability and peacefulness of Glaister's patient.

Alfred Worcester's Challenges to Modern Physicians: 1928–1935

To the depths of his soul, and with all the powers of his intelligence, Alfred Worcester (1855–1951) believed that modern physicians should recover professional duties regarding expert and personalized care for persons who are dying. In one of a high-profile series of lectures at the Harvard Medical School, he asserted in 1928 that palliative care had become "sidetracked"—set aside for other pressing priorities that betrayed medicine's historic attention to the personal well-being of dying patients. He said the sidetracking of palliative care was occurring because the progress of medical science presses practitioners to show interest only in the diseases of their patients, such that they "find little that is noteworthy in [patients'] dying beyond ... the possible opportunity of verifying their diagnosis." He says that far too often physicians continue aggressive treatments when death's approach is inescapable. They give false hopes to patients and their families. When they think they can no longer extend life, they surrender the care of dying patients to nurses and sorrowing relatives. To Worcester, these developments amount to medical malpractice.[79]

These are harsh and public judgments on Worcester's part. They appear to be particularly harsh for a physician who graduated from Harvard Medical School in 1883; developed a successful medical practice in Waltham, Massachusetts; became a professor at Harvard; organized nursing training programs; and was elected president of the Massachusetts Medical Society.[80] But Worcester's deeper preparation for his lecture spanned decades. He traveled to Europe in 1895, where he consulted with Florence Nightingale and stayed for a season in Paris to study the work of the Augustinian Sisters who had been caring for poor, sick, and dying persons for over 600 years.[81] When he gave his lecture, he had been practicing family medicine for over 40 years. And, pivotally, 16 years prior to his lecture he published an article in the *Boston Medical and Surgical Journal* that set forth his fundamental criticisms of modern, hospital-based medical education and practice.

He began his 1912 article by briefly describing scientific medicine's "rapid succession of brilliant discoveries regarding the causation of diseases" and how that led to the extermination of epidemics of infectious diseases. He ends by recognizing the amazing successes of modern surgery. Between these pages, he praises the "most admirable opportunity for the study of disease" in modern medical schools and hospitals.[82]

These accolades set the stage for Worcester's counter-perspective: "There is ... a radical difference between the science of medicine and the art of medical practice."

> In the modern medical schools science is enthroned. Carried away by the brilliance of etiological discoveries, the whole strength of the schools is devoted to the study of diseases. The art of medical practice is not taught; even its existence is hardy recognized. And in consequence the graduates of the medical schools of today are not properly fitted for the practice of their profession.[83]

Worcester asserts that scientific practitioners are often ignorant of human nature. When dealing with the mysteries of life, science fails them. They are not being taught about the therapeutic value of sympathy and encouragement. Their training does not prepare them to be patients' *physicians* in the full sense of the term. The successes of modern surgery are startling, and no one should belittle the fame of modern surgeons. But the "grievous wrong of unnecessary mutilations" is occurring in surgery, followed by a "hell of pain and misery." Should not modern surgeons, he asks, "also be taught the art of relieving, of soothing, and comforting those who suffer"? Should they not also steady and support those who are walking through "the valley of the shadow"?[84]

Worcester's 1928 lecture on "The Care of the Dying" is, therefore, rooted in long-standing concerns. It is also informed by a timeless, often-quoted lecture and essay by Francis Weld Peabody, in whose memory the entire Harvard lecture series was dedicated. The year before Worcester was invited to speak, Peabody delivered and published his lecture on "The Care of the Patient." Peabody critiqued modern practitioners for practicing as though their patients were bodies beset with diseases. Patients, he asserted, are persons with bodies, minds, personalities, and unique, fascinating, and influential social backgrounds that must be taken into consideration by physicians dedicated to patient care. Medicine focused on diseases and treatment alone is not scientific enough. Fully scientific medicine combines the science and art of medicine, inescapably embracing the whole relationship of the physician and the patient. Peabody concluded his address with this famous sentence: "One of the essential qualities of the clinician is interest in humanity, for the secret of the care of the patient is in caring for the patient."[85]

These backdrops set the stage for Worcester's 1928 lecture and publication. He revised the first two pages of his lecture and published it in 1935 as a book named *The Care of the Aged, the Dying, and the Dead*.[86] His book was republished in 1940, 1945, and 1950. In these publications Worcester displays his indebtedness to Francis Bacon, Florence Nightingale, William Munk, and a number of physicians whom Munk relied upon. Worcester's publications are finely crafted classics in the story of the quest for a good death.

Early in his essay Worcester observes that when the death of their patients becomes apparent, many doctors assume that it is proper to leave the dying in the care of nurses and sorrowing relatives. He asserts, "This shifting of responsibility is unpardonable."[87] Worcester greatly appreciates and admires the work of nurses, from whom he learned so much and for whom he expended great energy and support. His mother's influence surely contributed to his appreciation of nurses. She had been a gifted and devoted "old time neighbor nurse" who assigned her eleven-year-old son Alfred the duty of watching all night over one of his dangerously ill classmates.[88] Worcester observes that with the proper direction, nurses can give most of the service that is needed for dying persons, but he considers it unfair to expect them to carry out the burdens of palliative care by themselves and with little or no direction from informed physicians.[89]

For Worcester, the overwhelming scientific focus of modern medicine pressures practitioners to dismiss palliative care as one of their duties, thus accounting for the lack of knowledge and expertise. Like John Ferriar 130 years earlier, Worcester wryly comments, "Inasmuch as all our patients, as well as we ourselves, must die sooner or later, it might naturally be supposed that the care of the dying would receive more attention."[90]

Worcester knows that his criticisms of many of his scientific peers are unwarranted if he cannot convince his hearers and readers that physicians devoted to both the science and the art of medicine are able make invaluable contributions to dying patients. His essay underlines those contributions. Like William Munk, Worcester outlines the components of terminal care for all physicians and nurses, but he especially wants to educate medical students. Students should be instructed in what they ought and ought not to do with dying persons, and they should be required to hand in several reports of their experiences at the bedsides of the dying.[91] His emphasis on students' writing about their experiences was far ahead of his time.

Like earlier physician writers, he holds that physicians should know when the actual process of dying has begun, at which point "the treatment of the patient must then be radically changed." Further efforts to restore life are "worse than useless."[92] Surgeons, for example, are performing unnecessarily mutilating operations.[93] Worcester exclaims that

> all these modern methods of resuscitation, which of course are obligatory where valuable lives might thus be saved, are decidedly out of place where by disease or accident the body's usefulness has ended. Especially is this true where resuscitation would only renew the patient's sufferings....
>
> Efforts for prolonging life when the inevitable approach of death [occurs] offers merciful release.... [T]oo many of our profession seem to believe themselves in duty bound to do their utmost. They ought to know better.[94]

Attempts to extend life should be replaced with well-established, symptom-easing palliative measures: keeping the throat and mouth moist and clear of obstructions, arranging pillows and posture to enhance breathing, lightening bedcovers, and providing abundant fresh air, quietness, even music if wanted.[95] Worcester references the work of physicians who wrote about palliative care, and he regularly relies on his own experiences and insights (which, at times, serve as correctives to previous authors). He will also demonstrate why physicians should be in charge of the care and treatment of dying patients, with nurses as essential assistants.

Worcester emphasizes that at the end of life death is not wrought with agony. During the early stages of dying, however, discomfort and suffering are all too possible. But in contrast to S. D. Williams, who equated countless deaths with terrible tortures, Worcester found that

> the discomfort and suffering of the dying almost always can be relieved by medical treatment.... Opiates are indispensable. If morphine fails to give comfort, a hundred to one it is either because too small doses have been given or because it has not been successfully introduced into the enfeebling circulation. Large and frequent doses may be needed.... Its main effect is its soothing influence.... All the usual heart stimulants on these occasions are worthless. Massive doses of morphine given to the dying[,] instead of hastening the end[,] more often seem rather to postpone it.[96]

Palliative care competency also includes the physician's appreciation of each dying patient's personality, which is the foundation of the art of medical practice and distinguishes the physician from the veterinarian.[97] Worcester therefore writes at length about the varying mental conditions of dying patients. He agrees with Munk and Munk's scholarly sources that although some dying persons may seem to be in a state of complete stupor, their minds are actually active to the point of death. He also describes the visions some persons experience at the end of life and describes three fascinating cases from his practice. One involves a hospitalized patient who, as Worcester entered the room, was propped up in bed, smoking a cigarette, and reading the morning newspaper.

> As I left his room the nurse stopped me to report that the patient had been talking to some visitor invisible to her, who he said was dressed in white. I went back to ask him about it. "Oh, it was only my sister," he answered casually and went on reading the newspaper. His sister had died previously, yet her presence seemed to him merely a natural fact. A few hours afterwards, without any other warning, his heart suddenly stopped beating.[98]

Worcester believes in the consolation afforded by faith in divine forgiveness and a future life, and he observes that dying persons do not always recognize the differences between the clerical and medical professions. In almost total contrast to Hermine Kane's pronouncement that "no adult wants to die," Worcester speaks of the "general ignorance of the fact that death is almost always preceded by a perfect willingness to die." Based on his broad experience, he asserts, "I have never seen it otherwise."[99]

William Munk had pointed out that patients sometimes know they are about to die. Worcester extends that to say, "Most dying patients have the feeling that death is near." This, however, does not settle the issue of what the doctor should say about the patient's terminal condition because some patients want nothing said to their families. Others want complete frankness, which will enable religious patients to prepare their souls for death and which will surely be comforting to the family after their loved one's death. Worcester adds that after the doctor has decided that the process of dying has begun, he should voice that view in all but the most exceptional circumstances. The doctor's devotion to the truth does not require him to tell all that he believes he knows, but it requires him to give timely notice of the patient's danger. The positive consequences of truth revealing are extensive. "The physician ought not to find it hard to establish with his dying patient and family absolutely frank relations which will be of immense advantage in carrying out the proper treatment."[100]

Undergirding all the particularities of comfort-directed care are doctor-patient and doctor-family relationships based on experience and empathetic presence. Worcester's emphasis on these relationships continues throughout his essay and starkly contrasts with the widespread neglect of attention:

> The physician must not underrate the help that his mere presence may afford in steadying and comforting both the dying patient and the family.
>
> Until the doctor has had the sad experience of standing by to very last those nearest and dearest [to the patient], he can only imagine the heartache of his dying patient's family and their sore need of sympathy; nor until he himself has been nigh unto death[101] can he ... imagine the comfort that even the firm clasp of a friendly hand can give to one in such extremity.
>
> No small part of the physician's duty and privilege in attending the dying is to steady and comfort the stricken family. This can best be done by giving each one some share in the nursing service.... [W]hat ever they can do they should be allowed to do.
>
> In the practice of our art it often matters little what medicine is given, but matters much that we give ourselves with our pills.[102]

Alfred Worcester's essays honor the historic legacy of the palliative care tradition by adopting its fundamental elements and principles, updating them with his own experience, and speaking to the needs of the time. Like Simeon Baldwin and Harrison Sainsbury, he forthrightly opposes scientific practitioners who believe they are duty-bound to do everything possible to prolong the lives of dying patients. But far beyond bemoaning how palliative care is being neglected, he blames that neglect on an egregious professional flaw at the core of scientific medical practice: the loss of the therapeutic power of deeply personal and caring relationships with patients and their families. He passionately believed that the recovery of that relationship would profoundly benefit dying patients, as well as bring pleasure and meaning to medical practitioners.

Nurses praised Worcester's 1928 original lecture on "The Care of the Dying." A reviewer of the original collection of lectures at the Harvard Medical School singled out Worcester's essay as one that "should be adopted by schools of nursing as essential materials in their teaching."

> Wise, sympathetic, comprehending, Dr. Worcester has most beautifully illumined the way for those with the sensitive perception to follow his teaching whether they be clinicians or whether they be nurses.[103]

In contrast, an unknown number of Worcester's physician contemporaries were neither moved nor interested in what he had to say. Dismissive of Worcester's arguments about the therapeutic value of doctor-patient relationships, the writer of a short, single-paragraph review of Worcester's 1935 book in the *Journal of the American Medical Association* stated that Worcester's points are "obvious when attention is called to them" and "in a way [they are] extra-medical." They only pertain to sympathy and comfort, and the author—Worcester—has a "sympathetic disposition." In emotional situations "where sympathy is useful," his book "ought to be appreciated." It's "a wholesome little book" that physicians and laypersons will find worth reading.[104] Thus ends the review that relegated Worcester's concerns to the periphery of medical attention.

Concluding Perspectives

Between 1895 and 1935 a new "heroic age" appeared in the history of medicine and surgery.[105] In contrast to the heroic remedies used by medical practitioners in the first half of the 19th century, which fell out of favor after the 1850s, the new era of ingenious and bold interventions would characterize modern medicine's expanding goals and capabilities up to the present time. These new interventions were greeted with great enthusiasm. They became entrenched in modern hospitals and gave birth to a new medical imperative on the part of many doctors—prolonging human life to the point of death. In 1798 John Ferriar credited unavailing attempts to stimulate the dissolving system to "ignorant practitioners." But in the new heroic age, attempts to sustain failing life were being made by the best-educated and most highly trained doctors the world had yet known.

Those who promoted care for the dying in the new age had the winds of progress in their faces. They had to maintain anew that death is natural and that death should be fought only if there were, in the words of Harrington Sainsbury, "reasonable probabilities" that life could be won. But when death seemed certain, defenders of palliative care argued that the fighting should end.

In the new age of medicine, palliative caregivers knew that they must become informed, skilled, and experienced in the science and art of palliation. Toward those ends, J. Norman Glaister modeled how psychiatrists might attend to the mental turmoil of inoperable cancer patients. Alfred Worcester likewise modeled the importance of palliative care on the part of physicians in medicine's revolutionary new era, and he sought to extend that legacy to new generations of medical students. Professionals devoted to palliative care upheld these legacies in order to ease the sufferings of dying persons, to comfort and counsel them and their stricken families, and to give of themselves along with their pills.

6

Never Say Die Versus
Care for the Dying

1935–1959

Tensions over how to treat dying persons increased to the breaking point between 1935 and 1959. Physicians who sought to rescue persons from the jaws of death clashed with peers who sought to soothe suffering, provide counsel, and enable dying persons to enjoy creature comforts as long as possible.

The ongoing progress and cultural power of scientific medicine can hardly be over-estimated: its diagnostic brilliance, its therapeutic triumphs over historic scourges of infectious diseases, its awesome surgical successes, and its entrenched institutionalization in medical and surgical training and practice in modern hospitals.[1] Increasingly, citizens believed that scientific medicine was rescuing humanity from the clutches of death. Chapter 5 showed how these vital forces emboldened efforts to prolong human life and eroded attention to palliative care.

Excitement over the continuing and amazing therapeutic advances between 1935 and 1959 paralleled, or perhaps even exceeded, the optimism of the previous fifty years. The following partial listing of medical and surgical breakthroughs in this time period indicates why the optimism continued among practitioners and in the minds of the public[2]:

- Discoveries of vitamins and treatment of diseases such as beriberi and pellagra during and after the 1930s, and the discovery of vitamin B12 as treatment for pernicious anemia in 1948.[3]
- An identification of blood compatibility groups, followed by blood transfusions and Red Cross donor programs in the 1940s.
- Sulfa drugs for pneumonia in 1939 and 1940, penicillin in 1941, heparin as an anticoagulant in 1942, and streptomycin for tuberculosis in 1944.
- Expanding programs of research sponsored by the National Institutes of Health during and after the second world war (1939–1945).[4]
- Cardiac resuscitation via defibrillation of the heart in 1947 and open-chest defibrillation beginning in 1955.[5]
- The first kidney transplants in the 1950s and the discovery of cyclosporine and other immunosuppressive "wonder drugs" thereafter.

- Development and use of the iron lung (Dinker's tank ventilator) in 1952, Engstrom respirators in the early 1950s,[6] and the refining of modern respirators/ventilators thereafter.[7]
- The first open-heart bypass surgery in 1953 via an artificial heart-lung bypass device that replaced heart and lung functions during the surgery.
- Development and testing of the first vaccine for poliomyelitis by 1955, followed by campaigns to eradicate the crippling disease.[8]
- The first fully staffed intensive care units for patients with various types of organ systems failure in 1958.

New curative treatments were saving countless lives. This further inspired efforts to prolong the lives of grievously and fatally ill patients.[9] In 1957 a physician exclaimed, "Truly, we are in the golden age of medical miracles."[10] A year later a notable internist spoke of the sequel to that excitement—the profession's "extravagant and ridiculous ... maneuvers aimed at keeping extant certain representative traces of life, while final and complete death is temporarily frustrated or thwarted."[11]

Behind medicine's technological breakthroughs lay a spirit of fighting optimism. That optimism became infectious both within and outside hospitals, and also within the hearts and souls of healthcare professionals and the public. Like the victories of the Allied powers during World War I (1914–1918) and World War II (1939–1945), the advances of medical science were hard fought. They were the products of preparation and planning, ingenuity, brilliance, dedication, unremitting work, cooperation, and keen competition. The world of medicine mirrored the world war victories and the vast resurgence of competitive sports after the wars.

Beginning in the 19th century and continuing into the 20th century, medical break-throughs made the news, creating great expectations in the minds of the public. The growth of the popular media coincided with the emergence and dominance of scientific medicine.[12] Media sources—newspapers, magazines, film, and television—covered newly discovered cures, medical research, and stories of famous and heroic physicians. Imbued with "epistemological authority," physicians were portrayed as modern-day heroes rescuing victims from various diseases and injuries with the marvels of modern technology and the latest pharmacological discoveries.[13] A prominent physician spoke of "the public's naïve acceptance of scientific medicine as magic, as being able to do all things for all men."[14]

Therapeutic optimism gave birth to a rationale that overtly *opposed* any suspension of attempts to prolong life for numerous patients. The rationale against stopping treatment partly rested on the conviction that if grievously ill patients were kept alive long enough, they might be saved by a suddenly discovered remedy.[15] "Tomorrow may bring news of the discovery of an effective treatment for cancer ... possibly for the very kind that will deliver a given patient.... The humane course is to hold to such a hope, slender as it is, and help the patient to live on."[16] "We never know just what [therapeutic cure] is around the corner."[17] This rationale, combined with the life-saving successes of existing medical treatments and the pressures to continue to sustain life, created physician opposition to replacing curative measures with palliative care.

For well over a century, physician proponents of palliative care had opposed an uncritical allegiance to medicine's therapeutic imperative. From John Ferriar in 1789 through Alfred Worcester in 1928 and 1935, these physician advocates actively stepped forth as countervailing voices against the therapeutic excesses of their times. Worcester's criticisms had targeted scientific, hospital-based practitioners. Sometimes inspired by Worcester, ever-increasing numbers of physician and nurse authors published articles on palliative care in the 1940s and 1950s, and explosively so thereafter.[18]

Between Alfred Worcester and Walter Alvarez: Increasing Interest and Controversies, 1935–1952

Of the dozen or more articles and book discussions about palliative care published between 1936 and 1952, none approached the power and relevance of Walter C. Alvarez's "Care for the Dying," published in 1952. Alvarez's article is another benchmark classic in the 400-year history of the quest for a good death.

The articles and book chapters on terminal care between Worcester's publication in 1935 and Alvarez's in 1952 are nevertheless significant, for they show that palliative care was beginning to attract renewed attention. They further consolidated the principles of comfort-centered care into a more coherent body of literature with a standard set of themes. Seven themes were advanced in the increasing literature of palliative care during these years.

The first theme underlines the great value of palliative care for providers, patients, and families. Dr. W. N. Leak from Great Britain reaffirmed that physicians have a duty to care for patients up to the time "the last breath has been taken and the flickering pulse is still."[19] Drawing upon the convictions of William Munk and Alfred Worcester, a nurse named Virginia Kasley said that expert care for dying persons and their families is "a great accomplishment, if not a rare gift," that brings "untold satisfactions" to caregivers: "It is our sacred duty and highest triumph to make dying as beautiful and meaningful" as possible.[20] The second theme lamented lack of attention to terminal care. Writing in 1944, Clifford Hoyle, for example, said that care of fatally ill persons is important both in its own right and because it receives so little notice in professional training and medical literature.[21] A third response opposed excessive preoccupation with disease diagnosis accompanied by unwarranted attempts to cure and prolong the lives of terminally ill patients. Doctors are charged with the moral duty to do no harm, which forbids "the subjection of dying folk to dramatic but indulgent surgery, or to investigations of no practical value."[22] Updated discussions of pain-relieving and peace-producing opiates, the treatment of bed sores, nurses' responsibilities, minor surgeries to relieve pain, and other matters constituted a fourth theme.[23]

Discussions and evaluations of the respective places where dying persons were cared for—hospitals, patients' homes, and nursing homes and institutions—were the fifth theme.[24] Some writers stressed the need to separate dying persons from other hospital patients,[25] a practice that appears to have been in place by 1952 in many hospitals.[26] Due to patients' desires not to be relegated to chronic or "dying wards" in hospitals, home care movements explored ways to enhance the care of terminally ill patients in their own homes. Home care included special training and regular home visits on the part of nurses, medical students, and physicians.[27] Within many hospitals, nurses, social workers, and chaplains were giving far more attention to the physical and emotional needs of the terminally ill patients than were physicians, who reasoned that their therapeutic responsibilities excused them from caring for dying patients.[28]

The sixth theme centered on the controversy over concealing, rather than revealing, the truth about patients' dire and/or terminal conditions. Clifford Hoyle noted, "Although some patients become aware of the imminence of death, to a great majority it seems to be denied."[29] Writing in *Annals of Internal Medicine*, Charles C. Lund broached the topic of what to reveal to cancer patients when cancer was considered unmentionable.[30] He held that before operating on the cancer, only the words *cyst, nodule, tumor*, and *lesion* should be used. But after the operation and in spite of resistance on the part of relatives, the patient should be told exactly what was found and what was done during the operation.[31] Lund's view contrasted starkly with others, who counseled outright concealing and lying, lest cancer patients become psychotic or commit suicide.[32] Reflecting upon his thirty years of medical practice, W. N. Leak observed that many patients ask whether they are dying and many doctors evade the question, but that he personally believed "a quiet straight answer with a clear look in the eye is as a rule the best reply." He added that his honest answer was usually greeted with a quiet "Thank you, Doctor," or "I knew it."[33]

Spokespersons for the seventh theme emphasized how effective terminal care should comprise joint contributions on the part of doctors, nurses, and clergy, which Alfred Worcester also endorsed.[34] Fifty years ahead of her time, Virginia Kasley spoke of the need for health professionals to become familiar with the beliefs and practices of different faiths and to be able to recognize when the patient would welcome a visit from a minister, rabbi, priest, or spokesperson from another faith tradition.[35]

In spite of the greater interest in palliative care seen in these themes, other physicians spoke out against them. In March 1952, E. M. Bluestone published an article that portrayed the beliefs and passions of modern, hospital-based practitioners to a group of hospital executives. "Death," Bluestone contends, "must be prevented and postponed at all costs, even if it sometimes thwarts our efforts after a long and costly struggle, since it is an insidious, ever-present, and implacable enemy." The struggle for prolonged existence is being fiercely carried on in hospitals, where "patients and their families will clutch at a straw in a frantic attempt at survival." While some patients prefer to die at home surrounded by family members, this is only their personal preference, over which hospitals have little control. For hospital executives, "eternal vigilance" must continue, and anyone who is too tender-hearted should step aside for the doctor "who is fearless in a good fight and never says die."[36]

And should patients be told they are fatally ill? No, Bluestone answers. Because "the incurable patient of today may be the curable patient tomorrow," a diagnosis of incurability should never be made, "lest we convert a possibly hopeful and curable patient into a hopeless and incurable one."[37]

Walter C. Alvarez Updates "The Excellent Little Book" by Alfred Worcester: 1952

In his essay "The Care of the Dying," published in the *Journal of the American Medical Association* (*JAMA*) in September 1952,[38] Walter C. Alvarez (1884–1978) disagreed with everything Bluestone said six months before. He opposed the extent of fiercely fought struggles over death waged in general hospitals. As opposed to Bluestone, he believed that the time comes when the never-say-die doctor should step aside for an honest, informed, self-assured, and caring physician who will give comfort-focused care.

Alvarez's article displays all of the previously outlined seven themes, but beyond his predecessors, he conveys these ideas with unique degrees of literacy, plain speaking, humor, pathos, and a cultivation of the art of telling memorable stories and crafting word pictures.[39] He is writing in the tradition of medical humanism that takes us back to Thomas Browne in the 17th century.[40]

That his article was published in *JAMA* seventeen years after a *JAMA* editor/author gave Alfred Worcester's book a one-paragraph cold-shoulder review partly testifies to a renewed interest in palliative care. Alvarez reverses the virtual dismissal of Worcester in *JAMA*. He refers to Worcester's counsel five times, and in a sixth reference he says, "An excellent little book on the medical care and nursing of the dying is the one by Worcester. Every physician in the land should read and re-read it."[41]

The son of a physician, Alvarez practiced medicine in Mexico and San Francisco before he joined the Mayo Clinic in Rochester, Minnesota, in 1926 and achieved a national reputation for excellence in research and clinical care. After he retired from the Mayo Clinic in 1950, Alvarez enjoyed a world-renowned career as the author of best-selling books for non-physicians and the writer of syndicated columns that appeared in over 80 U.S. and Canadian newspapers and 20 publications across the globe. His article on palliative care displays Alvarez's intimate acquaintance with the worlds of dying patients and their families in both homes and hospitals. He takes his readers inside these worlds.

This background sets the stage for the probable reasons why the editors of *JAMA* saw fit to print Alvarez's lengthy essay. His accomplishments as a physician were outstanding, and he was becoming all the more famous. He appeals to William Osler, who represented the ideal physician to everyone in the profession.[42] He gives attention to the interplay between terminal care and major types of fatal diseases identified by scientific researchers and practitioners. He discusses the best drugs to use for different types of pain, as well as the latest forms of surgical and radiological treatments that can modify symptoms.[43] He praises the virtues that physicians commonly treasure—being wise, kind, philosophical, observant, professional, and aspiring leaders.[44] And he writes as an experienced, articulate, no-nonsense practitioner.

Rather than lament the lack of attention physicians are giving to palliative care, Alvarez forthrightly discusses why many physicians are forsaking terminal care. He draws his readers into his topic by honestly and personally testifying that accepting that calling is not easy. All physicians realize how trying it is to walk into a room or home "shadowed by sorrow and fear." Once there, it is not easy to find words that are helpful and comforting, rather than banal or upsetting. "It is also not pleasant for the physician to have to admit his inability even to do much in the way of prolonging life, and it is not easy to have to stand by ... for weeks or months watching the invalid as he slowly dies."[45] These factors explain why some physicians dodge talking with dying persons and their relatives and sometimes refuse to go to their bedsides.

Alvarez contends that all slowly dying patients can be enormously helped by caring physicians. They can be comforted, supported, and encouraged. Their physical pain can be relieved, their mental stress and anguish lessened, and their lives often lengthened and made worthwhile. They should never be shunned and neglected because they can no longer be cured.[46] Reversing the dread and dodging, he exclaims, "How wonderful it is when a physician, by his kindness and devotion to a dying person, obtains the deep affection of the family."[47] Time and again Alvarez illustrates that wonder in his stories.

Talking with Persons Who Are Terminally Ill

Knowing that many modern doctors are uncomfortable with what to ask and what to say to terminally ill patients, Alvarez lays out do-and-don't instructions about how to form personal relationships with these patients and their family members: Talk and act naturally. Don't try to appear to be kind and sympathetic by becoming "sugary and Pollyann-ish." Don't treat the situation so lightly that the patient becomes disgusted and feels like she is being treated like a child. Avoid words of pity because most sick persons don't like them. Instead, they want physicians to express sympathy through demeanor and behavior.[48]

Doctors should also speak truthfully. Family members often want physicians to deny that there is anything to worry about, and most physicians are trained to go along with that denial. But "most such medical lying is wrong, usually futile, and even harmful. The patient is seldom so stupid that he is deceived. He knows that he is seriously ill, and he would prefer to have the physician talk honestly with him."[49]

Alvarez explains what his readers already know if they think about it—dying patients in hospitals have many ways to discover the seriousness of their conditions: They can read their medical records. They hear medical staff talking about their illness. They may have had an unsuccessful operation. They may see spouses weeping over their dire conditions. Furthermore, Alvarez observes that when charades of denial are maintained, patients are beset with feelings of great loneliness and isolation. He exclaims,

> Hundreds of times during my medical life I have talked frankly with dying persons and have thereby gained their lasting gratitude. Often, too, I have said to a husband and wife, "You two either know or strongly suspect what this disease is, so why should you now be lying to one another.... Why not now face this hardest of all things together?" Always they have been grateful to me for speaking in this way.[50]

Silence and denial about the realities of patients' conditions force them to walk through the valley of the shadow of death alone.

Beyond contributing to the well-being of terminally ill persons, physician-patient communication, according to Alvarez, relieves physicians from the stilted burdens of disingenuousness, fakery, and lying. Talking naturally frees them to become involved in terminal care, rather than escape its responsibilities. Truth telling is the companion to interpersonal truth acting. Concerning truth telling, he adds that all the truth need not be told. The truth about one's illness should not be forced on patients. What the physician says or does not say depends on the doctor's sense of each patient's courage and willingness to hear and face the truth. But when a man or woman looks him in the eye and asks, "What did you find?" Alvarez says a physician must tell the truth.[51]

Historic Themes Aligned with Experience

Like his historic palliative care predecessors beginning with Carl F. H. Marx in 1826, Alvarez also laments the fact that caring for slowly dying patients is rarely discussed as a subject in medical schools, medical meetings, or medical journals. As stated earlier, he recommends Alfred Worcester's book as an essential source of information, and in accordance with the recommendations of Worcester, Alvarez at one point in his teaching career required students to write papers about their experiences with dying patients.[52]

In agreement with Worcester, Alvarez adds his experience to the theme that most patients are not fearful of death. He testifies that hundreds of patients have told him that their fears pertain to a protracted and painful process of dying. Others worry that medical procedures may exhaust life savings they'd rather leave to their family.[53] Nevertheless, he observes that some persons do fear death immensely. Upon hearing of his inoperable cancer, one of his physician acquaintances became so fearful and demoralized that he could no longer work. And one of his women patients with a failing heart had an overpowering fear of death due to her dread of endless years in the fires of hell.[54]

Similar to his palliative care predecessors, Alvarez opposes overly aggressive and futile attempts to prolong the lives of dying patients. This was all the more problematic when Alvarez was writing. He believed that when persons approach death, the family's wishes should be ascertained after the physician describes what is likely to happen if resuscitation with oxygen, injections with stimulants, or surgeries are tried. To enable family members to express their wishes, the physician must talk with them frankly.[55]

Alvarez notes that physicians are of two minds on this matter. Some are guided by the wishes of the family. Others believe that they have no option but to try to prolong life. The actions of those bent on extending life can end tragically. He has known older men who, on being brought back to life, are distressed to think that they will have "to go through the miserable job of dying all over again." He has no doubts about where he himself stands:

> [S]ome day when I myself lie dying, I hope that I will have by me some wise and kindly physician who will keep interns from pulling me up to examine my chest. Or constantly puncturing my veins, or putting a tube down my nose, or giving me enemas and drastic medicines. I am sure that at the end I will very much want to be let alone.[56]

Another historic theme pertains to caring for persons with various types and severities of incurable disease. For example, persons with chronic leukemia and other forms of cancer need empathetic and realistic bolstering. They should be encouraged to cease endless preoccupation with their disease conditions and go on with their usual business, as others under the doctor's care have learned to do. Patients with other terminal conditions—such as those suffering from a series of minor strokes—need the caregiver's aid in explaining to family members that their fatally ill relative is acting normal for a patient with that illness. A wise older woman suffering from minor strokes told Alvarez, "Death keeps taking little bites of me." Alvarez recommended that her family members should accept her dizzy spells, confusion, and weight loss as normal, rather than resist or and rail against them. And the family may need to be told to cease telling a husband or father to "snap out of it" when his condition makes that impossible.[57]

Unlike many of his forerunners, Alvarez does not discuss the signs of death, nor does he survey essential components of terminal care near the end of life—bed coverings, light, the need for quiet, and so on. He mentions that nurses are capable of handling such things well. Good nursing should continue to life's end.[58]

He does discuss dietary and other restrictions forced on aging and slowly dying persons by well-meaning spouses and family members. He tells the story of two women in their fifties who brought in their 80-year-old, well-groomed father. Because the father had hypertension, his daughters had stopped him from smoking, drinking Scotch at bedtime, eating red meat, or even taking strolls around town. Their father had rebelled. He was smoking behind the garage, so they wanted Alvarez to upbraid him for such behavior. "I told them that my sympathies were all with their father.... I was sure he would live longer without that form of persecution.... I told them that some day I was going to found a society for the prevention of cruelty to aged parents by their loving and overly solicitous children![59] Alvarez also remarks that at the time of his writing there were no statistics on whether persons will live longer without their favorite pleasures.[60]

Caring for Patients with Different Ages and Temperaments

Unique in the story of the quest for a good death up to the time of Walter Alvarez, Carl F. H. Marx had written about palliative treatment and care in relation to patients of varying ages and temperaments in 1826.[61] Alvarez observes, "The problems of the physician vary according to whether the person who is dying is young or old, easily frightened and fearful, or stoical and acquiescent."[62] In his experience, children usually adjust to grave illness rather quickly. Physicians with the support of families generally keep fighting for a cure until the end of the child's life because children's powers of recuperation are great. Teenagers and young adults, however, often experience far more emotionally trying struggles with terminal illness. Women and men in the prime of life are often deeply distressed both for themselves and for their dependents. But some middle-aged persons make no great protest. He illustrates this by giving his readers the lines of a beautiful sonnet that the bacteriologist, Hans Zinsser, wrote to his wife when Zinsser was faced with approaching death due to leukemia.[63]

In Alvarez's experience, aged persons who find they are beset with slowly progressive fatal illnesses are generally less distressed than younger persons. Yet their responses to terminal illness vary. Some have lived well and are ready to die. Some have experienced so much failure, disappointment, sorrow, and bitterness that they are ready to die. Others would prefer to live longer so they can continue to enjoy life, and they want to watch their grandchildren grow up. Still others are willing to die after suffering the torments of a failing heart, crippling joints, or consecutive strokes. Others greatly fear death. Caregivers should discover how all these persons think and feel. Naturally, physicians should adjust what they say to the varying personalities of patients.[64] Caregivers should also confer with the relatives of older persons concerning the natural effects of their fatal illnesses. Aging patients should never be ignored, nor should they be burdened with excessive restrictions. He remarks that forced inaction and boredom "can only hasten the coming of childishness."[65]

Alvarez draws two main conclusions. First, all dying persons can be helped by caring physicians. Their suffering can usually be lessened. They can be comforted. And life can often be lengthened and made more worthwhile. Second, when the end of life approaches, all persons should be freed from futile attempts to extend life. He also suggests that educated physicians should know to ask dying persons and their relatives whether they desire the ministrations of priests and other clergy.[66] Beyond these conclusions is the transformative spirit of Alvarez's article: care for persons of all walks of life who are nearing the end of life can be deeply fulfilling.

Responses to Alvarez

Twelve years after his article was published, Alvarez said he received more reprint requests for his "Care for the Dying" article than any other he had written. He also observed that the popularity of his article proved that many physicians were greatly interested in the "problem of handling the patient who is headed for the grave."[67]

The wide reception of Walter Alvarez's article is not surprising. Through his stories, memorable style of writing and spirit, he humanized the widely avoided and widely presumed-dreadful topic of terminal care. He made the care of dying persons challenging, multifaceted, and, at points, captivating. He rendered palliative treatment and care relevant to medical practice in his time. He appealed to the underlying virtues of medical practitioners—honesty, insight, kindness, decision making predicated on experience, desire to ease suffering, and duty to prolong life within the constraints of meaningful life prolongation.

Concerning the historic story of palliative care, Alvarez mainly appealed to the work of Alfred Worcester. Yet much that he said was in keeping with the concerns of others in the tradition. Like Harrison Sainsbury in 1906, Alvarez held that decisions regarding life prolongation for patients in danger of dying should be brought before the family.[68] And whether he realized it or not, he fully agreed with J. Norman Glaister, who in 1921 depicted how hiding the truth about terminal conditions leaves patients with a feelings of loneliness and isolation.[69] Alvarez's unique emphasis on the do's and don'ts of effective and natural communication with fatally ill patients would become a central theme in palliative care beginning in the late 20th century.

By 1960 Alvarez was widely known and respected across the Western world. He began his career as a country doctor, and then rose to the top ranks of his profession and became the whole country's doctor.

Turning Points: 1952–1957

From 1952 through 1957, more books, book chapters, and articles were published on death and care for the dying than during the previous seventeen years. The formal presentations and panel-audience discussion about the treatment of dying patients that occurred in an annual medical meeting of the American Society of General Practice were printed in a medical journal in 1956.[70] One of the speakers, a clinical professor from the Harvard Medical School, commented that the topics were unusual for such a meeting, that he and his colleagues had just met with their students to discuss the topic, and that the discussion "mark[ed] a real advance in this problem."[71]

The increasing attention reflected both uncertainty and controversy over how to treat dying patients. The prevailing convictions and practices of many newly trained, cutting-edge practitioners clashed with promotion and practice of palliative care.

Death continued to loom as an affront to scientific medicine, a symbol of physicians' helplessness and an implacable enemy that could be defeated with invincible heroism and weapons of newly discovered medical technologies.[72] In 1957 a department chief in the University of Illinois' College of Medicine, William F. Mengert, offered his readers an insider's understanding of the new generations of medical interns and residents. He wrote that young physicians were unwilling "to acknowledge defeat" in the war against disease.[73] They were being taught and "have come to believe in the invincibility of the healing powers of modern medicine and surgery."[74] Mengert personally believed "in shooting the works when there is a fighting chance" to save the patient, but not when death can only be briefly postponed for six months or less at the cost of great pain and expense.[75] Even though Mengert disagreed with his medical residents' insistence on another intestinal operation for a patient who was virtually moribund, he permitted them to proceed with what they "almost unanimously demanded." The patient died during the surgery.[76]

Other authors recounted their own stories of invasive and sometimes mutilating, but eventually fruitless, efforts to prolong life.[77] Earl M. Chapman's analysis before an assembly of physicians in a medical meeting profiled the age:

> The surgical attacks on disease have produced brilliant results in our time, and we have seen hopeless cardiacs restored to work; we have seen lung cancers removed; and we have seen vascular systems repaired, and we have watched the brain pierced with percentile improvements. But, now and then this enthusiasm to destroy disease has led to such mutilation of the person and a consequent dependency on society that I cannot assign it to an ethical place in medical practice.[78]

Those who believed the diagnosis terminal disease should usually be revealed also encountered headwinds in hospitals. In 1955 Donald C. Beatty, a hospital chaplain, observed, "There is a hardened convention, a conspiracy of silence that makes it difficult if not impossible for the critically ill person to talk about his impending death."[79] He spoke of other chaplains who reported that the hospitals they served did not allow doctors and nurses to tell critically ill patients that the end of life was probably near. Beatty opposed the common notion that death is an "unrelieved calamity." He told the story about a visiting member of the clergy, who, apparently unaware of reigning hospital policy, said to one his hospitalized parishioners, "Well, Bella, I understand that you're not going to get well." Bella responded, "Oh, do come in and sit down. You're the first person I've been able to talk to in the longest time! They keep telling me how much I'll enjoy my garden in the spring. But I'm not going to be *here* in the spring!"[80]

Others also spoke of the "conspiracy of silence regarding the hopeless prognosis and the nearness of the end."[81] As is evident in the words and practices of physicians, nurses, and clergy who continued to champion palliative care, the conspiracy was extensive. But it was not all-embracing. A groundbreaking study of 444 physicians published in 1953 indicated that 70 percent of the questioned physicians either never told patients they had cancer or usually did not tell. The other 30 percent either always or usually told. Both sides voiced strongly held positions.[82] Ironically, a study of 500 patients that same year confirmed the then-surprising results that a large majority of patients felt that they could not be fooled—that they wanted to know their diagnosis, and wanted their families to know.[83]

The conspiracy was fostered for several reasons. First, silence was being maintained to keep patients from losing hope. Second, a number of psychiatrists fervently held that if a patient learned she or he was terminally ill or had cancer, the results would be catastrophic—personal guilt, denial of diagnosis, hostility, withdrawal, agitated depression, hopelessness, paranoia, suicide ideation, and sometimes suicide itself.[84] And third, death was widely construed as a cultural taboo, as unmentionable and distasteful a topic of conversation as sexuality had been in the Victorian age.[85]

Morally, the conspiracy of silence denoted the persistence of physician paternalism and authoritarianism. Near the end of his article on "Care for the Dying," Walter Alvarez said that older patients with widespread cancer should be given the facts and then allowed to decide on a course of action for themselves. That position had been taken by Harrison Sainsbury in 1906.[86] A majority of doctors between 1935 and 1960 felt otherwise. Like John Gregory, Thomas Percival, Christoph Hufeland, and many other authors of the past, they believed that their parent-like duty to protect patients from grievous emotional harm justified keeping patients from knowing the truth about their medical conditions. Family members often agreed that their loved ones should remain unaware of their terminal conditions.[87] That was a beginning point for exponentially greater levels of physician authoritarianism. Patients who were not told were excluded from decisions about their treatment options. Depending upon the physician's judgment, family members might or might not be informed about the patient's prognosis or allowed to express their preferences.[88] It followed that many doctors took it upon themselves to treat patients with whatever interventions they deemed justifiable. This cascade of convictions was about to be confronted.

Two pivotal turning points occurred in 1957, both of which took place outside of the medical literature. The first was brought forth by an anonymous woman who moved the long-simmering, in-house disagreements between the contending voices recorded above into the public arena. Her story, titled "A Way of Dying," was published in a distinguished national journal and sparked a medical and moral revolution.[89] She begins:

> There is a new way of dying today. It is the slow passage via modern medicine. If you are very ill modern medicine can save you. If you are going to die, it can prevent you from doing so for a very long time…. Enter the sickroom and sit with your beloved, and

endure the long watch while an incredible battle between spirit and medicine take place. It may take weeks ... but the victim is going to die.

The widow's husband survived one surgery, leaving him "just barely there." No one thought he could survive another surgery; yet days later she arrived to find that he had been taken to surgery again, this time without anesthesia. The news was nauseating. A doctor told her not to go see him, as he would not recognize her, but she resisted, saying that "if we were nearing the end of our time together, I must memorize every detail of this scene." Unfortunately, the scene revealed carnage from the surgical battlefield—her husband sitting straight up in bed, imprisoned by metal bedsides. His eyes and face were crazed, his arms bruised. He ranted senseless words. "Choked with anguish and horror," she could do nothing to help him.

After three days of torture, during which time he repeatedly cried out to her, the widow's husband awoke from his delirium and asked to speak to the doctor. He said, "Doctor.... I realize how badly off I am, but you must give me help." When the doctor's only reply was that they "were doing for him what they could," her husband lamented, "They just don't care."

The suffering continued, mitigated only by sedatives. Finally, the widow's husband went into a coma. News of the coma evoked differing responses. The hospital staff countered, "We are doing all we can." Registering relief that the suffering might end, the widow responded, "Amen." But even the coma brought no real relief. The widow watched for hours as her husband sat curled up, connected to tubes and oxygen and "breathing a noise of horror." The next morning she "begged [the doctor] to cease this torture." The doctor replied that "except under most unusual circumstances they had to maintain life while they could."

With the knowledge that he couldn't last much longer, the widow stood by her husband's bedside, watching her "beloved as he attempted to cross the great divide." Her prayer asking God to take him ended abruptly when a nurse burst through the door with a doctor-ordered injection. Shocked, the widow "staggered out the door; there was nothing else to do."

The next day her husband finally died. The widow experienced "calm, knowing he deserved to be released."

An unknown woman had pulled back the curtain hiding the Wizards of Oz from public view. Here, unvarnished, was a loving spouse's experience of the savage days that her beloved husband endured under the knives of uncommunicative surgeons and the impersonal and routine practices of nurses in a modern hospital.

This anonymous writer does not single it out, but her final journey with her husband was exceedingly lonely. They could barely communicate with each other. Both were offered spoonfuls of information by the hospital staff, but in fact they only had each other in this foreign and uncommunicative world of the hospital. She also does not single out the backdrop for the horrors she experienced—the foreign culture of the hospital. The phrase "a new way of dying" in the first sentence of her article might well have been subsumed under the title "A New World for the Dying." It was a strange, disturbing, and dehumanized world, in total contrast with the familiar worlds of Walter Alvarez and his patients or of the visiting pastor who spoke warmly and truthfully to his terminally ill parishioner.

The second turning point was anything but anonymous. It was initiated publicly by Pope Pius XII in response to questions posed by a group of world-renowned anesthesiologists. As noted in the list of amazing therapeutic advances at the beginning of this chapter, iron lungs that enabled persons enduring respiratory failure to breathe mechanically were being used up to the 1950s, after which C. G. Engstrom and others developed new types of sophisticated ventilators/respirators that would control ventilation and anesthesia gases at comfortable rates. As specialists in life-supportive measures, anesthesiologists supervised the use of these and other life-extending techniques.[90]

Aware of Pope Pius's intense interest in the rights and wrongs of many medical innovations, and possibly also aware of the long tradition of Roman Catholic reflection on medical-moral questions, the anesthesiologists asked the Holy Father to address three questions pertaining to acceptable and unacceptable uses of the new resuscitation and life-prolonging technologies[91]: First, do physicians have the right, if not the obligation, to continue maintaining life with artificial respiration even when they believe the case is hopeless? Second, does the anesthesiologist have the right or obligation to remove artificial life-supportive measures when the patient is in a state of deep unconsciousness and blood circulation will quickly end if these means are withdrawn? Accompanying this question, should doctors heed the requests of family members who are urging that life support end? And third, does the Catholic Church consider the patient dead when he or she is in a state of compete and irreversible unconsciousness?[92]

Speaking authoritatively for the Roman church, Pope Pius XII responded, "We are pleased, gentlemen, to grant this request."[93] After describing the tasks of anesthesiologists and surveying the way lives can be saved and extended, the pope set forth three basic principles: First, natural reasoning and Christian morals prove that in the face of serious illness, it is the duty of seriously ill persons "to take the necessary treatment for the preservation of life and health." But, second, normally sick persons are required "to use only ordinary means" to save or extend life—that is, "means that do not involve any grave burden for oneself or another." Third, sick and injured persons are "not forbidden to take more than the strictly necessary steps to preserve life and health."[94]

Then Pope Pius answered the first two questions posed to him by the anesthesiologists. He did this by setting forth a moral rule that opposes doctors who claim they are duty-bound to extend a patient's life—even to the point of death—without the express permission of the patient and/or family members.

> The rights and duties of the doctor are correlative to those of the patient. The doctor, in fact, has no separate or independent right where the patient is concerned. In general he can take action only if the patient explicitly or implicitly, directly or indirectly, gives him permission. The technique of resuscitation ... does not contain anything immoral in itself. Therefore the patient, if he were capable of making a personal decision could lawfully use it and, consequently, gives the doctor permission to use it. On the other hand, since these forms of treatment go beyond the ordinary means to which one is bound, it cannot be held that there is an obligation to use them nor, consequently, that one is bound to give the doctor permission to use them.[95]

Patients, therefore, have a right to refuse or choose life-sustaining resuscitation treatment. Furthermore, the rights and duties of family members depend upon "the presumed will of the unconscious patient" if he is of legal age to make such decisions. And if life-prolonging measures are deeply burdensome to families, they have the right to insist on discontinuing these attempts, and doctors are morally permitted to comply with the family's requests. So, yes, under these conditions families have a right to request and expect that such attempts should be discontinued.[96]

Concerning the third question about when death occurs, Pope Pius said that generally the Catholic Church holds that death occurs when the vital functions of human life end, not when a body's organs cease to show signs of life. He added that questions surrounding life and death "remain open," such that doctors, especially anesthesiologists, need to give "a clear and precise definition of 'death' and the 'moment of death.'"[97]

These pronouncements are decisive and, given their source, revolutionary. They affirm the rights and preferences of grievously sick and dying patients with respect to accepting or refusing life-extending medical treatments. Equally revolutionary, Pope Pius' affirmations directly oppose physicians who believe that their medical expertise and authority justify imposing treatments on patients without patients' express permission. The moral standoff occurring between physician proponents of palliative care and authoritarian physicians armed with new technical means of possibly extending life and advancing modern medicine was being shifted toward patient-desired palliative measures.

The first healthcare "rights movement" thereby broke forth in the late 1950s, not the late 1960s or early 1970s.[98] Appeals to patients' rights during and after 1957 suited the times. It harmonized with the emergence of the civil rights movement that year in Little Rock, Arkansas. It also called constitutional law into play. Indeed, in 1957 the term "informed consent" was adopted in U.S. case law and brought to the attention of the American medical community.[99] Morally, patients' rights began to trump the authoritarian paternalism of physician enthusiasts.

Intra-Professional and Public Warfare: 1957–1960

The story of widow's ordeal and that of her husband immediately secured the attention of medical journals and popular publications. A 1957 editorial in the *New England Journal of Medicine* noted that the woman's story "should be required reading for physicians" whose dignity was in danger of decreasing "in inverse proportion to the efficacy of the medical sciences to prolong life." The widow was battling for "the right to die" against the "ghastly reality" of her husband's treatment.[100] William F. Mengert used the widow's story as the theme of his presentation at the annual meeting of the Illinois State Medical Society, in which he described two similar stories that constituted "a plea to the physician to refrain from unnecessary heroics."[101]

Quoting from both the woman's story and the editorial in the *New England Journal of Medicine*, John J. Farrell said in 1958 that "the right to die with the dignity which is the right of every man" had become a serious problem that was being discussed in the wards of hospitals, in medical meetings, and in the lay press.[102] Citing his forty years of hospital experience, R. Ruff contrasted the physically comfortable and spiritually peaceful death of a physician friend who had declined hospitalization with the horrifying death of a man with inoperable bowel cancer who, despite his protests, was subjected to numerous costly treatments until he lay exhausted, financially depleted, and close to death. Ruff added,

> I've seen any number of patients who, in the opinion of the referring physicians and consultants, were beyond hope. Yet they were rarely permitted to die in peace. They were hospitalized, given this and that expensive medicine, transfused, X-rayed from head to foot, subjected to costly chemical examinations and often painful surgery, and made thoroughly miserable.[103]

These are among the 28 or more articles, books, and book chapters on the right to die and care for the dying published from 1957 through 1960—in contrast to 12 publications during the previous fourteen years.[104]

Edward H. Rynearson on the Should Nots and Shoulds of Terminal Care: 1959

No publication by a medical professional between 1957 and 1960 matched the influence and creativity of an article by Edward H. Rynearson (1901–1987) in 1959. Rynearson joined the Mayo Clinic in 1932. He authored and co-authored numerous articles on endocrinology in *JAMA* for decades thereafter. Unafraid of controversy, he famously called popular American dietary schemes "hogwash," and in front of thousands of physicians and their guests in 1963, he discussed the roles of religion and medicine with the outspoken and controversial American Roman Catholic bishop Fulton J. Sheen.[105] After Rynearson was killed in an automobile accident in 1987, the writer of his obituary in the *New York Times* noted that he had become nationally prominent when he published his article on terminal care in 1959.[106]

To engage physicians as individual decision makers, Rynearson titled his article "You Are Standing at the Bedside of a Patient Dying of Untreatable Cancer."[107] He begins with unvarnished criticisms:

> There are too many instances, in my opinion, in which patients ... are kept alive indefinitely by means of tubes inserted into their stomachs, or into their veins, or into their bladders, or into their rectums—and the whole sad scene thus created is encompassed within a cocoon of oxygen which is the next thing to a shroud.
>
> The present piece has nothing to do with euthanasia,[108] nor am I talking about any patient in whom there is any question as to the diagnosis. I refer to the patient who is almost in extremis ... and there is no question in anyone's mind as to the prognosis.... Despite all "the impressive ministrations science can provide," he is still dying and is still suffering.[109]

Rynearson contends that when the attending physician and his or her colleagues agree with the above, they should stop life-extending measures and talk frankly with the patient and her or his relatives. He observes that the patient by now knows about her situation and is usually asking for pain relief, not a prolongation of distress. The relatives "almost never ... wish to have their loved one maintained indefinitely in a tragic interlude of more and more suffering." So, if neither the patient nor the relatives want any further heroic measures, who wants them to be used? Rynearson states that no representatives from Roman Catholic, Greek Orthodox, Jewish, or Protestant faiths believe "physicians should try extraordinary means to keep life going when every process of the body is bent toward extinction."[110] To prove his point, Rynearson, a lifetime member of the Methodist church, innovatively summarizes the 1957 address of Pope Pius XII to anesthesiologists.[111]

Who, then, is causing extraordinary medical life-extending measures to be continued virtually indefinitely? Rynearson asserts, "In most instances it is the physician himself, and thus this presentation of mine is address to members of my own profession."[112] He adds that death is "a social event," not merely a doctor's event. Therefore, care for dying persons implicitly includes the dying person, family members, friends, and society. Reprehensively, he argues, too many doctors are disregarding that encompassing reality. They fail to recognize that dying involves "the philosophies of the one who is dying, of the living family, and of the medical attendants," as well as traditional society values. Dying and death also include "unconscious elements, such as the feeling on the part of some relatives that they are somehow guilty," as well as remorse, anxiety, and many religious values and rituals interwoven in the dying process.[113]

What, then, should be the components of the care of the dying patient? Rynearson reasons that these components should include both immediate and overarching features. More immediately, physicians should attend to historic concerns in palliative care advocacy. "When a doctor and his consultants have sincerely judged that a patient is incurable, the decision concerning further treatment should be in terms of the patient's own interests and reasonable wishes, expressed or implied." He adds that appropriate treatment also includes the use of ordinary means of preserving life (such as food and drink), as well as good nursing care, measures to ease physical and mental suffering, and preparations for death.[114]

Creatively, Edward Rynearson steps back from the specifics of palliative care to outline the overarching components of end-of-life care predicated on his understanding of dying and death as socially and culturally rooted realities. The essential components of care for each dying person include the following:

1. He should die with dignity, respect and humanity.
2. He should die with minimal pain.
3. He should have to opportunity to recall the love and benefits of a lifetime of sharing; he and his family and friends should visit together, if the patient so wishes.
4. He should be able to clarify relationships—to express wishes—to share sentiments.
5. The patient and relatives should plan intelligently for the changes which death imposes upon the living.
6. The patient should die in familiar surroundings, if possible; if not ... in surroundings made as near homelike as possible.
7. Finally, but importantly, there should be concern for the feelings of the living.[115]

Returning to his censoring of physicians intent on keeping patients alive indefinitely, Rynearson points out that most incurably ill physicians want nothing more than kindness and comfort. They likely oppose heroic measures for themselves. He asks how doctors would want their family members to be treated. Rynearson then answers his own question by describing the care of a member of his immediate family: "We kept her in her own bed in her own home and made certain she suffered as little as possible until she was released by death." He ends with a confession and challenge: "I make the decisions I have recorded here." His readers who are standing at other patients' bedsides must now make their own decisions.[116]

When Rynearson wrote, the tide was beginning to turn toward greater attention to palliative care. The anonymous woman's story and stories from physicians were calling for a right to die peacefully. Rynearson held that patients "should die with dignity, respect and humanity," the meanings of which he sought to capture in his list of moral components of terminal care.

The year after Rynearson's article was published, a psychiatrist named Paul Chodoff defined the meaning of the phrase "opportunity to die with dignity" through a list of should nots and shoulds. Dying with dignity opposes the physician's presumed omnipotence, refusal to accept the inevitable, and engagement "in an onslaught of desperate measures which have no realistic hope of staying the disease process or effectively prolonging life." Emotionally mature physicians will abandon those measures, develop strong and trusting relationships with dying patients, and enable them to become as comfortable as possible at the end of their lives.[117]

Responses to Rynearson: Accolades and Drawn Swords

Responses to Rynearson's article extend beyond the time frame of this chapter by two years. The responses of 40 physicians, nurses, reporters, and others were soon printed in the American Cancer Society's journal, in which Rynearson had published his article. Most were positive—some extremely so. A physician from the Scott and White Clinic in Temple, Texas, commented that he believed a majority of physicians in America would go along with Dr. Rynearson's philosophy. A physician from the Wayne State University College of Medicine in Detroit, Michigan, felt that Rynearson's approach to this difficult subject was excellent and made it the topic of discussion in a staff conference. A doctor from Toms River, New Jersey, commented that little provision had been made for the matters Rynearson discussed, so could the American Cancer Society please supply reprints of his article for "distribution to physicians on request, or perhaps a few reprints each to physicians generally?"[118]

But all the swords had not yet been turned into plowshares. Charles S. Cameron, dean of the Hahnemann Medical College in Philadelphia, wrote that he "disagreed most violently" with what Rynearson had written. He therefore asked to be relieved from his duties as a consulting editor for the journal. Four years earlier in that journal, Cameron had defended the view "that the doctor should never abandon the fight" to prolong the lives of incurable cancer patients.[119] A brief survey of opinion in 1960 proved that Cameron was not alone.[120]

Siding with Cameron, David A. Karnofsky objected to the "ethically wrong" tenor of Rynearson's publication. It is the doctor's duty, he said "to sustain [life] as long as possible." The patient "entrusts his life to his doctor." To stop treatment and allow persons to die is a step in the direction of the extermination policies of Nazi Germany. Doctors can make compromises to their duties to prolong life if patients reject further treatment or relatives take them home to die, but the achievements and triumphs in the fight against cancer come from doctors "who continue to treat the patient when the odds may appear overwhelming."[121]

Dr. Karnofsky took his never-say-die message before 1,500 persons at the annual meeting of the American Cancer Society in 1961, a summary of which was printed in *TIME* magazine. To his list of reasons for not letting the patient "go quickly, with dignity and without pain," Karnofsky added that life must be prolonged because there is always a chance during a temporary reprieve that science will find a more effective, long-lasting treatment. "When," he asked, "should the physician stop treating [the] patient?" He answered, "I believe he must carry on until the issue is taken out of his hands."[122] Death must do the taking.

The issue of treating or not treating fatally ill patients with life-saving attempts was brought before the broader public by an article in *Reader's Digest* in 1960. The reporter, Lois Mattox Miller, said she had been handed a folder of letters by an unnamed medical educator who told her the letters dealt with the "most difficult problem the doctor must face: whether to prolong life—and suffering—in the face of inevitable death." Miller cited three cases from the folder of letters and said she had interviewed numerous physicians, nurses, and hospital administrators. She summarized the views of Edward H. Rynearson, Pope Pius XII, Alfred Worcester, and Walter C. Alvarez. "We had better get somewhere and soon," a geriatrician said. "This problem is getting more pressing all the time."[123]

Concluding Perspectives

The increasing therapeutic optimism after 1935 gave birth to a rationale that overtly opposed any suspension of attempts to prolong life for numerous patients. This rationale reflected enthusiasm over the amazing advances of modern medicine listed at the beginning of this chapter and in the first pages of Chapter 5. It also rested on the assumptions that death is an implacable enemy, that failing to prolong life symbolized medical surrender and failure, and that postponement of death demanded heroic, often painful interventions.

To embed these assumptions into medical practice, many doctors relied upon authoritarian paternalism. If patients and family members were informed about their treatment and non-treatment options and then allowed to state their preferences, the war against death would be delayed. Cameron, Karnofsky, and like-minded colleagues believed that the achievements and triumphs of modern medicine could not be maximized if patients and their families stood in the way of medical progress. Triumphs of modern medicine were being used to silence the wishes and choices of patients and families.

Informed by voices from their heritage and common moral conviction, palliative care practitioners opposed that worldview. They accepted the naturalness and inevitability of death. They were familiar with how dying persons could be comforted and took it upon themselves to do the comforting along with family members and clergy. They ventured into the worlds of patients described by Alvarez. Those who read the anonymous woman's story in the *Atlantic Monthly* became even more outspoken. Those who discovered that their views were affirmed by Roman Catholic medical moralists and the authority of Pope Pius XII found that their personal moral compasses were aligned with a long-standing tradition of ethical reasoning.

So palliative care proponents continued to battle physician adversaries. They spoke of the personal rewards of caring for dying persons and their surrounding family members. They fought for greater truth telling instead of truth concealing, for the beneficence of replacing aggressive treatments with personalized end-of-life care, for the rights of terminally ill patients to refuse aggressive curative treatments, and for the moral right to die as naturally and peacefully as possible. The fighting brought palliative care advocacy out of the shadows, and it would contribute to the birth of a culture-wide death and dying movement.

7

Times of Momentous Transition

1960–1981

Between 1960 and 1981 palliative care finally secured far stronger cultural foundations. Beyond the expert and devoted attention of individual physicians and nurses that it had received for over 250 years, end-of-life care received support from hospice programs, bioethicists, and law and legislation. These new cultural foundations did not fall from the sky. They were built in response to a combination of factors that demanded their construction—public exposés of the oftentimes dehumanizing inner dynamics of hospitals, continuing stories of dreadful attempts to prolong lives of terminally ill persons, and the emergence of the death and dying movement that made it impossible to hide from the reality and roles of death in human life.

All the while, stunning new discoveries were occurring in scientific medicine, and enormous popular enthusiasm accompanied these advancements. So the 22 years from 1960 through 1981 were times of momentous change on two fronts: innovations in curative and life-saving medical procedures, on the one hand, and breakthroughs in supportive care for dying persons, on the other.

Amazing Medical Advances

The high hopes engendered by remarkable medical discoveries continued into the 1960s and beyond. The following list of medical advances and discussion of the revolutionary discovery of cardiopulmonary resuscitation (CPR) reveals why the public, the national media, and sponsors of medical research displayed abounding enthusiasm over the promises of modern medicine. These advances forged major changes in medical specializations and the structuring and dynamics of hospitals.

- 1960: The development of the modern CPR protocol—closed chest cardiac resuscitation that replaced the invasive cut-open chest resuscitation used during surgery between the 1930s and the 1950s[1]
- 1960: First heart bypass surgery
- 1960s: Development of new ventilators for patients undergoing surgery and/or CPR, experiencing respiratory distress, and being kept alive when comatose[2]

- 1960s: Establishment of respiratory care units
- 1962: First kidney transplant
- 1962–1970: Coronary care units established in large hospitals[3]
- 1967 and thereafter: Development of successful coronary bypass surgeries using patients' leg veins as replacements for blocked coronary arteries
- 1967: First heart transplant by Claude Bernard in South Africa
- 1968: Founding of the American College of Emergency Physicians
- 1970: Discovery of cyclosporine, an immunosuppressive drug that became a powerful impetus for organ transplants
- 1972: First programmable implanted cardiac pacemaker replaces first reliable 1970 pacemaker, followed by further pacemaker innovations between 1973 and 1981 and their expanding usage[4]
- 1972: Emergence of public health campaigns to promote CPR training for millions of police officers, firefighters, flight attendants, and other non-medical personnel[5]
- 1974–1977: Balloon angioplasty (opening of blocked arteries) for persons with angina and other cardiovascular problems
- 1980: Publication of the invention of the percutaneous endoscopic gastronomy (PEG) feeding tube for supplying artificial nutrition and hydration to the stomach through the abdomen[6]

Modern Cardiopulmonary Resuscitation (CPR)

In 1960 Drs. William Kouwenhoven, James R. Jude, and G. Guy Knickerbocker began a medical revolution. They published a description of 14 out of 20 (70 percent successful) resuscitations of patients whose arrested hearts were restarted by means of closed-chest cardiac massage.[7] Attempts at resuscitation began in the 18th century and included discoveries derived from medical trial and error, followed by research on animals and humans starting in the last decades of the 19th century. Drawing upon eighty years of experimental attempts to restore and extend life, Kouwenhoven and his colleagues created a new, definitive, step-by-step CPR protocol.[8]

The new protocol included the following steps: (A) Free mouth and throat for breathing. (B) Inflate the lungs with mouth-to-mouth breathing or by ventilation via tubes inserted into the trachea (windpipe). (C) Begin blood circulation with manual chest compressions. (D) Inject drugs, especially adrenaline and sodium bicarbonate. (E) Monitor electrocardiography via EKG machines that record normal and abnormal heartbeats. (F) Conduct electrical defibrillation—external electric shocks to restore the beating of stalled hearts or reverse heart fibrillation.[9] Refinements of these steps were made over time, but the basics remain intact.[10]

Modern CPR emerged as the definitive means for either reviving dying patients or certifying their deaths. John Anthony Tercier, a historian-defender of CPR, praises it for three reasons: it might restore life, it diagnoses the cause(s) of death, and it certifies death. "There is some point," he says, "in beating a dead horse—to ensure that it *is* dead." Tercier acknowledges that CPR "leaves the living with various degrees of loss, grief, anger, and guilt," but argues that its benefits far outweigh these effects.[11]

Having become a fellow in the American College of Emergency Physicians, practiced emergency medicine for seventeen years, and seen a "thousand or so deaths," Tercier characterizes CPR as violently invasive and often a violation of the patient's or "victim's" autonomy. He calls resuscitation "a deathbed ritual" that "transgresses the body's boundaries," and then remarks, "Few corpses go to the grave unbeaten."[12] Occasional complications of CPR include broken ribs, lacerations of the liver and spleen, cardiac trauma, and gastro-esophageal damage.[13] But the many persons rescued from cardiac arrests, near drownings, electric shocks, and traumatic injuries rightly regard its value as incalculable.

Excitement over modern CPR became infectious and transformative. In the eyes of many, it ascended to the realm of the miraculous, the means by which the dead would be raised, the symbol of the science of "reanimatology."[14]

Emblematic of modern Western medicine, CPR constituted "the supreme medical emergency having priority over all other medical maneuvers and ailments."[15] "Code Blue, room 202!" over loudspeakers calls for immediate action by all members of the CPR team. CPR led to rebuilding and reorganization in hospitals, redesigned with coronary care units (CCUs) and multi-disciplinary intensive care units (ICUs). Hospitals were restructured for the rapid mobilization of equipment and newly established resuscitation teams to the sides of persons in cardiac arrest. CPR and artificial ventilation became ubiquitous in the treatment of cardiac arrest and arrhythmias, electrocution, poisoning, near drownings, hemorrhages, head trauma, seizures, organ transplantation, and renal, liver, and neurologic failure.[16]

CPR created new medical disciplines and revolutionized anesthesiology. Its wondrous possibilities spurred its American physician innovators to take their message and methods to the ends of earth. Between 1960 and 1968 Kouwenhoven gave some 53 lectures and demonstrations to distinguished medical audiences. Five thousand physicians attended his lecture in St. Louis in 1961. He and his staff produced numerous films, one of which received an award from the British Medical Association.[17] Between 1965 and 1973 the American Heart Association widely dispersed CPR programs and training materials. After 1973 the American Red Cross and other agencies began training the lay public to assist in life-saving CPR. The third national conference on CPR held by the U.S. National Academy of Sciences in 1979 recognized the "growing worldwide enthusiasm."[18]

CPR became and still remains a cultural icon. Popular journals and TV programs (such as *Emergency!* and *ER* in the United States and *Casualty* in the United Kingdom) gave full-fledged depictions of CPR by emergency personnel for the purposes of promotion, entertainment, and education.[19] For its practitioners, the resuscitation experience has been described as an emotional high, the ultimate adrenaline-stoked rush, which also confers a sense of power.[20]

Modern external CPR conferred a jeweled crown on the king of life-saving technologies. The shocking stories in the last two chapters described how patients, in spite of their dire diagnoses, were subjected to life-prolonging medical interventions until they reached death's door. The development of CPR kept thousands of patients in the throes of death from reaching that door.

So why didn't the newly crowned king of technology, combined with other amazing medical advances, further marginalize palliative care? Why, instead, did proponents of supportive care become more numerous, determined, and influential? Why did comfort-focused care find new institutional foundations in hospices, secure the support of influential non-physicians, and build upon protections provided by law and legislation?

Four Forces Foster Concern for Palliative Care

Answers to those questions are supplied by a constellation of forces that began to reverse the struggling fortunes of palliative end-of-life care and treatment. This constellation included the following four factors: continuing alarm and contention over excessive attempts to prolong life; disturbing book-length studies and ever-increasing periodic literature on the plights of patients within hospitals; sobering findings about CPR; and the birth and growth of a multi-disciplined, culture-wide death and dying movement.

Alarm and Contention Over Excessive Attempts at Life Prolongation

Chapter 6 detailed graphic stories of heroic, often futile attempts to prolong the lives of catastrophically sick patients and how these stories seized the attention of the public and created intra-professional disputes among doctors. Moral dilemmas over whether to prolong life (and, if so, for how long) continued to preoccupy the attention of medical personnel throughout the 1960s and beyond.[21] Uncertainties over the time of death encouraged attempts to extend patients' lives, including those who were diagnosed as terminally ill. Sometimes family members would insist that the patient should be kept alive by all available means. The ideal of prolonging life at all costs would sometimes press a doctor "to continue an all-out effort to save a lost patient even though he [the doctor] is dimly aware that there is no hope."

> In one emergency case a patient who was not very sick, and certainly was not expected to die, suddenly had a seizure and stopped breathing. The doctor in charge made a heroic effort to revive him with chest massage, but finally another doctor asked gently, "Do you want to continue that if his pupils are fixed and dilated?" That query brought the intense doctor to his senses; he said, "No, I guess not," and stopped the chest massage.[22]

In addition to administering CPR, last-ditch surgery for patients who were not likely to survive would be tried on those who were willing to take the 10 percent chance of survival.[23]

After three years of systematically exploring how dying patients were being treated in hospitals, two sociologists, Barney G. Glaser and Anselm L. Strauss, published their landmark book, *Awareness of Dying*, in 1965. They observed that the degrees of life prolongation most frequently occurred in particular hospital contexts and with particular doctors.[24] Young doctors "fired with the ideal of saving" were often unable to "bear the thought of losing a patient," and they felt that their professional competence might be called into question if they did not persist in life prolongation.[25] Nurses also were involved in numerous attempts to rescue patients, "however senseless it may seem."[26] Distressingly, explicit requests of some patients to end life-prolonging efforts should they become comatose were sometimes ignored by doctors, who occasionally would renege on their promises to honor the patient's wishes.[27]

The medical literature confirms the findings of Glaser and Strauss. The egregious story of a doctor patient who was "Not Allowed to Die" was published in the *British Medical Journal* in 1968.[28] A 68-year-old doctor retired from medical practice after a severe heart attack reduced his ability to work. Worried that he might also have cancer, surgeons opened his abdomen and found that cancer had indeed invaded his lymph nodes and liver. A surgeon colleague removed part of his stomach in hopes of preventing his tumor from metastasizing further; yet the patient "suffered constantly with severe abdominal pain and pain resulting from compression of spinal nerves by tumor deposit." Ten days later, the patient collapsed due to a massive lung obstruction, so the surgeon removed the obstruction.

> When the patient had recovered sufficiently he expressed his appreciation of the good intentions and skill of his young colleague. At the same time he asked that if he had a further cardiovascular collapse no steps would be taken to prolong his life, for the pain of his cancer was now more than he would needlessly continue to endure. He himself wrote a note to this effect in his case records, and the staff of the hospital knew his feelings.
>
> His wish notwithstanding, when the patient collapsed again—this time with acute myocardial infarction and cardiac arrest—he was revived by the hospital's emergency resuscitation team. His heart stopped on four further occasions during that night and each time was restarted artificially. The body then recovered sufficiently to linger for three more weeks, but in a decerebrate [unconscious] state, punctuated by episodes of projectile vomiting accompanied by generalized convulsions.[29]

On the last day of the patient's life, preparations were being made to put him on an artificial respirator, but his heart stopped before this could occur.

Physicians voiced several, often radically differing opinions about these efforts to maintain life. Upon recounting stories similar to that of the 68-year-old doctor, some physicians asked how to prevent such cases. Others ardently approved of CPR whenever the details and final outcomes of the case were not known.[30] Physicians who struggled with what to do sometimes agonized over what they themselves would prefer after taking the wishes of family members into consideration.[31]

One doctor commented in 1963 that efforts to maintain life were being stigmatized as prolongation of dying. He then listed ten reasons for erring on the side of active treatment. They included the fallibility of the physician's prognosis, the medical tradition of "*active* contention with disease," the possibility that a new curative agent might be discovered, and the possibility that extraordinary treatment might result in a cure. He asserted, "There are no 'hopeless' patients, only hopeless doctors."[32] In 1971 another doctor argued that for the sake of some family members, he would keep the patient alive by means of respirators, CPR, and other procedures, even if the patient's brain had irretrievably lost its higher functions. He added that if the patient was still a functional human being, "I would have done my best to see that she got them, until the issue was taken out of my hands."[33] Dr. David Karnofsky used that last phrase in 1960.[34]

Other physicians duly recognized the brilliantly successful reversals of sudden death by CPR, but held that doctors "are widely guilty today of assault upon the dignity" of consciously dying patients. CPR is acceptable when the diagnosis is uncertain, they argued, but surgery is impermissible if it will not save life or relieve pain. Last-chance gastrostomy, colostomy, and tracheotomy procedures also constitute no less than an assault upon the patient. And if the hopelessness of the disease is established and no meaningful surgical palliation is possible, the surgeon's duty is to avoid operating.[35] In their zeal to preserve life, too many doctors were neglecting their obligations to relieve suffering and allow patients to die.[36] Quoting extensively from the 1958 article by Edward H. Rynearson, John McClanahan held that "many of the so-called extraordinary measures are not often indicated." Despite all "the impressive ministrations science can provide" for patients *in extremis*, they will continue to suffer and inevitably die.[37]

In an influential article written in 1968, Charles D. Aring drew upon the long tradition of palliative care promotion. He confessed, "I am not among those who strive officiously to keep [patients] alive.... Death and dying can become natural if you and I make it so. Those unable to face death have not begun to face life. Death is not a taboo surrounded by disapproval or shame."[38]

By 1968, 59 percent of a group of 418 physicians surveyed indicated that they would omit major life-resuscitation procedures and medications for dying patients if they were given a signed request to that end from the patient's next of kin.[39] Physicians were going through a period of uncertainty and turmoil, and the growing opposition to uncritical life prolongation forecast greater support for palliative treatment and care.

The Plights of Dying Patients in Hospitals

During the 1960s and 1970s humane care for dying persons achieved a new and powerful sense of urgency due to exposés of the plights of fatally ill patients in hospitals—their isolation, profound loneliness, social alienation, and assigned inferiority.[40]

In addition to an ever-increasing number of articles published by physicians and nurses on end-of-life care between 1960 and 1981, the impressive studies by the Glaser and Strauss displayed the degrees to which the entrenched and systematic dynamics of hospitals brought about the isolation and dehumanization of dying patients.[41] Isolation and inhumanity had been displayed by the poignant and powerful story of the anonymous woman writer in 1957. The influence of Glaser and Strauss's participant-observation and interview study was also far reaching, in part because the percentages of deaths in hospitals rose from 39.5 percent of the American population in 1949 to 53 percent in 1964 and 54 percent in 1980. In England 50 percent were dying in non-psychiatric hospitals in 1965, rising to 54 percent in 1970. In Western Europe well over 50 percent of dying patients were spending their final days in hospitals.[42]

In *Awareness of Dying*, Glaser and Strauss explore the intricate interactions between physicians, nurses, patients, and family members with respect to patients' awareness or lack of awareness of their terminal conditions. The standard mode of interaction involved "closed awareness," whereby "the patient does not recognize his impending death even though the hospital personnel have the information" and are determined to keep the patient from getting it.[43] Less frequently there is "suspicious awareness," when the patient does not actually know his diagnosis but suspects that hospital personnel believe him to be dying. The interaction of suspicious awareness "can be described metaphorically as a fencing match, wherein the patient is on the offensive and staff members are carefully and cannily on the defensive."[44]

The two additional modes of awareness explored by Glaser and Strauss are mutual pretense and open awareness. Mutual pretense occurs when the patient and the staff know the patient is dying but pretend otherwise. The pretense is "like a masquerade party, where one masked actor plays carefully *to* another as long as they are together, and the total drama actually emerges from their joint creative effort." The hospital's numerous props support the staff's side of the masquerade—thermometers, baths, meals on time, and so forth. Both parties follow rules of avoidance regarding the dangerous topic of the patient's death, and each party pretends that nothing has gone awry. "One terminal patient told a friend ... that she suffered from isolation and feeling as if she were trapped in cotton batting." The mutual pretense eliminated the need for staff members to attend to the emotional needs of dying patients.[45]

Open awareness—staff and patients' overt recognition of the terminal prognosis— occurs when pretense collapses due to the patient's obvious physical deterioration, increasing pain, and/or increased sedation, or when a chaplain might convince the patient that it's better to bring realities out into the open, rather than remain silent. Nevertheless, certain implicit rules of patient behavior must be maintained in open awareness situations—composure, cheerfulness, cooperation with staff members, and no wailing, accusations, or apathy. Glaser and Strauss found that only a few doctors spent time getting to know terminal patients well enough to judge their desire for disclosure or capacity to withstand the expected shock of disclosure.[46]

All was not impersonal. Some doctors would reveal the prognosis in order to avoid losing a patient's confidence; be able to manifest an honest, rather than a cheerfully false front; and enable patients to attend to their legal and financial affairs.[47] Some nurses actually preferred open awareness, which offered them the personal gratification of being able to work with patients and help them face death. Better than all other staff members in the study by Glaser and Strauss, a chaplain was able to converse freely, openly, and humanely with some patients who knew they were dying.[48]

To preserve the standard mode of closed awareness, the medical staff would "*act as though they were still trying to save the patient's life*"—that is, persist in "do-something" care. Do-something care included physician visits to the bedsides of some fatally ill patients who would receive brief medical examinations. At times it included surgery intended to make the patient more comfortable, but which was presented to family members as a means of helping the patient recover.[49]

In contrast to do-something care, the staffs in all the hospitals studied by Glaser and Strauss used the phrase "nothing more to do" for patients who were diagnosed as unsalvageable, especially those who knew they were dying. Nurses became the main custodians of what was being called comfort care for these patients—pain relief and routine bodily care filled with "expressive avoidance"—that is, avoidance of personalized interaction, bland facial expressions, and evasive conversation.[50] Kept from communicating genuinely, many nurses frequently felt helpless as they worked with "nothing more to do" patients.[51]

Patients in great pain were at times allowed to end their own lives, which was termed "auto-euthanasia." These patients would be left unwatched in a separate "dying room" with a lethal bottle of pills at the bedside.[52] Upon the deaths of most patients, the staff experienced a collective mood of relief and *"gladness* that the ordeal is over for themselves, the patient and the family."[53] Consigning patients to separate dying rooms had been done since 1952, but what occurred in them is not known.[54]

The dynamics and emotional consequences of the most common mode of systematic interaction—closed awareness—were predicated on the fact that a majority of physicians (between 69 and 90 percent, depending on the study)[55] favored not telling patients about their terminal illnesses. Additional implicit social dynamics kept patients unaware of their fatal conditions. These included limited disclosures to family members who would guard the secret if told. It also included close-knit and intricate teamwork by the medical staff "against an opponent" (that is, the patient) who had little experience in interpreting signs of death and "who is usually without allies." Patients' symptoms were often explained away, discounted, or falsely interpreted with inaccurately optimistic statements by staff members.[56]

All these factors, along with highly limited visiting hours for family members, increased fatally ill patients' isolation. Under these circumstances, the patient begins to "understand very well that staff members are not interested in [her] awesome problem or cannot grasp its nature even if they wished to."[57] She is facing death. She is becoming weaker and more dependent. She is about to experience leave-taking of all she ever experienced and loved. Except perhaps for a chaplain or a beloved and intimate family member, she must undertake that journey alone—alone in this strange new world of pretense, impersonal and disingenuous interacting, and carefully honed, multi-layered deception.

The accuracy and power of Glaser and Strauss's findings are confirmed in the writings of doctors and nurses from both before and after *Awareness of Dying* was published in 1965. In 1962 Thomas P. Hackett and Avery D. Weisman wrote that fatal illness increases the patient's alienation to a sense of profound loneliness because the false hope and optimism of physicians undermine meaningful communication and force the patient into exile.[58] Deception only increases the distance between physicians and patients. Here is Hackett and Weisman's story of a reversal of roles:

> The easiest course for the physician to follow in treating the dying is to withhold the truth and support the patient's use of denial. There probably are cases where this policy must be used, but we have not as yet uncovered one valid contraindication to the use of truth.... A case in point was that of a charming and worldly man dying of tongue cancer.... He was considered an excellent denier. A few days before he died, the tumor suddenly enlarged and swelled his tongue to such an extent that he could not speak. On the night of his death, his psychiatrist visited him, but could think of nothing to say. So he sat on the bed and put his arm around the patient's shoulder. The patient reached for a pencil and pad and wrote, "Don't take it so hard, Doc." He had known the prognosis throughout those many months of conversation.[59]

Hackett and Weisman add that the physician's attitude defines how he relates to the patient's family and friends: "When he advises them not to disclose the grim truth, a lie is born. To act out a lie requires acting ability."[60]

A year later two nurses—Joan M. Baker and Karen C. Sorensen—displayed several of Glaser and Strauss's themes by listing strategies nurses were using to terminate conversations with irreversibly ill patients. These included the following: moralizing to the patient saying, for example, "You shouldn't talk that way, Mr. Jones, no one knows when he will die"; denying directly the fact that the patient may die with such words as "No, I don't think you'll die today or even tomorrow"; philosophizing to the patient with the words "No one really knows what the future holds for him"; changing the subject by asking, for example, "Who's that in the picture on your night stand?"; and either remaining silent or turning away from the patient.[61] Baker and Sorensen observe that these responses force the patient to face death alone. Too often nurses only deal physically with dying patients, which keeps them from being able to discuss their concerns. Against the grain of that tradition, Baker and Sorensen suggest ways to communicate more meaningfully.[62]

In a 1966 article titled "Let's Talk about Death: To Give Care in Terminal Illness," another nurse, Ramona Powell Davidson, faced resistance to the title of her article, which she first presented at the University of Florida Health Center. She was warned, "Nurses do not usually talk about death and, above all, would not talk about a patient's death with him." Davidson described her open communication with five patients and their families in order to counteract their sense of overwhelming loss and feelings of entrapment, as well as "make as meaningful as possible the life that is left."[63]

Informed by Glaser and Strauss's *Awareness of Dying*, Dr. Charles D. Aring penned a classic essay on the care of dying patients in 1968. "The immediate threat of dying is isolation," he said. "Hospital personnel generally are cold [and] so busy taking care of routines they learn nothing about a process they themselves will eventually experience. It is startling to find repeatedly the primacy of hospital routine over dignity, respect, and humanity." Aring held that hospital staffs "assign inferiority to the dying." They die—"ergo, they ... *are* inferior."[64]

These studies, stories, and journal articles recall earlier articles and stories—notably, J. Norman Glaister's description of the atmosphere of unreality surrounding a cancer patient in 1921, Walter Alvarez's 1952 discussion of the loneliness and isolation dying persons feel when they are being deceived, and the horrible experiences of the anonymous woman and her husband in 1957. Beyond these historical precedents, the descriptions and stories about how dying persons were being disrespected, neglected, and deemed inferior in hospitals during the 1960s became momentous calls for reform in their own right.

Sobering Findings about CPR

The third element of the constellation that would reverse the fortunes of palliative care involved sobering data about the actual success rates of CPR. Regrettably, the 70 percent survival rate of 20 patients reported by Kouwenhoven and his colleagues in 1960 was never again duplicated, or even approximated.[65] The five-year study of a far greater number of patients—552 patients altogether—by A. L. Johnson and his Canadian colleagues in 1967 showed that 32 percent of the patients receiving CPR were alive after 24 hours, but only 14.9 percent survived past the time of being discharged from the hospital. No patients with sepsis, cancer, or gastro-intestinal hemorrhage survived post–CPR hospital stays. Only 3 percent of patients in renal failure survived at discharge. And 2 percent of the patients became permanently comatose and died from four days to six weeks thereafter. The great news within these sobering statistics was that the 14.9 percent survival rate was "remarkably constant" over the five-year period. Had these patients not been given CPR, they would "have been included in the hospital mortality statistics" instead of remaining alive and active for many months after their resuscitations.[66] Three additional studies between 1965 and 1969 reported even lower survival rates of resuscitated patients after discharge—between 8.8 percent and 8 percent.[67]

The incongruity intensified. As CPR became increasingly used and fervently praised, its success rates became increasingly dismal.[68] In the midst of that incongruity lay irreversibly ill and dying patients. When their hearts failed, should they be subjected to CPR or allowed to die more peacefully? Additional data that undermined survival rates included the percentages of patients who died during attempted CPR (74 percent, 67.8 percent) or before they might have been discharged from the hospital (85.1 percent, 91.8 percent, 80.9 percent, 86 percent, 91.2 percent).[69]

One of the reasons for defending CPR offered by Tercier was its possible restoration of life. Unfortunately, restoration of life is a broad category that includes patients who survived less than 24 hours after CPR and patients who survived longer than 24 hours, but died 2 to 14 days later—usually in an intensive care unit—without ever leaving the hospital.[70] Furthermore, a study published in 1976 noted that 10.4 percent of initial survivors of CPR ended up in chronic vegetative states.[71] By 1978 two German researchers asserted that "to prolong life often means only to prolong dying."[72]

Studies about the harms and limitations of CPR proved that it was often being used on terminally ill patients. Stories of these patients added to the shocking stories about how dying patients were subjected to life-prolonging medical interventions. So, in spite of its manifest successes, CPR's excesses fostered, rather than marginalized, the promotion of palliative care and treatment.

New questions were raised and fervently discussed. Which populations of patients should be spared the invasiveness of CPR? Who and what forces would bring about that deliverance? And how should those who are not medically suitable subjects of CPR be cared for within different settings?

The Death and Dying Movement

The death and dying movement served as the fourth force that reversed inattention to palliative care and led to stronger cultural foundations for this aspect of medicine. Early signs of the movement appeared at the end of the 1950s, and it began to flourish and become influential by the mid–1960s and thereafter. Its complexities and influence are deserving of full-scale investigations.

Chapter 6 revealed how concerns over excessive attempts to prolong the lives of terminally ill patients became newsworthy in the late 1950s. Newsworthiness emerged as one of several contributing factors to a cultural infatuation with the meanings of death and the circumstances of the dying. In 1964 a world bibliography on death and dying contained some 400 items. By 1973 that literature had expanded to over 2,600 references. Four years later a bibliographical guidebook of 3,848 annotated books and articles on death and dying was published and organized according to the following headings: general publications, the humanities, medicine and nursing, religion and theology, the social sciences, and audiovisual media.[73]

Accompanying the literature were local and national conferences and a number of new journals (such as *Omega* beginning in 1970 and the *Journal of Thanatology* in 1971). Newly founded organizations included the Foundation for Thanatology (first established in 1968), the Forum for Death Education and Counseling, and the Equinox Institute. TV programs also dealt with topics on death and dying. Courses, teaching materials, and textbooks in death education ensued. Educational aids were prepared for all grade levels, from elementary schools through high schools, colleges, adult education programs, and professional schools of law, medicine, nursing, and theology. In 1974 the *New York Times* reported that more than 165 colleges offered courses on death and dying.[74]

Death education also found links to sex education. As early as 1955 T. O. Elliot opined, "If good sex education is important, delicate and subtle, so is proper 'death education.'"[75] The far greater candor about death in the early 1970s led Peter Steinfels to remark, "Death may never become as popular as sex, but as a topic of public discussion it is certainly not doing badly."[76]

The linkage between sex and death was due in part to the often-quoted 1965 essay by Geoffrey Gorer, who claimed that death, like sex during the Victorian age, had become a modern taboo, a forbidden subject of conversation.[77] The first of the realistic goals for death education outlined by Daniel Leviton in 1974 was to "gently remove the taboo aspect of death language so students can read and discourse upon death rationally without becoming anxious."[78] The thesis of Gorer's article had been set forth by Herman Feifel in 1959, in the first of Feifel's two edited books, which served as standard multidisciplinary texts in the death and dying movement:

> In the presence of death, Western culture, by and large, has tended to run, hide, and seek refuge.... Concern about death has been relegated to the tabooed territory heretofore occupied by diseases like tuberculosis and cancer and the topic of sex....
> [P]rofound contradictions exist in our thinking about the problem of death.[79]

Two best-selling books contributed to the notion that death had become a taboo in Western cultures, and they also advanced the movement to nullify the taboo by facing death far more forthrightly. In 1963, Jessica Mitford's book, *The American Way of Death*, was published. Mitford contrasted the 19th-century tradition of laying out the bodies of the dead by friends and family, who then bore plain coffins to the grave, with the modern funeral director industry that whisked the dead away, used cosmetics to make them appear life-like, and then aggrandized the dead in expensive coffins. In 1969 Elisabeth Kübler-Ross's *On Death and Dying* appeared. Kübler-Ross contrasted the peacefulness and dignity of family-surrounded deaths of loved ones in their homes in earlier eras with dying in the 1960s, "in which death is viewed as taboo, discussion of it is regarded as morbid, and children are excluded with the presumption and pretext that it would be 'too much' for them."[80] Beginning in 1965, Kübler-Ross became a famous and tireless advocate of meaningful communication with terminally ill hospitalized patients.

The depths of the death and dying movement should not be underestimated. Beginning in the early 1960s, reflections on death included sophisticated, sometimes Pulitzer Prize–winning studies about the meanings of and responses to death in religious and cultural traditions and in the fields of philosophy, psychology, and theology.[81] Innovative explorations of ethical and legal issues surrounding terminal care loomed just over the horizon.

As evidenced in the studies of Glaser and Strauss and others, empirical and clinically relevant studies of death and dying in hospitals appeared in the 1960s. Critiques of the over-treatment and dehumanizing circumstances of terminally ill patients in hospitals undoubtedly contributed to the growth of the death and dying movement, but an explanation of why Americans and other Westerners became transfixed by death exceeds those critiques and accompanying demands for reform.

The successes and pervasiveness of science presupposed a secular worldview that deeply challenged beliefs regarding eternal life in religious orthodoxies. What, indeed, is the meaning of human existence if death totally annihilates "all the devotion ... all the noonday brightness of human genius" in a vast and indifferent solar system?[82] The assassination of John F. Kennedy in November 1963, the Vietnam War between 1963 and 1973, the assassination of Martin Luther King, Jr. in January 1968, and television's fixation on violent death also contributed to the culture-wide preoccupation with death and finitude.

The death and dying movement critiqued the view that death is only an enemy to be fought to life's inevitable end without patients' and/or family members' knowledge or consent. The movement's leaders explored death as a foreboding reality that should not merely be fought but also faced in all of its complexity, including its fostering of genius, creativity, devotion, honor, celebration, philanthropy, sympathy, nurturing, and sorrow. Death must be defanged enough to render it discussible. Suffice it to say, the more death and dying became common topics in popular culture and the classroom, the less they could be neglected in medical institutions.

Historic Breakthroughs in Palliative Care

Linked together, the four previously described forces empowered programmatic changes in the treatment of dying persons. Glaser and Strauss fully realized that their sociological analysis of the plights of dying patients in hospitals cried out for systematic reforms. At the end of their second book, they revealed their reformist agenda. They titled the last chapter of *Time for Dying* (1968) "Improving the Care of the Dying," which set forth the urgency of the situation:

> Our research has radical implications for changing, and perhaps improving, the nursing and medical care given to the dying. No reader can have read the foregoing chapters without drawing such conclusions.... One can neither read nor write such chapters without responding critically to what transpires in our hospitals....
>
> We believe that tampering with the present system of terminal care merely to institute a specific change here and there, without consideration of systematic correction to the whole system, will do little to improve today's terminal care.... There is need for a

systematic, comprehensive, concentrated, and determined effort to reform contemporary modes of caring for the dying.[83]

They correctly pointed out that "provisions for terminal care" already existed in the organized work of hospitals, but those provisions paled in the face of the overarching social dynamics of healing and saving. While these provisions seemingly made dying persons as physically comfortable as possible, they remained socially and psychologically deficient (*deficient* is a neutral term for being impersonal and dehumanizing).[84]

In their book, Glaser and Strauss call for four tough-minded and comprehensive reforms. First, greatly amplified terminal care training in schools of medicine and nursing is mandatory. The training should include how to disclose news of impending death to patients and family members, how to organize terminal care so that more attention will be given to the psychological and social needs of patients and families, and how and when to teach about these matters. Second, clear levels of accountability must be identified, reviewed, and established. Explicit rules of accountability should replace reigning ad hoc personal discretion, incidental reporting, and makeshift inter-staff communication. Third, systematic connections must be made between the care of terminal patients in hospitals as they transfer back and forth from their homes. And finally, public discussions must occur regarding the grave problems frequently debated but often left to the personal decisions of doctors and nurses based on their assumptions about professional responsibility and estimates of public opinion. The two most pressing specific problems are worries over the addiction of patients to pain-relieving drugs and the "senseless prolonging" of life.[85]

Joined by a nurse, Jeanne C. Quint, Glaser and Strauss had published all these critiques and recommendations virtually word-for-word four years earlier. To help people "die gracefully," they argued, nurses and doctors must become accountable for their psycho-social-ethical actions and interactions. Perhaps workshops and in-service courses and training sessions, "at which personnel can at least air and talk openly together about their problems and usual tactics," would serve as beginning points. "Conceivably, the personnel—including house physicians—might be taught greater psychological sensitivity" through role playing and programs that would include advice from chaplains.[86]

Quint, Strauss, and Glaser republished their recommendations for nurse practitioners, administrators, and educators in 1967. Again they called for comprehensive reform that would bring about rational and compassionate care for patients, which would surely benefit staff members also. Strauss republished the recommendations yet again in 1969.[87] Agreeing that the "whole system" of the existing approach to dying patients must be changed, a nurse from British Columbia illustrated the system's depersonalization with this story:

> Not long ago I sat at the bedside of an 84-year-old dying patient ... very close to death. A staff member came into the room and cheerily said, "Well, Mrs. J., how are we today?" ... Mrs. J. moved herself up in bed with her elbows and said in her most regal best British accent: "Well, my child, I don't know how **we** are feeling but I am doing something I shall not do again. I am dying."[88]

Training and teaching about death, dying, and personalized palliative care began to increase in nursing and medical schools and in hospitals after the mid–1960s, but these changes fell far short of the reforms Quint, Strauss, and Glaser envisioned. They were 30 years ahead of their time.

Important breakthroughs in palliative care began on two levels—reforms in hospitals and reforms in newly established hospices. Chronologically, hospice care began first, but to continue with this chapter's focus thus far, we will begin with hospitals.

Elisabeth Kübler-Ross's Innovativeness and Influence: 1965–1995

As a notable participant in the death and dying movement, Elisabeth Kübler-Ross (1926–2004) devoted her career to the emotional well-being of persons with incurable illnesses within hospital settings. Trained as a psychiatrist, Kübler-Ross became an instructor at the University of Chicago's Pritzker School of Medicine in 1965. That year, in spite of hostility from a number of doctors and nurses, she began an interview-based seminar on the experiences of dying patients with a group of Chicago seminary students at the University of Chicago's Billings Hospital. Within two years the seminar became an accredited course in the medical school and the theological seminary. Physicians, nurses, orderlies, social workers, and clergy attended these courses.

In another two years Kübler-Ross published her best-selling book, *On Death and Dying*, which was based on her counseling with dying patients and their responses in her seminars. Lonely, isolated, and sometimes wishing to offer a lasting gift to posterity, the overwhelming number of patients Kübler-Ross approached welcomed the chance to speak with empathetic counselors and learners. Many nurse attendees became far less fearful of spending time with fatally ill patients, and hospital chaplains served as models of effective listening and communication.[89]

Although *On Death and Dying* was questionable with respect to its particular theoretical framework, its radical innovativeness should not be overlooked. Elisabeth Kübler-Ross's fundamental approach reversed the pretenses and paucity of communication with terminally ill hospitalized patients that Glaser and Strauss had unveiled. The reigning assumptions Glaser and Strauss uncovered were that medical personnel believed that fatally ill persons by and large should, and could, be fooled. They were second- or third-class human beings. They had nothing meaningful, or wise, or wry, or humorous to say. For Kübler-Ross, these patients were normal human beings who were grappling with death. Patients stepped forth as unique sources of insight and wisdom in their walks through the shadow of death.

With respect to her theoretical concerns, Kübler-Ross explored the coping mechanisms of patients who became aware of their terminal conditions. She identified a sequel of five psychological stages that last for differing periods of time, by and large replace one another, sometimes exist side by side, and ultimately display degrees of hope. These five stages are shock and denial, rage and anger, bargaining, depression, and final acceptance.[90] In the minds of numerous authors and counselors, these stages achieved the status of an orthodox creed that greatly facilitated provider-patient communication. Oftentimes the stages were used as proof that patients should be told the truth about their terminal prognoses because that would allow them to "progress toward a peaceful and dignified death."[91] Over time, however, Kübler-Ross's stages were questioned as ambiguous, based on intuition rather than systematic research, and lacking in predictive value. One psychiatrist praised her for greatly popularizing concern for the dying, but held that dying persons vacillate emotionally and respond according to the manners in which they lived.[92]

The fame that Dr. Kübler-Ross acquired from *On Death and Dying* was fully matched by her own unrelenting efforts and resourcefulness with respect to addressing the emotional needs of persons grappling with death. She was featured in a major article in *LIFE* magazine; gave magnetic lectures throughout the United States and Western Europe; taught seminars in colleges, seminaries, schools of social work, hospitals, and medical schools; and received 20 or more honorary degrees.[93] She also continued to publish books on palliative care: *Questions and Answers about Death and Dying* in 1976, *To Live Until We Say Goodbye* in 1978, and *Living with Death and Dying* in 1981.

Courses in Nursing and Medical Schools

In 1964, the year before Elisabeth Kübler-Ross taught her first series of seminars, Bernice M. Wagner described the course she was teaching to nursing students at the University of Kansas. Designed to enable nurses "to face up to death vicariously" before their involvement with dying patients and their families in the wards, the course included a variety of readings (including the anonymous widow's story from 1957), a student essay, and classroom discussions.[94]

In 1972 David Barton and others published a detailed description of their elective course on death and dying for third- and fourth-year medical students at the Vanderbilt University School of Medicine. Three clinical professors and one philosophy professor taught the sixteen-week, one-and-a-half-hours-per-week course that included patient presentations, readings from literature and medical periodicals, and presentations from nurses, chaplains, and the instructors. The course was uniformly well received as a probing study about "an integral part of life."[95]

A 1972 survey of U.S. medical schools indicated that 49 percent of the responding institutions had formal courses on the psychological care and understanding of patients with fatal illnesses, 64 percent of which were required. An additional 14 percent of respondents said the subject matter was being dealt with via rounds, informal discussions, and lectures. A study in 1981 found that 58 percent of the responding medical schools included death education in the curriculum, and it concluded that death education "is increasingly becoming a part of the curriculum."[96]

Cicely Saunders's World-Wide Contributions to Palliative Hospice Care: 1958–2004

As foundations for her lifelong and ultimately transforming care of patients within homes for dying persons known as hospices, Cicely Saunders (1918–2005) earned a degree in nursing from Florence Nightingale's training school in London's St. Thomas' Hospital, a degree in medical social work from Oxford University, and an MD from St. Mary's School of Medicine. From the time she began training as a nurse in 1940 to

1952, when she decided to study medicine, Saunders cared for patients in hospitals. Her nursing care and loving relationship with a terminally ill patient, David Tasma, a Jewish survivor of the Warsaw ghetto, led to their discussing the creation of a combined hospital-home for dying patients. When Tasma died in 1948, he left Saunders a gift of 500 pounds sterling for establishing such a home. Their covenant of hope became reality when Cicely Saunders, with financial backing from many others, established St. Christopher's Hospice in 1967.[97]

Hospices have a long history dating all the way back to the 12th century, when they were established as places of refuge for homeless and hungry wayfarers, women in labor, needy poor persons, orphans, lepers, and sick persons. Hospices founded by Roman Catholic, Anglican, Methodist, and other groups' religious charities included beds and wards for incurably ill persons suffering from tuberculosis, cancer, dementia, and other conditions. They were widely established in the nineteenth century and early decades of the twentieth century in Great Britain, Ireland, the United States, Canada, Australia, and other nations.[98] Like medieval hospices, these institutions provided food, lodging, personalized care, and spiritual succor for persons whose medical, financial and physical conditions made home care impossible—persons who were frail, chronically ill, and dying.[99] These hospices were almost entirely staffed by nun and deacon nurses with limited visitations by doctors during eras when many physicians were deserting patients approaching the end of life.[100]

Saunders served as a nurse volunteer in St. Luke's, a home for dying persons, before she pursued medical training. After receiving her MD in 1958, she conducted clinical research for six years as a research fellow at St. Joseph's Hospice in Hackney, England. As a devout Protestant working with Irish Catholic nuns, Saunders soon discovered her lifelong calling—the calling to become the first modern physician dedicated to caring for terminally ill persons.[101] Between 1958 and 1959 she published seven articles on the care of fatally ill patients, the first of some 220 publications. Her first publication drew upon the writings of a number of notable proponents of palliative care, especially Alfred Worcester.[102] Beyond all indebtedness, however, her publications embody Saunders' abiding personal involvement with and attention to dying patients—their pain, sleep, bed sores, mental distress, emotional needs, and frequent desire for pastoral care.

Saunders's commitment to building out-of-hospital communities where dying persons would feel neither strange nor neglected would bring modern hospice care into being.[103] Fundamentally, and in accord with her training and years of experience, she united the care of incurably ill and dying patients in traditional religious-sponsored hospices with the scientific contributions of modern medicine. Her expertise in modern medicine enabled her to further develop methods of symptomatic treatment for bed sores, bowels, sleep, mental distress, anorexia, and other problems. She also conducted creative research on the control of mild to severe pain.[104] Her medical training and experience led her to believe that doctors should be at the center of palliative care teams that work together to instill hope and consolation at the end of life.[105]

Saunders's approach to comprehensive terminal care opposed the isolation, loneliness, and dehumanization of persons dying in hospitals. In 1965, the same year that Glaser and Strauss's *Awareness of Dying* was published, Saunders wrote in the *British*

Medical Journal that doctors need to enable fatally ill patients to talk openly and freely. And "listening," she said,

> has a therapeutic effect on many symptoms, and it is then that the doctor will also give the patient what he may need most of all, the chance to talk as and when he wishes. Anxiety and depression can be helped by drugs, but it is the true listener who helps most of all.... At St. Joseph's Hospice we do not see intractable fear and depression but rather the growth of acceptance and serenity.[106]

Expanding on her philosophy of palliative care, she spoke candidly about how dying persons were being mistreated and about the attitudes that accompanied that treatment:

> Death is feared, all thoughts of it are avoided and the dying themselves are often left in loneliness. Both in their homes and in the hospital, they are emotionally isolated even when surrounded by their families or involved in much therapeutic activity. When we come near to them we tend to look at them with that pity which is not so far removed from contempt.[107]

"This should not be so," she declared. "The last stages of life should not be seen as defeat, but rather as life's fulfillment. It is not merely a time of negation but rather an opportunity for positive achievement."

This vision about the last stages of life shaped Cicely Saunders's expansive approach to palliative care and treatment: "The care of the dying demands all that we can do to enable patients to *live* until they die. It includes the care of the family, the mind, and the spirit as well as the care of the body." With every new visit with the patient, the caregiver should determine what the patient wants to talk about. Jokes, too, are welcomed, just as they are between members of families.[108] Effective pain control is essential. If needed, large doses of opiates can be used for months. Her research showed that only 2 percent of some 1,100 St. Joseph's patients became addicted to them.[109] She later emphasized in an impressively researched article that all the doctors who have written on these subjects have emphasized the great importance of frequent visits to terminally ill patients and families. "Suffering of all kinds is greatly intensified by isolation," such that the omission of physicians' visits is desperately felt.[110]

The opening of St. Christopher's in 1967 represented the fulfillment of eight years of planning by Dr. Saunders, and it mirrored all that she believed about the science, art, institutionalization, and promotion of hospice care: a multi-disciplinary, supportive, and devoted community of caregivers; a setting for innovative research in pain management and mental distress; and a place that freely welcomed the visitations and assisting activities of family members. The hospice care she fostered also included the presence of children, playgrounds, gardens, celebrations, spiritual counseling, worship services, and the prized possessions and continuing activities of terminally ill persons. Hospice communities were encouraged to extend their services to surrounding homes or domicile settings. She envisioned St. Christopher's as "a city on a hill" that through its programs of training, lecturing, and conferences would take its message to the world.[111]

Unafraid, Saunders spoke mystically and theologically about death:

> It is the very intensity of the moments of parting, the weakness and weariness of the end of a long illness and the problems endured together, that give these moments their

depth and power. We see people go through a lifetime of experience in a few weeks.... They seem to know a timeless "Now" when all the moments of time are held in stillness.[112]

St. Christopher's became a city on a hill, a city bound together as a close-knit community in which individuals were drawn together as one in heart and purpose.[113] It inspired a world-wide movement in palliative care that encompassed free-standing hospices, home care, and "translatable" care in hospitals.[114] Twenty-three free-standing hospices were established across England by 1973, and 50 hospice groups had been formed in the United States by 1977.[115] Hands-on physician and nurse visitors described their experiences at St. Christopher's in *The Lancet, JAMA,* the *American Journal of Nursing,* the *CMA (Canadian Medical Association) Journal,* and other publications. On the tenth anniversary of the founding of St. Christopher's, its staff reported that 418 doctors, medical students, and multi-disciplinary teams had visited and studied there during the previous year, some of whom stayed well beyond their participation in its week-long intensive course.[116]

Cicely Saunders served as the medical director of St. Christopher's for its first eighteen years, after which she became the chair of St. Christopher's, while continuing to teach, write, speak nationally and internationally, and give TV interviews. She relished international lecture tours. Her tours to the United States, Canada, and other nations began in 1963 and continued for decades. I was privileged to spend time with her at the medical school in Galveston, Texas, in January 1977 and could only marvel at how much she had influenced medical and nursing pilgrims at St. Christopher's. The import of her discoveries and commitments continued to empower the expansion of palliative care. The awards and prizes she received (including the title of Dame Commander of the Order of the British Empire in 1979, the Templeton Prize in the United States in 1981, the Order of Merit from Queen Elizabeth II in 1989, and the Conrad N. Hilton Humanitarian Price in 2001) attest to her towering fame.[117]

Additional Modern Hospice Programs

Rather than pressing for a replication of St. Christopher's free-standing hospice and home-outreach services, its staff held that "what we do must be translatable into general hospital and home practice."[118] And so it happened. Having spent three months of life-transforming training in St. Christopher's, and acutely aware of the limited outreach and costs of free-standing hospices, Dr. Belfour Mount established a palliative care program at the Royal Victoria Hospital in Montreal, Quebec. It was designed to serve a large population of patients via an in-hospital palliative care unit (PCU); an extensive home-care program serviced by trained physicians, nurses, and a host of volunteers; and in-hospital consultation services.[119] At the opening of Royal Victoria's PCU in 1975, Elisabeth Kübler-Ross gave an address to an overflow audience.[120] Signaling the development of international networks of comfort care advocacy, Cicely Saunders spoke at the first International Seminar on Terminal Care in Montreal in 1976.[121]

Mount's program exemplified the way others applied the principles of St. Christopher's to their own settings after the needs of their settings were extensively researched. These included the home-based Hospice, Inc., project in New Haven, Connecticut, in

1974, which was followed by the building of a creatively designed free-standing hospice in New Haven; the development of an interdisciplinary hospice team that cared for patients throughout St. Luke's Hospital in New York; the use of a death and dying specialist in the Harrisburg (Pennsylvania) Hospital; and the free-standing Hill Haven Hospice and home-outreach program similar to St. Christopher's in Tucson, Arizona.[122]

By 1980 Constance Holden wrote that hospices "have become a fast-growing American phenomenon" that included some 150 organizations in 40 states and an equal number in the planning stages. She contrasted the two-day symposium on the care of the dying sponsored by the National Institutes of Health (NIH) in 1979 with a similar NIH symposium that took place three years earlier. The large audience of the 1976 symposium was almost entirely female—predominantly nurses who were on the front lines of tending to the dying—and it included a presentation by Dr. Cicely Saunders, "the matriarch of British hospices." The 1979 meeting featured "health professionals of every stripe" and displayed three basic models of American hospices: home-care services that include medical supervision, counseling, and visits to patients whose families can take care of them at home; free-standing facilities; and hospice care within hospitals similar to St. Luke's Hospital in New York.[123]

Other palliative care programs were developed apart from explicit ties to hospices. As if they had been mentored by Francis Bacon or John Gregory, Melvin J. Krant and Alan Sheldon considered treatment and care for the dying as a branch of medicine—a body of knowledge, special skills, and research initiatives that would enable patients to "die well" and provide a deep sense of personal fulfillment to caregivers.[124] Capturing the spirit of change under way by 1972, Krant commented, "In recent years, we have come to appreciate that dying is an inherent part of the life cycle, rather than just a failure in medical technique." Krant spearheaded a highly organized program at Boston's Lemuel Shattuck Chronic Disease Hospital, affiliated with Tufts University Medical School. It was designed to overcome the abandonment of dying patients and included interdisciplinary staff conferences two mornings a week, teaching and training sessions for medical students at Tufts, and a home-outreach program serviced by family physicians and visiting nurses.[125]

Greater familiarity with death and dying on the part of healthcare professionals and the lay public, as well as involvement of nurses, trained volunteers, and family members in home care, contributed to renewed interest in caring for dying family members at home. In 1979 a nurse named Carol Goffnett told how she and her family freed her terminally ill, outdoors-loving father from the rules, routines, confinements, I.V.s, and respirators of the hospital, all of which he hated:

> Besides controlling his own life, Dad had a chance for privacy with his family. Once he spoke to me about how much he was suffering and how he would just as soon have it over. I asked him if he was afraid to die. He looked at me wide-eyed and said, "Well, I'm not exactly looking forward to it, Carol, but no one's escaped it yet."
> Near Dad's end, he resembled a skeleton more than a man.... Still, his grandchildren continued to climb on his bed, and he continued to laugh and tell them, "Get me a drink of water" or "You're the best nurse I ever had."
> Dad's dying was filled with laughter, sorrow, neighbors and relatives coming and going, and children crying, fighting and playing.
> Our family's way of dealing with a loved one's death won't be the right way for every-

one. But the point is, we all need to examine our present ways of handling the dying and the dead.[126]

Others told similar stories of the home dying of parents and children, one of which was a photography book titled *Gramp*.[127]

Specifications for Permissible Life Prolongation

Modern medicine's increasingly elaborate and invasive ways of prolonging expiring life posed this question: Which patients should be spared from invasive CPR and other life-saving and life-prolonging interventions and provided, instead, with expert and personalized terminal care?

Long-standing medical precedents, the institutionalization of CPR, and the law maintained that all medical emergencies involving undiagnosed patients and patients with potentially reversible conditions should be treated aggressively.[128] This rule of thumb opened doors of uncertainty regarding definitive diagnosis and the use of long-shot treatments to extend meaningful human life. Even patients with end-stage diseases might be brought back from cardiac arrests for a few more days of consciousness, semi-consciousness, and unconsciousness.

Made clear in the discussion above, some physicians advocated aggressive treatments for all patients with signs of mental and physiological function, while others opposed the overuse of CPR and life-prolonging surgery. In a 1973 survey of physicians in Iowa, 44 percent of the 1,600 respondents answered that they "frequently omitted life-prolonging measures when caring for terminally patients." Only 6 percent claimed they never omitted those measures. Most of the physicians polled saw a need for change. Two internists contended that the "practice of maintaining life at all costs with complete disregard for function and for the agony of a prolonged struggle with death is senseless and uncivilized."[129] In 1974 a doctor wrote that only a minority of physicians were routinely resorting to heroic treatments for all dying patients regardless of the underlying diseases.[130]

In the face of too-frequent and sometimes unbridled attempts to prolong life in the early 1960s, some physicians begin to specify when heroic life restoration and prolongation were or were not morally permissible. In 1962 Frank J. Ayd asserted,

> Only when there is a reasonable hope of sustaining life for several weeks or months, and if during this time the patient can be comfortable, should we exert every effort to delay death. Otherwise life-preserving treatment ceases to be a gift and becomes instead, a scientific weapon for the prolongation of agony.[131]

In 1965 an associate professor of surgery at the Johns Hopkins Medical School discussed at length when surgery was warranted. He held that "if the nature of the disease is established, its hopelessness demonstrated, and no meaningful palliation [is] possible it is our duty to avoid operating." The common argument, "He'll die if you don't operate, so you must try," is not valid in advanced and disseminated malignancy or a number of other conditions.[132]

Over time, these concerns became more specific and critical. In an article published in *JAMA* in 1968 Vincent J. Collins wrote that

On the basis of medical facts and good judgment, the physician ... must do those things which predictably result in improvement of his patient. The techniques of reanimation are proven sound, and legitimately can and do prolong life, **but** it must be determined that the nature of the resultant life is not mere biological existence of several organs but totally integrated functional existence at a rational human level. To continue an act or proceed with therapy which produces no improvement, which does not achieve or have the potential to achieve "full human life" ... **is** impudent, illogical, and irrational.

It is the physician's obligation to cease efforts early when they are determined to be ineffective in the total reanimation process and objectives. The patient should then be allowed to die. He has this right; he should not be cheated of a peaceful death when the physician is powerless to restore consciousness.

Approvingly, Collins quoted from a law professor at the University of Washington, George P. Fletcher: "The medical profession ... confronts the challenge of developing human and sensitive customary standards for guiding decisions to prolong the lives of terminal patients.... They should have a clear standard for deciding when to render aid, or not, to the dying patient."[133] Other doctors listed examples of corrective therapies that were no longer obligatory, such as blood transfusions for end-stage leukemia patients with slow gastrointestinal bleeding and pulmonary surgery for elderly terminal cardiac patients with obstructions in their pulmonary arteries.[134]

Bioethicists and Terminal Care

Bioethics emerged as a movement and disciplined scholarly activity in the late 1960s and early 1970s.[135] Bioethicists seek to find morally convincing answers to problematic, often complex decisions and procedures inherent in the practices of health care professionals; to set forth morally permissible uses of new medical and biological technologies (such as life-saving procedures, genetic engineering, reproductive technologies, and animal-to-human transplants); and to analyze ethically acceptable biomedical research on human subjects. By definition and in practice, bioethics demands interdisciplinary expertise. It requires moral philosophers, moral theologians, and lawyers to become familiar with each other's disciplines and deeply informed about the areas of medicine and technology they intend to analyze for the purpose of offering ethical insights and answers. In like manner, physicians, nurses, biological and social scientists, and others who wish to do ethics must become deeply familiar with the complexities, strengths, and weaknesses of traditions of ethical reasoning. They must also be able to identify and defend their chosen form of philosophical reasoning, as well as apply it convincingly, or at least challengingly, to the moral issues in question.[136]

Between the late 1960s and the early 1980s, most bioethicists were academically trained philosophers (e.g., Daniel Callahan, Robert Veatch) or moral theologians or specialists in religious studies (e.g., Paul Ramsey, Arthur J. Dyck, Richard McCormick, William May, Albert R. Jonsen, James Childress), all of whom became informed about medical training, medical procedures and technologies, and the thinking of medical professionals. Some of these bioethicists held degrees in the biological sciences. All had to work closely with health professionals, and they naturally became familiar with the social dynamics of medical treatment and practice. Bioethicists during these years also included physicians who worked closely with philosophers and theologians and did their own studying (e.g., Willard Gaylin, Andre A. Hellegers, and Erik J. Cassell), as well as lawyers (e.g., William J. Curran and George Annas) and medical historians (Stanley Joel Reiser).[137]

The work of bioethicists called for expertise in back-and-forth discussions between persons with different academic backgrounds. Facilitating shared decisions between such people required replacing established disciplinary rhetoric and modes of thinking with common, far more readily understood language.[138]

From its beginnings, leading bioethicists and institutions established for the study and teaching of bioethics[139] voiced increasingly publicized views about many of the hallmark ethics issues raised in this book—physician paternalism versus respect for patients' wishes, truth telling, issues regarding life-prolonging medical treatment, and types of care and treatment for terminally ill persons.[140] Under the gaze and in the minds of bioethicists, strongly voiced personal opinions of the past would not suffice. Deeply influenced by the rights movements of the 1950s and 1950s, bioethicists generally and strongly opposed physician paternalism and favored the rights of patients to make their own decisions.[141]

While many doctors were allowing family members and patients to play a role in decision making, the great majority shouldered the responsibility of making the final decision about whether and how to treat the patient or, alternatively, to cease aggressive treatment and initiate terminal care.[142] This moral paternalism on the part of physicians would be fought tooth and nail by bioethicists.

The Genius of Paul Ramsey: 1969–1971

Paul Ramsey (1913–1988), an articulate and tough-minded moral theologian from Princeton University, pioneered and modeled the training, thinking, and gifted scholarly discourse of a bioethicist in his groundbreaking 1969 series of lectures on bioethics at Yale University. In preparation for his lectures, Ramey spent two semesters as a visiting professor at the Medical School of Georgetown University, where he attended bi-weekly conferences and talked extensively with prominent members of the Georgetown faculty. He, as well as the major scholars who brought him to Yale, surrounded his lectures with the give and take of daily seminars led by prominent scholars from many fields. Ramsey published his lectures as a landmark exploration of bioethics titled *The Patient as Person* in 1970.[143]

Notably, one of the chapters in *The Patient as Person* focuses on the care of dying persons. Ramsey commissions doctors to move "beyond many present day efforts to rescue the perishing" and accept the "medical duty to (only) care for the dying."[144] He held that biblically rooted ethical perspectives resonate with all those who believe human relationships should manifest fairness, respect, loyalty, charity, and "steadfast *faithfulness*" toward fellow human beings.[145]

Paul Ramsey's goal in his chapter on terminal care was to argue convincingly about why there is a duty only to care for persons who are irreversibly dying. He spoke of the "solidarity in mortality" between dying persons and all of "us who also bear flesh."

The right medical practice will provide ... those who are dying with the care and assistance they need in their final passage.

Upon ceasing to try to rescue the perishing, one then is free to care for the dying. Acts of caring for the dying ... manifest that they are not lost from human attention, that they are not alone, that mankind generally and their loved ones take note of their dying and mean to company with them in accepting this unique instance of the acceptable death of all flesh.

Out of respect for the dying life as such, there arises a fresh understanding of the forbidden torturing of it; and, of course, from this same source springs the awesome understanding of the forbidden taking of life.[146]

Ramsey exclaimed, "We must not, as Dr. Karnofsky supposed, carry on our medical efforts to save life until the issue is taken out of our hands.... We must carry on our ministry of care and comfort and keeping-company with the dying until but only until *that* issue is taken out of our hands."[147]

An About-Face on Patient Rights and Truth Telling

Ethical and legal counterweights against the long-standing reign of physician paternalism coalesced after the mid–1960s. Bioethicists spoke with one voice about the rights of patients to be fully informed about the nature and seriousness of their illnesses and then be granted the power to choose the available treatments they wanted. Law and legislation both spearheaded and fully supported these rights of free choice—the story of which will follow.

Clashing convictions over concealing or revealing the truth about terminal illness are evident from the time Theophile Bonet defended truth revealing in 1683 up to the long period of time ranging from Samuel Bard in 1769 to the descriptions of hospital practices by Glaser and Strauss in 1965, when truth was by and large concealed. We have seen, however, that beginning with Thomas Gisborne in 1794, up to Walter Alvarez in 1952, as well as a number of physician and clergy spokespersons in this chapter, truth revealing was defended and practiced.

A revolution in favor of physician truth telling took place between 1961 and 1979. Evidence of the revolution is found in the contrast between the findings of an article published in *JAMA* by Donald Oken in 1961 and the findings in the article by Dennis H. Novack and his coauthors in 1979. Oken found that almost 90 percent of the physicians surveyed had a strong or general tendency to *conceal* cancer diagnoses, while only 4 percent said they often revealed that diagnosis. In 1979 Novack and his colleagues found that 98 percent of the physicians who were surveyed *revealed* cancer diagnoses, and 100 percent of those questioned thought patients had a right to know their diagnoses.[148] This assumes that significant parallels exist between cancer and terminal diagnosis. Novack and his coauthors concurred with these parallels.[149]

Multiple forces empowered this historical about-face. Before and especially after Oken's article appeared, a number of studies "dispelled the myth of the harm" inherent in patients' hearing the truth about their diagnoses. This revelation undermined the primary rationale behind physicians' paternalistic concealment and deception—the historic duties to maintain hope and protect patients from alarm and depressing influences that can shorten life. Other transformative forces included more teaching and training about provider-patient communication; the legal requirement of informed consent in medical practice and research; and convincing arguments from bioethicists regarding respect for the autonomous decisions of patients as an essential principle of medical ethics.[150] Many physicians and nurses concurred with that ethical conviction. In response to Novack's article, George L. Spaeth wrote, "The physician should be honest with the patient because it is the patient's right to be dealt with honestly. Other considerations are subsidiary."[151]

No bioethicist championed the dying person's right to know the truth and make her or his own decisions about whether to accept or refuse medical treatments more than Robert M. Veatch, whose *Death, Dying, and the Biomedical Revolution* was published in 1976. Veatch concludes his lengthy chapter "The Right to Refuse Treatment" with the assertion that "competent individuals may refuse any medical treatment they desire for whatever reasons they desire (unless they are prisoners) [even] if the treatment is offered for their own good." He adds that "refusal of a death-prolonging treatment is not in itself grounds for declaring a person incompetent." The overarching criterion for the right of competent persons to refuse treatment, including life-extending treatments, is whether the decision is reasonable—not reasonable to the physician, but reasonable to the patient with respect to physical or mental burdens or other objections such as religious opposition to blood transfusions.[152] This patient-centered framework for questions regarding rights of refusal is rooted in ethical principles involving freedom and responsibility for decisions with respect to treatments of one's own body and person. Patients' rights to refuse the initiation of medical treatments logically require their rights to withdraw from treatments that have already begun.[153]

These rights of refusal are predicated on the right to be told the truth about one's diagnosed medical condition and the treatments that pertain to those conditions. Consent to or refusal of treatment must be informed. In his chapter on truth telling Veatch refutes traditional beliefs that patients will be happier if they are never told. He defends the patient's right to be told the truth by analyzing and critiquing major modes of ethical reasoning. Having probed these modes, Veatch concludes that "only in extremely rare exceptional cases—whose gravity extends well beyond the ordinary sort where the physician feels that harm would justify withholding the bad news—can withholding information potentially useful or meaningful to the patient be condoned."[154]

Vanderpool on the Moral Essentials of Palliative Care: 1978

During and after the 1950s "death with dignity" became the popular symbolic title for how persons should be able to die. The ring of that phrase had, and continues to have, staying power. Yet multiple and ambiguous meanings were attributed to "death with dignity," and its bottom-line meaning denoted "death *without indignity*"—namely, without the indignities of systematic deception, isolated depersonalization, embarrassments over incontinence and other hygienic needs, and the agonies of heroic measures to the point of death.[155]

In the tradition of Edward H. Rynearson's summary of the moral components of palliative care in 1959,[156] this author's "The Ethics of Terminal Care" was published in *JAMA* in 1978.[157] The article critiqued the commonly used term "dying with dignity" as a short-hand title for meaningful terminal care, and it set forth guidelines designed to capture the moral breakthroughs that were occurring in the 1960s and 1970s. I argued that the term *dignity* had become a catch-all cliché for any number of actions, and that, linguistically, it primarily serves as a term of distinction reserved for individuals manifesting nobility and excellence. "Notable humans or martyrs may die with dignity, but death with fame or grandeur ... makes little sense for humans generally."[158] Furthermore, the term *dignity* is ill suited as a symbol for terminal care, because in modern culture it is manifestly undignified to be dependent, burdensome, needful, and unattractive. And, lastly, the phrase "dying with dignity" fails to call into play essential moral dimensions of good dying.

    This author therefore proposed that the terminology of dying with a sense of meaning or with a sense of personal worth should replace the commonly and uncritically used phrase "dying with dignity." Meaning and worth are suitable aims for persons in all stages of human life, including terminal illness. These words logically encompass four fundamental features of human life that serve as essential moral foundations for palliative care[159]:

> First, human worth is founded on the principle of respect for persons.... Respect for each person requires at least three concerns about individual choices and rights: (1) Each patient must be given truthful information about all decisions and procedures affecting his or her well-being and must consent to these procedures before they are performed. (2) The current belief that dying with peace ... necessarily includes passing through certain psychological stages needs to be [questioned]. (3) The autonomy and self-control that characterize Western individuality need to be preserved as much as possible. The sense of lost dignity resulting from excessive dependency and loss of control ... are major problems for the terminally ill person.
>
> Second, human worth is based on the individual's inclusion in a community ... characterized by communication, mutuality, and the ethical ideals of fidelity, gratitude, reciprocity, justice, and love. Persons who are terminally ill lose a sense of worth if they are left alone, if they are avoided and not touched. The strength and attractiveness of the hospice movement reflects this communal framework for human meaning.
>
> Third, human value is rooted in concern for the body. A person's sense of worth or well-being ... is affected by personal grooming, by the presence of pain, and by disfigurement or mutilation.... [S]elf-worth has extremely important physiological and aesthetic dimensions.
>
> Fourth, human worth is often maintained by considerations of a broader purpose.... This understanding of individual life as fitting into some ennobling destiny or some ultimate purpose can be framed in naturalistic or theistic terms.[160]

These broad and essential dimensions of life should serve as fundamental guidelines for palliative end-of-life care. Dying persons who are likely to feel their former dignity is being threatened should receive these comprehensively defined levels of care that reflect the inherent and incalculable worth of human beings to the end of their lives.[161]

Foundations in Law and Legislation

    Grounded ethically in each individual's freedom and right of self-determination, the legal doctrine of informed consent grants conscious patients the right to control how they are treated regardless of the convictions of the responsible physician. Changes in the law spawned state-based legislative initiatives designed to empower competent patients and their appointed surrogates with the right to accept or refuse life-prolonging treatments. These changes occurred against the cultural background of increasing institutional separation and alienation of non-physicians from physicians beginning in the 1960s.[162]

Between 1957 and 1972, consent became informed consent in American law. Legal precedents involving the right of self-determination began to require explicit disclosures of risks and alternative treatment prior to requesting the consent of patients. The standard for these disclosures began to shift from existing standards of disclosure in professional practice to information that reasonable persons would need to know in order to make decisions regarding their medical conditions. The penalties for failing to honor the reasonable-person standard were variously linked to penalties of negligence, malpractice, and/or assault and battery arising from touching persons without their legally valid informed permission.[163] Lawyers and bioethicists argued that these rights of self-determination should embrace the competent patient's decision to refuse life-saving treatment irrespective of the reasons for that refusal.[164]

Importantly, momentous changes in the law were reported in the medical literature. For example, Joseph E. Simonaitus's regular updates about the rulings of appellate and state supreme courts on informed consent were published in *JAMA* between 1970 and 1973. He noted how these court rulings held that the scope of disclosure "is not determined by the standards of the medical community" but by the patient's need, "and that need is whatever information is material to the patient's decision." Nevertheless, some courts said that situations "may exist in which disclosures should not be made because they might unduly agitate or undermine an unstable patient."[165]

A historic breakthrough occurred between December 1973 and February 1974. At its annual convention in December, the American Medical Association (AMA) "really faced up to the moral and legal implications of artificial prolongation of life" and "tried to establish a uniform policy concerning death." The assembly forthrightly recognized the widely varying hospital policies at the time, and prior to its December convention, the AMA had surveyed various religious organizations and found "strong support for allowing a patient to choose his own fate, once a doctor has carefully explained the options."[166] Three months later the AMA's House of Delegates, its principal policy-making body, adopted the following statement as a guideline for American physicians:

> The cessation of the employment of extraordinary means to prolong the life of the body when there is irrefutable evidence that biological death is imminent is the decision of the patient and/or his immediate family. The advice and judgment of the physician should be freely available to the patient and/or his immediate family.[167]

Despite the uncertainties surrounding what constitutes "irrefutable evidence," when biological death is "imminent," and how the decision to refuse treatment can be made by "the patient and/or his immediate family," this guideline recognizes that life prolongation can be refused and that the final decision to continue or end treatment does not belong to the physician.

Breakthroughs also occurred in state legislation. The bioethicist Robert Veatch critiqued legislative initiatives regarding legalizing "active euthanasia" (the physician intentionally ending the lives of terminally ill patients). He also championed the rights of competent patients to accept or refuse treatment, and he identified who should make medical decisions when patients are incompetent. In 1978 Veatch examined eighty-five pieces of legislation that addressed these issues. In 1977 alone, bills were introduced into forty state legislatures, and by 1977 eight states had passed death and dying legislation. Veatch commented, "The real breakthrough came in 1976, when California passed the Natural Death Act, the first piece of legislation of this kind in the United States." That bill specified that instructions regarding end-of-life care given by certifiably terminally ill patients would remain in effect after the patient lapsed into incompetency.[168]

While a first-of-its-kind legislation is certainly a breakthrough, the California bill was beset with problems. It held that what competent patients write down "may" be given "weight" by attending physicians who could justifiably consider other factors, including family wishes and the nature of each patient's illness. Reminiscent of the "irrefutable evidence" of "imminent" death phrases in the AMA's 1974 guideline, the California bill only applied to patients with "incurable" conditions "where the application of life-sustaining procedures serves only to postpone the moment of death."[169] Veatch gave greater praise to a bill that was introduced in Alabama in 1976. Evoking the individual's rights of privacy and self-determination, that bill declared that all patients, including the terminally ill, have the right to "make a declaration instructing any physician ... to cease or refrain from medical or surgical treatment ... as long as such demands do not result in undue harm to society as judged by court decision."[170]

Veatch then cogently outlined the essential elements of model legislation on the rights of patients, including terminally ill patients, to have their instructions followed in keeping with the ethical and legal foundations of informed consent. Veatch's comment that the movement to legislate "death with dignity" had gained momentum marks a legal culmination point at the end of the 1970s.[171]

Concluding Perspectives

The twenty-two years from 1960 through 1981 were full of tension, complexity, creativity, and change. Medicine made stunning advances with respect to sustaining life and overcoming disease. At the same time, fervent life-saving attempts, including the emotional highs and ecstatic rushes of those conducting CPR and other emergency measures, became constrained by doctors, nurses, bioethicists, lawyers, and legislatures.

These years engendered answers to the question: What should be done about the conflicts over excessive and paternalistic use of life-prolonging treatments of terminally ill patients? The answers set forth in this chapter are multifaceted: Learn when to stop attempts to prolong life. Discover what's actually happening to dying persons in hospitals. Learn to think and talk openly about death and dying. Build alternative programs to nurture dying persons and their families. And, flying in the face of the long tradition of authoritarian physician paternalism, adhere to the counsel of bioethicists and like-minded physicians and nurses, as well as to laws and legislation that uphold the rights of patients and their surrogates to make their own end-of-life decisions. These answers became breakthroughs that renewed and expanded the fortunes of palliative care and treatment.

Over these 22 years, two legitimate and contending forms of rescue took center stage. On the one hand, numerous catastrophically ill patients were rescued from impending death. On the other, increasing numbers of terminally ill persons were being rescued from institutionalized loneliness, neglect, and powerlessness in hospitals. Between 1960 and 1981, the interplay between these two contending forms of rescue began to shift toward the second. The foundations for fundamental reform in the care of dying persons were now in place, but what did the future hold? What obstacles remained? How powerful were these obstacles? What would it take to secure the promises of breakthroughs that were under way? Surprises remained.

8

Progress, Threatening Seas, and Endurance

1982–1999

The forces propelling better care for persons nearing the end of life became stronger and more pervasive after 1982. But the headway proved arduous beyond expectations.

The journey of proponents for palliative care from 1982 through 1999 recalls that of Richard Henry Dana, Jr. and his shipmates in *Two Years Before the Mast.* Under fair breezes as their sailing brig approached the tip of South America, Dana and his mates had "every prospect of a speedy and pleasant passage" around Cape Horn. But approaching the Cape,

> We found a large black cloud rolling on toward us ... and darkening the whole heavens. "Here comes Cape Horn!" said the chief mate. In minutes a heavier sea was raised than I had ever seen. The little brig plunged into it, and all the forward part of her was under water. The sea pouring in through the bow ports and hawseholes and over the knightheads, threatening to wash everything overboard.... The brig was laboring and straining against the head sea, and ... sleet and hail were driving with all fury against us. Here was an end to our fine prospects. We made up our minds to [endure] head winds and cold weather.[1]

The fine prospects envisioned by advocates of improved end-of-life care between 1982 and 1994 were confronted by the likes of Cape Horn in 1995. Many of the things they treasured were threatened with being washed away. Like those on board Dana's brig, they endured the heavy headwinds of 1995 and traveled with renewed determination to the end of the 20th century.

The story of more humane and acceptable terminal care from 1982 through 1999 is, however, more absorbing and multi-themed than that of a sailing vessel. This story includes the following major parts: "Progress in Palliative Care: 1982–1994"; "Continuing Excessive Efforts to Prolong Life and Their Counter-Measures, 1982–1994"; "Threatening Seas: 1995"; and "Endurance Beyond the Storm: 1996–1999."

Every era in the story of comfort-directed care was shaped by the medical practices of its times. Modern medicine became, as it were, the sea upon which palliative care inescapably traveled. Between 1982 and 1999 remarkable medical innovations continued to sustain faith in the seemingly miraculous power of modern medicine and to maintain the status and authority of its therapeutic-focused practitioners. These developments included the following:

- 1981 onward: Exponential worldwide use of PEG (stomach-inserted feeding tubes) for artificial nutrition and hydration for adults and children[2]
- 1981–1983: Era of computer-controlled (microprocessor) ventilators, which enabled single ventilators to be programmed to perform a wide variety of functions depending on each medical condition; another generation of ventilators became available in the 1990s, which provided respiratory assistance aligned with patients' spontaneous breathing abilities, increased patient survival, reduced use of sedation and muscle-paralysis medications, and decreased patient anxiety[3]
- 1983–1999: Intensive care for life-threatening conditions, including acute respiratory distress syndrome (ARDS),[4] chronic obstructive pulmonary disease (COPD),[5] congestive heart failure, sepsis (toxic infection), and end-stage renal disease (ESRD)[6]
- 1985: FDA approval of the first implantable cardiac defibrillator, and improvements in implanted cardiac pacemakers throughout the 1980s and 1990s[7]
- 1986 onward: American Society for Critical Care Medicine approval of specialized certification in critical care medicine for board-certified anesthesiologists, internists, surgeons, and pediatricians, and publication of guidelines for the training and administrative roles of these ICU "intensivists" in 1992[8]
- 1987: Successful implantation of intravascular stents following balloon expansion of blocked or partially blocked coronary arteries; explosive use of expandable stents thereafter[9]
- 1996: First commercially available and more effective automated external defibrillators (AEDs) for in-hospital and widespread out-of-hospital availability in airports and other public places[10]
- 1997: Three-dimensional magnetic resonance angiography for better view of heart blood flow

Progress in Palliative Care: 1982–1994

In the midst of major medical innovations before and during the 1960s and 1970s, the palliative care movement secured far stronger cultural foundations. With its momentum building in the 1970s, it continued to expand, achieve historic support from the public sector, secure greater attention from non–palliative care healthcare professionals, and become more visible in medical and nursing training from the 1980s through 1994.

This era in the narrative is multifaceted. Attention will now be given to the professionalization of palliative medicine, the public support and growth of hospice care, changes in medical and nursing education, heroic efforts to prolong human life despite outcries against these heroics, and four notable efforts to rein in treatment excesses.

The literature on all aspects of end-of-life care and treatment expanded enormously in medical, nursing, legal, and ethical journals, as well as in the news media and in books written for both academic and popular audiences. Along with the numerous sources referenced in this chapter, an exploration of the yearly multi-volume editions of *Index Medicus*—a listing of all the publications on medical and medical-related topics across the globe—testifies to the explosive growth of the literature.[11] Having passed rigorous screening criteria, the articles published in the category "Palliative Treatment" expanded from 72 articles in 1982 to 224 in 1990, and then 501 in 1999. Those on "Terminal Care" increased from 47 in 1982 to 114 in 1990, and 223 in 1999.

Professionalization of Palliative Care and Treatment

After 1982 palliative care became increasingly professionalized—that is, recognized as a medical subspecialty with its own body of knowledge, technical procedures, and training programs.[12] The professionalization of treatment and care for persons facing death after 1982 became a hard-fought battle. It began in earnest when physicians who devoted themselves to the care of dying patients in hospices recognized that great potential was at hand even though only a few of their peers were involved in hospice care.[13]

Inspired by the leadership of U.S. physician Josefina B. Mango, the International Hospice Institute (IHI) was formed in 1984. The IHI created a task force comprising presidents of medical societies and representatives of medical centers. The task force concluded that the reason for the widespread lack of hospice involvement by physicians could be summarized by one word: ignorance.[14] A typical example of a physician who did not know what hospice care was, but believed he did, was the chief of staff in a large municipal hospital. When asked what he knew about the hospice concept,

> His reply was a very confident "yes," he knew everything about hospice care. In fact, he said, one of his nurses had recently got sick, the hospice took care of her, the team held her hand and really loved her, and in eight days she had died.
> This physician, and probably many more like him, thought that hospice was nothing more than compassionate, loving care which he himself could provide. The physician later apologized, admitting he had realized that he really did not understand the hospice concept.[15]

That doctor, like numerous other physicians and non-physicians, falsely equated palliative care with palliative caring, not with expert medical attention and treatment combined with multi-dimensional caring. Some doctors castigated the entire hospice movement for promoting pre-modern approaches to care for dying patients.[16]

The ranks of physicians devoted to expert palliative care nevertheless expanded. The Academy of Hospice Physicians (AHP) was established in 1988 with 125 founding members. Its purposes included changing physicians' perceptions, providing academic forums, and rectifying the view that hospice physicians and physician-directors were second-class practitioners.[17] The rapid growth of membership in the AHP signified that palliative care was coming of age. Three years after its formation, the Academy had almost 1,000 members from all over the United States and in 14 other countries, and it became the main professional organization for physician specialists in hospice care and palliative medicine.[18]

U.S. physicians knew they could learn a great deal from Great Britain, where palliative medicine was more widely respected and accepted. Palliative care became recognized as a medical subspecialty in general medicine in Great Britain in 1987, in Ireland in 1995, in New Zealand in 1998, and in Australia in 2000.[19] In the United States two tiers of nurse-specialist training were proposed in 1990—hospice nurse certified (HNC) and hospice nurse advanced (HNA).[20] In Canada in 1999, an accredited one-year program in palliative medicine was approved jointly by the College of Family Physicians of Canada and the Royal College of Physicians and Surgeons in Canada.[21]

Professionalization proceeded hand in hand with internationalization. In addition to the world outreach of the AHP, St. Christopher's Hospice developed a world-wide network of hospices in 1999 that included over 89 countries.[22] The World Health Organization's (WHO) definition and promotion of palliative care after 1982 added to the international advancement of the practice and institutionalization of comfort-focused care.

International collaboration began with the First International Congress on the Care of the Terminally Ill in Montreal, Quebec, in 1979 and continued through international congresses held every two years thereafter. The European Association for Palliative Care was formed in Milan, Italy, in 1988 with 42 founding members. Establishment of the Eastern and Central European Palliative Force occurred in 1989, and the Foundation for Hospices in Sub-Saharan Africa followed in 1999.[23] These benchmarks were preceded by years of end-of-life care advocacy, and they were secured by overcoming continuing challenges.[24]

Expanding Hospice Care

By 1982 several types of hospice care existed in the United States, the United Kingdom, and Canada—free-standing community-based in-patient hospices, home care–based hospice care, hospital-centered care in separate units or as rotating teams, day-care programs, and medical school outreach programs.[25] In 1984, 1,429 hospice programs existed in the United States, 38 percent of which were hospital-based as separate units and/or rotating teams and 59 percent of which were community-based.[26] In keeping with one of Cicely Saunders's ideals, the care of out-of-hospital hospices was being translated into other settings.

Knowing that hospice programs took many forms, proponents of these programs began to emphasize that hospice referred to a philosophy of personalized medical care that would enable terminally ill persons to experience peaceful or good dying and death. As opposed to the way dying persons were often treated in hospitals, hospice embraced expert and compassionate attention to patients' physical, emotional, social, and spiritual needs by interdisciplinary teams of committed caregivers.[27]

Prior to 1983, U.S. home- and community-based hospice programs readily sent patients to in-patient hospital settings if symptoms could not be managed or if the fatigue and/or discord of family caregivers became oppressive. Once control and medical relief were reinstituted, patients would return to home and other out-of-hospital settings.[28] Trained volunteers were widely involved in both non-specialized patient care and a variety of supportive services.

In Great Britain 77 hospice programs were developed by 1985. Forty-two of these were in-patient programs like St. Christopher's Hospice, 23 were community-based home-care programs, and 6 were day-care focused.[29] These expanded to 428 teams of caregivers in the United Kingdom and Republic of Ireland in 1990. Teams consisted of nurses, physicians, and, frequently, chaplains, social workers, pharmacists, and occupational therapists who worked in free-standing hospices, home-care programs, and hospital in-patient units. Volunteers in out-of-hospital settings provided day care, fund raising, administration, and other services.[30]

The National Health Service (NHS) was created in Great Britain in 1948 to provide tax-funded healthcare for all citizens. Yet hospice care in Great Britain received and still receives most of its funding from charitable foundations and private donations. The NHS began to fund hospice care in the late 1970s, but continues to fund less than 40 percent of that care up to the present time.[31]

National Hospice Coverage in the United States in 1983

In 1982 President Ronald Reagan signed into law the Tax Equity and Fiscal Responsibility Act (TEFRA), which called for national Medicare coverage of hospice care. The legislation was introduced by Congressman Leon Panetta and Senator Robert Dole and was overwhelmingly approved by the U.S. House of Representatives and the Senate. After the final bill was signed by the president, hospice services became a covered Medicare benefit.[32] The passage of Medicare reimbursement was indeed "the single, most dramatic event impacting the widespread change in the organization and structure of hospices" in the United States.[33]

A combination of motivations prompted the historic passage of national funding for hospice care in the United States: ideals regarding home dying surrounded by family members and friends; increasing public support for around-the-clock, compassionate, symptom-relieving palliative care from teams of caregivers; and, especially dear to the hearts of numerous co-sponsors of the Medicare bill, expectations of cost savings when national health care expenditures were increasing by over $250 billion each year.[34] When the Congressional Budget Office reported in June 1982 that home hospice care would save the government some $1,120 per patient over conventional hospital care, virtually all remaining opposition to the bill vanished.[35]

Hospice care appealed to the hearts and minds of millions of Americans. The National Hospice Organization (NHO) became a powerful lobbying force behind the legislation. Formed in 1977 by founders of existing hospice programs, the NHO held its first annual meeting in 1978 in Washington, D.C., to attract federal attention to hospice care. With its headquarters near Washington, the NHO began to focus on quality standards for hospice programs, and between 1982 and 1983 it worked closely with the Joint Commission on Accreditation of Hospitals (JCAH) and other agencies to draft standards into the final version of the Medicare coverage bill.[36] The NHO changed its name to the National Hospice and Palliative Care Organization (NHPCO) in 2000 and remains the largest nonprofit organization representing hospice and palliative care programs in the United States.

Humanistic motivations infused the encompassing legislation: the constant availability of critical services, including physician and nursing care; all necessary medications; a variety of as-needed services, including an interdisciplinary group that must include a physician, nurse, social worker, and pastor or other counselor; medical supplies and appliances; physical and occupational therapy; payments for volunteers conducting in-patient care and administration; and menu planning and preparation in free-standing hospice programs.[37]

Medicare coverage, however, was constrained by four regulatory and cost concerns of the Health Care Financing Administration (HFCA) and the Office of Management and Budget (OMB), concerns that constituted essential components of the final bill.[38] First, Medicare coverage was available only to hospices that met the JCAH's certification procedures. The structure of all covered programs was strictly prescribed and required extensive record keeping.[39] Second, the legislation clearly favored home-based hospice care. The plan allowed enrolled patients to be sent to hospitals for only 20 percent of their total days as Medicare recipients. Hospice programs were required to fund all in-patient expenses that exceeded the 20 percent time limit. These criteria created disruptions in back-and-forth patient care from homes to hospitals, and severe problems for critically ill patients.[40] Third, as an armored fist behind the coverage, those enrolled had to relinquish Medicare for all curative treatment via a signed statement. Many patients and their families were unwilling to accept palliative care predicated on recognizing that no hopes for cure existed. Many physicians chose to continue curative treatment instead of conveying a hopelessly ill diagnosis to patients.[41] Cicely Saunders was shocked by this part of the U.S. legislation. She said, "Many patients in need would never reach a hospice team if such a stark directive were implemented."[42] In response to criticisms, the framers of the final bill altered its original wording about the patient's "acknowledgment of terminal illness" in a signed statement: patients must only acknowledge that they are electing to receive palliative care "in lieu of curative care."[43]

Fourth, hospice coverage was limited to six months. Initiation of coverage was contingent on certification by two physicians that the patient was terminally ill. Yet physicians knew that identifying the point at which patients had less than 6 months to live was extremely difficult, if not impossible.[44] Howard Brody and Joanne Lynn held that there were "no validated criteria for making such judgments, except when death is clearly imminent." The effect of this requirement would likely be that "the only patients referred to the hospice may be those who are so obviously close to death that the hospice's palliative care will be offered too late."[45] The requirement was not revised. And Brody and Lynn's predilections about late referrals proved to be true. By 1990 the median patient time in hospice was 30 days—a sixth of the six-month prognosis requirement. In 1994 a study found that 15 percent of hospice patients died within 7 days of admission.[46]

Hospice and Palliative Care After Medicare Coverage Began

Early responses to national funding for hospice in the United States were decidedly mixed. On the side of sunshine, a family physician proclaimed that the reimbursement legislation ensured hospice "a solid place in the evolving health system," offered leadership roles to family doctors, and represented "a rapidly expanding, vital trend toward home-centered, patient-family-directed, and cost-effective care."[47] On the side of gloom, a Robert Wood Johnson Clinical Nurse Scholar held that the humanistic motivations of the hospice movement had become distorted by the cost-effective alterations inserted by the HCFA and the OMB into the original 1982 bill. She regarded the bill as a "holy war" that undermined the spirit and purposes of existing hospices.[48]

The four above-listed regulatory measures did indeed initially exact a toll on many existing hospices and the early expansion of hospice services. Josefina B. Magno accurately observed that the rigid certification requirements, record-keeping paperwork, inadequate reimbursement rates, and long delays in processing reimbursement claims caused many hospice programs—particularly small ones—to eventually close.[49] The regulatory components of the legislation restricted early referrals and enrollments: 13,000 patients enrolled in the Medicare program by 1985 instead of the government's projected 40,000.[50] Once Medicare-certified hospices accepted patients, they had to be responsible for the patients' full range of care needs until death. Fears that they might be financially overwhelmed contributed to the fact that by 1984 only 10 percent of potentially Medicare-eligible hospice programs wanted to become enrolled in the Medicare program.[51]

Greater bureaucratization followed as managerial professionals focused on the hospice accrediting process, licensing procedures, and professional standardization. Some bemoaned the fact that the former missionary spirit of hospice founders and participants began to wane in the face of more mundane concerns over daily maintenance, regulatory requirements, and financial necessities.[52]

Despite the restrictions of the Medicare regulations, history sided with those who saw sunshine. The total number of hospices in the United States increased from 516 in 1983 to 1,529 fully operating hospices in 1989. Some 50 percent of these hospices were Medicare-certified. Thirty percent were hospital-based, and another 64 percent were community- and home health agency–based.[53] By 1995, U.S. mortality statistics indicated 17 percent were dying in hospices.[54] Writing in the *Journal of the American Medical Association* in 1990, Jill Rhymes noted that hospice care for dying patients had "grown from an alternative health care movement to an accepted part of the American health care field."[55]

Fervor increased in the hearts and minds of palliative and hospice care proponents. In a keynote address before the annual meeting of National Hospice Organization in 1989, Sandol Stoddard declared, "The truth is, that hospice as it is generally practiced today is a far finer program than the one described in Medicare—far richer, and far more seriously responsible, to patient and family." He added, "And please listen carefully to your language" to avoid technological jargon. "If your team had a 'patient care coordinator' last year and this year you have suddenly got a 'patient service manager,' watch out. You are turning into a gas station."[56]

Numerous others joined the chorus in support of palliative and hospice care, and large public organizations, such as the W. K. Kellogg, John A. Hartford, and Robert Wood Johnson foundations, committed millions of dollars to programs of study in hospice care.

The career of Porter Storey illustrates the promotion and medical professionalization of palliative care and treatment. Storey graduated from the Stanford University School of Medicine and received specialty training in palliative care at the University of Edinburgh, at St. Luke's Nursing Home in Sheffield, England, and in a certification program at St. Christopher's Hospice under the tutelage of Cicely Saunders. He returned to his home state of Texas in 1983 and served as the medical director of the hospice at the Texas Medical Center in Houston until 2000, when he founded the interdisciplinary palliative care consultation service at Houston's St. Luke's Episcopal Hospital. His extensive publications include the first three editions of the widely sold AAHPM-published *Primer of Palliative Care* in 1994, 1996, and 2004. The (now six) editions of this *Primer* track ongoing developments in palliative care through 2014.[57] Impelling Storey's work and that of many others were the hopes that they would help persons to experience "good" and "meaningful" pilgrimages at the end of their lives.[58]

In the early 1980s hospices mostly cared for patients with various types of cancer, but over the years they served an increasingly diverse mix of patients with end-stage neurological, cardiac, and dementia diseases.[59]

The outbreak of the AIDS epidemic in 1981 introduced a radically new set of challenges to providers of hospice care. These included caregiver fears of acquiring the new infectious disease; homophobia from hospital staff members; blurred lines between palliative and curative care; and the special medical problems and needs of the patients themselves, including depression, guilt, anemia, fatigue, and wasting syndrome.

A model program of AIDS home-centered hospice care was developed in San Francisco in 1984. Conferences and other programs on hospice AIDS care drew participants from across the United States and Canada.[60] Hospice leaders were deeply concerned about the AIDS tragedy and its financial impact, and they maintained that the fundamental principles of hospice called for the care of HIV-infected patients to the end of their lives. Sandol Stoddard remarked in 1989, "Front-line people have told me, from one end of the country to the other, that they intend to care for people who have AIDS, to the best of their ability. It has been a moving experience for me to hear this, in so many different voices."[61]

Medical and Nursing Education

Progress in hospice care faced the critical problem of an extensive lack of medical and nursing education and training in expert and sensitive end-of-life care. Jill Rhymes correctly observed, "Although courses or segments of courses on death and dying were being taught, most physicians and nurses have not been trained in caring for the terminally ill, and many are not comfortable in doing so."[62] A majority of physicians and nurses in Britain felt they had been inadequately trained to care for terminally ill patients.[63] A 1992 survey of medical students conducted in the United Kingdom, New Zealand, and Japan documented "the urgent need for better teaching in palliative care." Representative of others quoted in the survey, a student from the United Kingdom in the final year of medical training remarked, "Little is done to help us to become comfortable with death and the care of the dying. The total support and understanding a terminally ill patient desperate needs cannot be given by someone who is still frightened by death itself."[64]

Adding to the problem, the Medicare hospice legislation appointed physicians as gatekeepers for patients into hospice, but many doctors bore that responsibility reluctantly. Physicians displayed uncertainties over delivering a six-month terminal diagnosis, hesitancy over sharing patient control with team members, outright unfamiliarity with hospice care, and little or no training in the science of palliative medicine and the art of attending to and communicating with dying persons.[65] A comprehensive survey of U.S. medical schools in 1989 showed that of the 111 (out of a total of 124) schools responding, 30 percent had one or two lectures on death and dying as part of a larger course, 52 percent taught those topics as a module in a required course, 18 percent taught topics on death and dying as a separate course (half of which were required), and 11 percent offered no formal educational experiences.[66]

Nevertheless, several medical and nursing educators in the United States began actively dealing with training in "all of the ramifications of terminal illness" by the end of the 1980s and in the early 1990s.[67] Clear models about what that education and training should be for nurses were developed in the early 1990s.[68] Details about a full-semester elective course in hospice care for first- and second-year medical students at the University of Pennsylvania were published in 1989. The course included regular assignments to home hospice settings, weekly meetings with instructors, and an essay on each student's experiences. Students were moved and changed by what they learned individually and in meetings. They witnessed dying patients who were treated poorly and others treated with care and concern. They learned about the importance of verbal and nonverbal communication with dying persons and their families.[69]

The report of an elective semester course with similar aims for a similar student population taught at the Yale School of Medicine was published in 1991. The course attracted the participation of 35 percent of Yale medical students during its first four years. It utilized patients as teachers who spoke about their experiences with physicians, their images of caring physicians and nurses, the impacts of their life-threatening illnesses, their fears, their faiths, and their personal stories. Students found that many patients who did not participate as teachers did not want to discuss death and dying or see themselves as dying. Like all human beings, they wanted to live as fully as possible until they died. Dying became demystified as students learned to talk easily with suffering and dying persons and realized that they had broken past a major barrier to effective patient care.[70]

The Yale course became a model for medical education in palliative care. It highlighted the inadequacies of a by and large rational, unemotional, scientific approach to medical education and post-graduate training.[71] It also forecast the initiation of projects to improve end-of-life care, including one by the American Board of Internal Medicine (ABIM) in October 1993, the Open Society Institute Project on Death in America in 1994, and the Task Force to Improve the Care of Terminally Ill Oregonians in 1995.[72] Modest progress was under way.

Continuing Excessive Efforts to Prolong Life and Their Counter-Measures: 1982–1994

The discussions that follow about major initiatives to rein in excessive efforts to prolong life presuppose that the medical advances listed at the beginning of this chapter engendered ongoing life-saving efforts. Decreasing mortality rates for a variety of severe illnesses encouraged aggressive treatment. Before the 1990s, for example, mortality rates for patients with ARDS were between 40 and 70 percent, but in the United States and United Kingdom those rates dropped to 30–40 percent in the 1990s.[73]

In his prize-winning, best-selling book *How We Die*, Sherwin B. Nuland takes readers inside the world of curative, life-prolonging medicine up to the time of its publication in 1993. His book is not for the faint of heart. It is a cousin to the sociological studies of Barney G. Glaser and Anselm L. Strauss, but this time the participant-observer is an outstanding and outspoken surgeon. Knowingly or not, Nuland's book embodies a modern version of one of the central themes in the writings of notable figures featured in former chapters of this text: how persons die largely depends on what they die from.[74]

Nuland graphically describes physiological details of dying from congestive heart failure, pulmonary disease, kidney failure, strokes, sepsis, Alzheimer's disease, AIDS, cancer, multiple organ failure, and other life-ending conditions. He depicts the agonies of patients with congestive heart failure and other ultimately fatal illnesses. He tells of the arrogance of his brother's cancer doctors and Nuland's own perpetuation of the deception that his brother might be rescued with experimental drugs, all of which added to his brother's anguish. Nuland was enthralled by the beeping and squealing monitors, the hissing of respirators, and the seclusion and "high-tech hope within the citadel" of the surgical ICU.[75]

Modern physicians, Nuland conveys, search for "The Riddle"—the diagnosis and treatment that will enable specific cures. When it becomes obvious that there is no longer a riddle to solve, many physicians lose their enthusiasm and emotionally abandon patients who are beyond recovery. To maintain enthusiasm, "treatment decisions are sometimes made near the end of life that propel a dying person willy-nilly into a series of worsening miseries from which there is no extraction"—surgery of questionable benefit and prolonged periods in intensive care beyond the point of futility. "I have," Nuland confesses, "shared the excitement of last-ditch fights for life and the supreme satisfaction that comes when they are won. Knowing that, I will not allow a specialist to decide when to let [me] go."[76]

Because the rescue credo of high-tech medicine almost always wins out in the treatment of fatal conditions, the dying process is by and large "a messy business," Nuland argues. Dying is usually an undignified process that runs its natural course regardless of death-delaying interventions. Some lucky persons will consciously experience serenity as they die.[77] But "there is no dignity" in CPR that too often ends with a corpse lying in the center of devastation. Nor is there any dignity in dying from AIDS or many other terminal conditions. Few will ever experience dignity before the hour of death, which is "commonly tranquil and often preceded by blissful unawareness."[78]

Nuland wrote *How We Die* in order "to demythologize the process of dying" by telling the truth about clinical realities to a wide public audience.[79] Ironically, years before the publication of his book, a contrasting exercise in demystification was taking place where Nuland was a professor of surgery. Yale's medical school course on death and dying was enabling students to talk openly and easily with suffering and dying patients who, for whatever reason, were not being subjected to death-delaying interventions to the point of death.

The impact of *How We Die* far exceeded the public attention it received. It further encouraged increasing numbers of physicians, nurses, and others to make dying as tranquil and meaningful as possible through the medicine and art of palliative care—which Nuland asserted "is now mostly lost, replaced by the brilliance of rescue."[80] It also further urged physicians, ethicists, lawyers, and legislators to find ways to limit excessive, invasive, and fruitless life prolongation.

So oppressive efforts to prolong the lives of dreadfully and terminally ill patients were continuing. Nuland describes how these efforts were not rare, but rather normative. He tells how he convinced a 92-year-old woman to undergo high-risk abdominal surgery, which she initially refused on the grounds "that she had been on this planet 'quite long enough, young man' and didn't wish to go on." Musing about her case years later, Nuland says that if he'd thought more deeply and responded less paternalistically, he would not have pressed her to undergo extensive surgery, which caused her to spend the last days of her life in a surgical intensive care unit. Then Nuland catches himself. "There is a lie in what I just said," he confesses. "[I would] probably have done exactly the same thing again, or risk the scorn of my peers." He later adds, "These days many hospitalized patients die only when a doctor has decided that the right time has come."[81]

Outcries Against Treatment Heroics

Sherwin Nuland's stories were laments, rather than outcries. The stories of others protested against the treatment excesses. In 1983, in the *Journal of the American Medical Association*, a physician recounted his daughter's ordeal:

> My daughter, whom I shall identify as J.A., succumbed to disseminated metastatic carcinoma of the breast at the age of 34 years. I hope that her abridged case history will help to somehow temper the overaggressive treatment of the obviously and hopeless[ly] ill terminal cancer patient by both academic and grass roots physicians.... The prolongations of suffering by often heroic measures and academic successes defies the basic purpose of a physician—the relief of suffering.
>
> J.A. had the benefit of excellent services at a well-regarded teaching medical center.... The initial diagnosis of cancer was delayed because of multiple oversights and is another example of tragedy. She actually received the bad news by mail! She had surgery, chemotherapy, unsuccessful operative site reconstruction, subsequent chemotherapy with enervating side effects, and salvage protocol all at the same institution.... When the dissemination of her disease became inexorably advanced, she had several episodes of pneumonia and experienced semi-comatose states.... She would have mercifully died had not heroic measures been instituted.
>
> The house staff and medical students were most enthusiastic with the responses of J.A. to various heroic measures.

The physician admitted that he and his two physician brothers did not constrain the enthusiasm and hopeful prognoses of the treatment staff. Then he exclaimed through a question, "When will **mercy** enter into the aggressive protocols and permit the ravaged patient to die peacefully?" In other words, when will physicians in charge manifest mercy through therapeutic restraint?[82]

Others noted that in intensive care units life-sustaining measures were being instituted without sufficient thought given to the proper goals of treatment.[83] Cardiopulmonary resuscitation (CPR) was routinely performed on all patients suffering cardiac arrest regardless of their underlying medical conditions, unless, perchance, a do-not-resuscitate (DNR) order was clearly specified.[84] Unfortunately, throughout the 1980s patients' rights to refuse treatment often continued to be overridden by the therapeutic imperative of CPR. The study by Andrew Evans and Baruch Brody in 1985 found that "the goal of promoting patient self-determination regarding resuscitation is not really being implemented in resuscitation decisions. For the vast majority of patients who were to be resuscitated, that decision was made without either patient or family input."[85] In an editorial that would further turn the tide against the overuse of CPR, Leslie Black-hall observed in 1987 that "too often CPR just happens, without inquiry into the patient's wishes or consideration of its [often highly limited] chances of success."[86]

Numerous additional studies indicated that the rates of survival after CPR—that is, survival past the time of being discharged from the hospital—were dismal for severely ill patients with many types of medical conditions: 2 percent of patients with severe cardiac disease, and no patients with metastatic cancer, or sepsis, or other chronic, debilitating illnesses.[87]

Four Notable Efforts to Rein in Treatment Excesses

Attempts to rein in the overuse of invasive life-saving and life-prolonging interventions—including CPR—were under way in the 1970s.[88] Hopes that these interventions would be further constrained increased and strengthened between 1982 and 1994. Ethicists, lawyers, legislatures, doctors and others recognized the "right to die"—that is, the right of terminally ill patients not to have their deaths postponed by CPR or other attempted life-saving measures.

Reflecting the problems of overtreatment in hospitals, efforts to secure patients' rights of self-determination and to protect medical professionals from choruses of criticism were conducted by four notable initiatives: a national commission led by renowned doctors, ethicists, lawyers, theologians and sociologists; hospital guidelines pertaining to do-not-resuscitate orders and life-sustaining treatments other than CPR; discussion and debate over judgments of medical futility on the part of doctors; and new legislation to enable patients to set forth their autonomous choices through advanced directives embodied in living wills and appointed surrogate decision makers.

The President's Commission

In 1983 the President's Commission[89] published a 550-page report, the title of which centered on the problem of medical treatment excesses: *Deciding to Forego Life-Sustaining Treatment.* To summarize its central concerns and policy recommendations, the commission held that as long as patients express no clear opposition to the procedure, and even if the physician is uncertain as to whether CPR would be beneficial, there should be a presumption in favor of trying resuscitation.[90] It also gave conflicting perspectives about patient autonomy by defining autonomy as free choice respecting treatment options devoid of undue influence, and then holding that doctors should voice their disagreements with patients' choices and be free to examine patients' capacity to make decisions. The report promoted the need for explicit hospital policies regarding Do-

Not-Resuscitate (DNR) orders and strongly favored advance directives of surrogate decision makers over the directives of written living wills.[91]

The commissioners debated these issues extensively. They sought to find a balance between the authority of physicians and rights of patients, but sided with life-extending interventions: "Until it is quite clear that a patient is making an informed, deliberate, and voluntary decision to forego specific life-sustaining interventions, health care providers should look for and enhance any feeling the patient has about not yet acquiescing to death."[92] Their recommendations regarding advance directives are noted below.

Hospital Guidelines Regarding DNR Orders and Life-Sustaining Treatments Other than CPR

By 1990 increasing numbers of physicians believed that "one should not have to pass through the jaws of technology in order to die," and that physicians are responsible for making "sure that the path of dying does not necessarily include CPR as the last milestone."[93] DNR orders would enable doctors to spare patients from aggressive attempts to revive life in the face of imminent and inevitable death. Within four years, guidelines for these orders became commonplace in hospitals.[94]

Little attention has been given to the way hospital guidelines developed over time. Between 1982 and 1994, three levels of guideline development occurred: first, intra-hospital policies to standardize the use of DNR orders; second, policies concerning the use and limitation of a variety of life-supportive technologies; and, third, policies that focused on judgments of medical futility (discussed in the sub-section that follows).

The establishment of guidelines for these areas became imperative for a number of reasons. They would serve as ways of upholding patient autonomy and protecting patients from overtreatment.[95] They would increase uniformity and decrease confusion and conflict among caregivers. They would empower physicians to make decisions pertaining to these life and death issues without fear of legal liability—which some called "litigation anxiety."[96] And, for some authors, clear guidelines and policies would prove to be cost-effective.[97]

DNR orders are equivalent to "No CPR" orders, and they relate to patients with all types of severe and catastrophic medical conditions. Virtually all physicians agreed with the President's Commission's opposition to "reflex resuscitation efforts applied to all patients" undergoing cardiac arrest.[98] But uniform and effective intra-hospital policies respecting DNR orders became essential.

An outstanding example of the establishment of intra-hospital policies regarding DNR orders is that of the Yale New Haven Hospital (YNHH) in 1983. The YNHH's multi-disciplinary committee sought to overcome communication barriers to uniform and effective DNR decisions, which included the lack of an identified responsible physician and a lack of awareness by other caregivers that an order had been given. The committee set forth policies covering all its identified barriers. It delineated three categories of patients for whom their policies applied: no DNR orders for patients needing curative therapies (unless patients refused such therapies), possible orders for those with uncertain outcomes, and DNR orders for incurably ill patients as long as the patient or a guardian expressly authorized such orders.[99]

The second level of guideline development addressed the termination of a range of life-sustaining treatments, including ventilator use, dialysis, artificial nutrition and hydration, and antibiotics. Addressing this range of procedures, the Hastings Center (HC), an influential think tank of bioethicists, physicians, philosophers, lawyers, and theologians, published its *Guidelines on the Termination of Life-Sustaining Treatment and the Care of the Dying* in 1987.[100]

The HC *Guidelines* distinguished DNR orders from other life-sustaining treatments: "A DNR order should not be understood as an indication that other life-sustaining treatment should also be withheld or that the patient should not be admitted to the Intensive Care Unit." Nor should the patient's acceptance of, for example, ventilator use be construed as acceptance of all other forms of life-sustaining treatment.[101] That said, the HC *Guidelines* agreed with the YNHH's position—no withdrawal or withholding of life-sustaining medical treatment should occur without the patient's or a patient surrogate's informed consent.[102] Providers are not obligated to provide "clearly futile" life-sustaining treatments to patients, but those treatments should not be discontinued without the consent and permission of patients or their surrogates.[103]

The third level of guidelines began to emerge by 1994—practice guidelines on suspending CPR and other life-prolonging interventions that doctors judge to be therapeutically useless. To understand these guidelines, the topic of medical futility must first be explored.

Treatment Futility and Developing Guidelines

Discussions of medical futility moved far beyond the President's Commission's general appeal to physicians' duties to benefit and not to harm. In his pivotal 1987 "Sounding Board" essay, Leslie Blackhall argued that CPR should not be offered "as a sort of high-technology placebo" treatment option to desperately sick patients. "In cases in which CPR has been shown to be on no benefit, as in patients with metastatic cancer, it should not be considered an alternative and should not be presented as such." If CPR is offered to give the family members hope, it's a cruel and false hope that can only increase the patient's suffering. The issue of patient autonomy, Blackhall added, "is irrelevant when CPR has no potential benefit."[104]

Extensive debate ensued. Blackhall's phrase "has no potential benefit" captured the core meaning of medical futility—interventions that will not benefit, "that will fail and that ought not be attempted," and "that cannot achieve the goals of the action, no matter how often repeated."[105] Positively, futility served as another means of limiting excessive attempts at life prolongation in clinical settings. Negatively, it could be viewed as encroaching on the nearly sacred principle of patient autonomy. Physicians differed on what probabilities of treatment success they had in mind when they considered treatments futile: 0 percent, 5 percent or more? Futility judgments were also beset by uncertain prognoses that called into question whether various interventions would in fact be useless.[106]

In spite of disagreements and uncertainties, the concept of ceasing futile treatments had staying power. It brought quantitative and qualitative judgments into play. Lawrence Schneiderman and others defined a futile effort as one "that will only promote vegetative survival, and "that reasoning or experience suggests is highly improbable and that cannot be systematically produced." They defined "highly improbable" as an arbitrary judgment based on clinical experience and data showing that in the last 100 cases the potential treatment was "useless."[107]

Many proponents of patient autonomy argued that futility determinations on the part of physicians undermine patient consent and reinstate physician paternalism.[108] Against that view, Tom Tomlinson and Howard Brody argued that doctors who refuse to allow patients to request and receive treatments that have no reasonable chance of benefit are rightly maintaining their professional integrity. Rather than undermining patient autonomy or rendering it irrelevant, physicians who act in accordance with their fiduciary obligations *protect* patient autonomy. "It is inherently and unavoidably misleading to offer a futile treatment" as if it will benefit, when the physician believes it will not. Rather than offering futile CPR as an option, doctors should inform patients and the family that CPR should not be attempted and explain the medical facts to support that decision.[109]

Given the importance of and disagreements about futility decisions, hospital guidelines were needed. In 1992 Steven Miles noted that medical futility was one of the most important and contentious topics of that time. He argued that without professional consensus, futility would be both legally powerless and ethically suspect because it could be viewed as devaluing respect for patient autonomy and human life. Medical associations would need to empower futility judgments with published guidelines. These guidelines would provide procedural oversight for decisions to discontinue futile care and confine those decisions to interventions that "a vast majority of persons would not accept for themselves."[110]

The editor of the *Journal of the American Medical Association* agreed with the need for futility-of-treatment guidelines. In 1993 he urged every hospital in America "to define futile care and develop guidelines that will identify and eliminate futile treatments." These guidelines should reflect the convictions of physicians and the wishes of patients and families. They should be approved by hospital ethics committees and hospital attorneys. When guidelines are developed and implemented, "everyone wins—the patient, the family, and society as a whole." They would also save billions of dollars annually.[111]

By 1994 formulations of futility-of-treatment policies were under way in the states of Colorado, California, and Washington. In Denver, Colorado, for example, the organizers of a project called Guidelines for the Use of Intensive Care in Denver (GUIDE) were developing a consensus that included community input. GUIDE would rule out aggressive treatment for certain specified conditions, as well as encourage healthcare teams to provide palliative care at the end of life.[112]

New Legislation on Advance Directives

The final major attempt to rein in excessive life-sustaining treatments pertained to the legal and ethical rights of patients to refuse unwanted medical interventions should they become incapable of making their own decisions. The last pages of Chapter 6 describe how rights to refuse unwanted treatment were first secured in the 1970s.

By 1983, 45 states in the United States had passed Natural Death Act legislation that included two types of advance directives giving patients the "right to die"—that is, the right not to have their lives prolonged should they become incapable of making their own treatment-refusal decisions. The first were written directives or living wills (LWs) that identify unacceptable medical interventions; the second were durable power of attorney (DPA) statutes that enable patients to appoint a surrogate to carry out their wishes. By 1983, 43 states had enacted DPA statutes, and 12 of the 43 had both DPA and LW laws in place. The complexities, strengths and weaknesses, and tentative nature of these directives are topics in themselves.[113]

LWs and DPAs were widely praised as protecting patient autonomy and securing informed consent. The President's Commission commended their use and, like the Yale New Haven Hospital, strongly encouraged living wills as "the most clear and unambiguous expressions of the patient's values." The New York Academy of Medicine affirmed the rights of patients who lose decision-making capacity to have their previous instructions honored through written directives and DPAs. The Hastings Center held that one of the major goals of its guidelines was to encourage patients to develop advance directives. And a unanimous report of England's House of Lords called for a national code of practice that would make an advance directive the "authoritative, respected statement of a patient's wishes regarding treatment."[114]

But a serious disconnect between those rights and clinical realities continued. CPR was frequently attempted without the input of patients or family members. In 1989 Sidney Wanzer and his coauthors flagged the "considerable gap between the acceptance of the [advance] directive and its implementation," between "what the courts now allow with respect to withdrawal of treatment and what physicians actually do." Only a few patients were setting forth advance directives, and a minority of physicians were having "timely discussions with patients about life-sustaining treatment and terminal care."[115] Furthermore, physicians continued to fear legal liability for withdrawing life-sustaining measures.[116]

Public support for advance directives nevertheless increased. The saga surrounding Nancy Cruzan focused national attention on these directives. After being resuscitated by paramedics at the scene of her auto accident in 1983, Nancy remained in a state of permanent unconsciousness, kept alive by a feeding tube for almost eight years. In 1987, when no hopes for her recovery remained, her parents went to court to ask that she be allowed to die by removing the feeding tube. The Supreme Court of Missouri disallowed the removal on the grounds that Nancy had not given clear and convincing evidence that she would have wanted to die. In June 1990 the U.S. Supreme Court upheld that judgment, but in her concurring opinion, Justice Sandra Day O'Connor said an advance directive would have dispelled uncertainty over Cruzan's wishes. Within a month, the Society for the Right to Die received nearly 300,000 requests for advance directive forms.[117]

In the wake of the Supreme Court's *Cruzan* ruling, the U.S. Congress implemented the Patient Self-Determination Act (PSDA) in December 1991. "*Finally ... the first federal* legislation to ensure that health care institutions inform patients about their rights ... to accept or refuse medical treatment and to formulate advance directives" had been passed.[118] The law required that all hospitals, hospices, and home health agencies receiving Medicare and Medicaid funding must develop written policies on advance care documents; must provide patients—upon admission to these facilities—with information about their rights to complete advance directives and refuse medical care; and must educate staff about advance care planning. A lawyer-bioethicist exclaimed that "the vast majority of physicians will welcome the ability to discuss treatment options with a person chosen by the patient who has the legal authority to give or withhold consent."[119]

Ezekiel J. Emanuel and colleagues published an impressive study on the consequences of the *Cruzan* ruling and the PSDA. Before *Cruzan* about 10 percent of the American population had formal advance directives. That number increased to between 20 percent and 24 percent of the population in the months following *Cruzan*, and then to 25 percent five months after implementation of the PSDA. The impact of the PSDA had been less than expected, but change seemed certain.[120]

Threatening Seas: 1995

Like sailors on board the brig in *Two Years Before the Mast*, some palliative care specialists saw a black cloud rising. Sean Morrison and others in 1994 questioned the assumption behind the Patient Self-Determination Act—that the use of advance directives would greatly increase if patients received information about them and had the option of filling them out. They found that physicians rarely initiated discussions about end-of-life decisions, often did not fully understand what advance directives were (or viewed them as unnecessary), and even in "catastrophic situations" rarely used them as guides for treatment decisions.[121] Ann Fade and Karen Kaplan warned, "Even if an individual completes an advance directive, there is a possibility that his or her wishes still may not be honored." Healthcare providers voice objections to advance directives, worry over the legality, and often manage "to avoid discussing and reaching a decision on a patient's care."[122]

The treacherous seas that threatened to wash away the fine prospects of limiting overtreatment, respecting patient self-determination, and improving palliative care in hospitals arose in the third week of November 1995. The threats were revealed in a study designed "to improve end-of-life decision making and reduce the frequency of a mechanically supported, painful, and prolonged process of dying." The study's authority was based on millions of dollars of funding from the Robert Wood Johnson Foundation, six years of research in five medical centers, some 100 investigators, and 9,105 patients who volunteered as study subjects.

The publication of the SUPPORT study (an acronym from its title) described the design and results of its two phases.[123] Both phases enrolled patients with advanced stages of one or more of nine life-threatening conditions, including acute respiratory failure, multiple organ system failure, metastatic colon cancer, and chronic obstructive lung disease.

Phase I, the observation phase, studied the frequency of aggressive treatment, the characteristics of hospital deaths, and the nature of physician-patient communication. It lasted 2 years and included 4,301 patients. Epitomizing understatement, Phase I "confirmed substantial shortcomings in the care for seriously ill hospitalized adults." Only 47 percent of physicians knew when their patients did not want CPR; 46 percent of the

DNR orders were written within 2 days of death; 38 percent of the patients who died during the study spent at least 10 days in an ICU, where 31 percent received mechanical ventilation within three days of death; and family members reported that 50 percent of their loved ones who were able to communicate experienced moderate to severe pain at least half of the time.[124]

Phase II was called the "Intervention Phase" because it was designed to alter the disturbing findings of Phase I. The study's leaders met with physicians at the five medical centers who wanted to effect changes in hospital end-of-life care. The group discussed the findings of Phase I and agreed on a plan that would enhance doctor-patient communication, honor patient preferences, result in earlier non-aggressive treatment decisions, and reduce the time patients would spend in undesirable states before death. All agreed that physicians lacked information about patients' prognoses and lacked time to discuss treatment alternatives.

Phase II would surely improve terminal care by providing physicians with timely and reliable prognostic information, by eliciting and documenting patient and family preferences based on a better understanding of patients' medical conditions and treatment options, and by utilizing specially trained and committed nurses. The nurses would spend time with patients and family members, provide emotional support, and then convey important information to physicians in meetings and discussions.[125] All these changes occurred according to plan.

But the Phase II interventions proved to be "completely ineffectual"![126] The number of days patients spent in the ICU remained the same in Phase II as in Phase I. No change occurred in the use of mechanical ventilation before death. DNR orders were not written sooner. The same percentages of patients experienced moderate to severe pain. Physicians' lack of awareness of their patents' preferences not to be resuscitated remained the same. And of the patients who did not have discussions about CPR with their physicians, 41 percent in both phases said they wanted such a discussion.

The investigators of the SUPPORT study exclaimed, "In conclusion, we are left with a troubling situation. The picture we describe of the care of seriously ill or dying persons is not attractive." The study "certainly casts a pall over any claim that, if the health care system is given additional resources for collaborative decision making ... improvements will occur." Physicians were clearly entrenched in their "established patterns of care," and their behavior was unchanged.[127]

More graphically put, the pall cast by the SUPPORT study was like a black cloud darkening the heavens over all dimensions of palliative end-of-life care in hospitals. The entrenched dynamics of medical culture—its patterns of doctor-patient interaction, the extent of its reliance on curative and life-prolonging technologies, its assigned low status to terminally ill patients—were now clearly revealed, now clearly proven to be threatening to proponents of palliative care.

Consternation and criticism ensued. The Hastings Center immediately published a special edition of its journal on the import of the SUPPORT findings. The aftermath of the study consumed the energies of additional authors and organizations for years. Bernard Lo, a prominent physician-ethicist, remarked, "The findings do not depict gentle, peaceful death, but high technology run amok with poor communication, inadequate relief of symptoms, and little respect for patient preferences." Dramatic changes must be made in the entire "health care system." Doctor-patient discussions about life-sustaining care must occur more frequently, he argued, but improving them "will be a difficult challenge."[128]

Patricia A. Marshall said that the study "illustrates profoundly the force and tenacity of Western biomedical culture": its hierarchy of social dominance; its typical casting of nurses in the role of talking with patients and families, and then relaying their messages to physicians in charge; its fundamental orientation toward the preservation of life; and its view of patients as "foreigners in biomedical territory" even though mechanisms ostensibly champion autonomy and more compassionate care.[129]

The lawyer-bioethicist George Annas evinced sound and fury. In an article titled "How We Lie," Annas played off the title of Nuland's *How We Die* to declare that "physicians simply have never taken the rights of hospitalized patients seriously." Their primary values are action- and technology-oriented. According to Annas, doctors are uninterested in having discussions with patients or families about death or pain. The problems are so pervasive "that the only realistic way to improve the care of dying patients in the short run is to get them out of the hospital, and keep them from going [back]." Living wills and healthcare proxies have failed to affect treatment or outcome. They cannot be expected to actually change physician behavior "in the absence of a change in physician culture." Doctors should have their medical licenses suspended for incompetently managing patients and not honoring their rights in hospital settings.[130]

Headwinds increased with the study of James A. Tulsky and others on the realities of discussions of Do-Not-Resuscitate orders between resident physicians and their patients. Tulsky and his co-investigators recorded 31 interviews between medical residents and mentally competent, seriously ill patients regarding whether they wanted DNR orders instated. This study demonstrated that even when physicians discussed resuscitation with patients, the goal of enhancing patient autonomy and informed decision making was not achieved. Only 13 percent of the physicians discussed the likelihood of survival after CPR, and none gave numerical estimates of survival or death. The physical problems of those who survived were rarely mentioned; 32 percent spoke of the almost inevitable need for intensive care, but only one described the potential for a prolonged stay in the ICU; only 16 percent mentioned CPR-related medical complications. On average, the interviews lasted 10 minutes, with physicians talking 73 percent of the time. Only 10 percent initiated discussions about the patient's values, goals, and life preferences.[131]

The ship of hopes filled with expectations of limiting overtreatment, improving care for patients at the end of life, and respecting patient self-determination now had to either turn back or labor and strain against the worsened conditions.

Endurance Beyond the Storm: 1996–1999

Dealing with the threatening seas would be daunting. Change physician *culture*? Make dramatic changes in the entire health care *system*?[132] Where would the inspiration, energies, and resources for effecting such changes come from? Why not accept the realities of modern hospital dying described by Sherwin Nuland as a by and large undignified and messy business? Why not follow the advice of George Annas—get dying persons who want to experience some measure of peace out of the hospital and keep them from going back?[133]

All the chapters in this book tell why resignation and flight were not viewed as viable options. How persons die—and live to the point of death—seizes everyone's attention, tapping into the roots of expressed and unexpressed concerns. For generations, stories of bad deaths continued to haunt and horrify, even as the visions and promises of better, if not good, dying continued to appeal and inspire. For generations the promotion of palliative end-of-life care and treatment continued.

So the threatening conditions inspired endurance, not resignation. In late 1995 Patricia Marshall expressed gratitude for the SUPPORT findings, which she said called for pursuing new, vigorous, extensive, and alternative interventions than those undertaken in Phase II of SUPPORT. In 1996, Kathryn Koch charged her physician colleagues with the tasks of developing the emotional ability to resist imperatives to treat incurable conditions and accepting the duty "to ensure as gentle a death as possible." In 1997, Joanne Lynn, the director of the Center to Improve Care of the Dying at the George Washington University Medical Center, outlined the components of excellent end-of-life care and exclaimed, "A health care system that cannot support excellence at the end of life isn't worth sustaining." In 1998 Ezekiel and Linda Emanuel outlined a comprehensive, multifaceted, framework for a good death that is "within our grasp."[134]

From late 1995 through 1999 major initiatives were undertaken to improve end-of-life care. These included efforts on the part of major organizations and medical groups, expansion of palliative care and hospice programs, discussions of good death, further limitations of CPR, additional guidelines on treatment futility, new hopes for reforms in professional education and training, and new textbooks on comfort-directed care.

Initiatives by Organizations and Medical Groups

The range and power of redetermined efforts to effect change are embodied in the 437-page publication of the Institute of Medicine's (IOM) *Approaching Death: Improving Care at the End of Life* in 1997. Founded in 1970 under the congressional charter of the U.S. National Academy of Sciences, the IOM and other national academies rely on workforces of unpaid experts to provide unbiased, evidence-based and authoritative information and advice on critical challenges and problem areas. Funded by a variety of sources, the IOM's reports focus on biomedical science, medical practice, and health. Reports include lists of action-oriented recommendations.[135]

The committee of 12 that generated *Approaching Death* began its deliberations in January 1996, conducted public meetings, commissioned papers from experts, heard statements from 36 groups, and held a workshop at the George Washington University Center to Improve Care of the Dying. The report noted that the SUPPORT study's disappointing results stimulated consideration of new strategies that would change the system—the practice patterns in the medical culture responsible for end-of-life care.[136] On its first pages the report asserts,

> A humane care system ... honors and protects those who are dying, conveys by word and action that dignity resides in people ... and helps ... to preserve their integrity while coping with unavoidable physical insults and losses. Such reliably excellent and respectful care at the end of life is an attainable goal, but realizing it will require many changes in attitudes, policies, and actions. System changes—not just changes in individual beliefs and actions—are necessary.[137]

Approaching Death is critical, thorough, informative, and action-oriented. It asserts that "very serious problems remain" in the current system of care for those with life-threatening and incurable illnesses. Too many people suffer needlessly at the end of life. Organizational and economic obstacles "conspire to obstruct reliably excellent care." The education and training of healthcare professionals is poor. Public perception is marked by a combination of fear, misinformation, and naiveté. Decent or good deaths are free from avoidable distress and suffering, accord with patients' and families' wishes, and reflect ethical and cultural standards. They result from thoughtful and expert attention to all the intertwined dimensions of critical illness and dying—physical, psychological, spiritual, and practical. "A bad death is characterized by needless suffering, disregard for patient or family wishes or values, and a sense ... that norms of decency have been offended."[138]

The Institute of Medicine's seven recommendations reflect the content and conclusions of its ten chapters. First, all persons with advanced, potentially fatal illness and those close to them should receive reliable, skilled, and supportive care. Second, all healthcare professionals must commit themselves to improving end-of-life care. Third, policymakers, consumer groups, and medical organizations and professionals must seek to rectify system problems through organizational, financial, and legal strategies. Fourth, changes should be initiated at all levels of professional education to enhance commitment, knowledge, and skills. Fifth, palliative care should become, if not a medical specialty, then a defined area of expertise and research. Sixth, the nation's research establishment should expand the knowledge base of end-of-life care. And seventh, widespread public discussion is essential.[139]

Valuable specific recommendations are embedded in the IOM's agenda of topics. For example, within the third recommendation is the critical point that drug prescription laws must be reviewed and revised to enable practitioners to improve management of patients' pain. Attached to the fourth is an impressive outline of the fundamental elements of professional preparation for end-of-life care. The committee offered its recommendations with optimism, declaring that heeding them would strengthen the public's trust in the healthcare system. The time was ripe for fundamental change.[140]

Other organizations greatly contributed to the cause. *Approaching Death* described 42 initiatives to improve end-of-life care. These and additional initiatives included documents and films by the American Board of Internal Medicine, programs in major medical centers, national conferences, contributions from religious charities, and nationally broadcast TV programs, including *Before I Die: Medical Care and Personal Choices* (broadcast in April 1997). The multi-year, multi-million-dollar initiative funded by the Robert Wood Johnson Foundation (RWJF) that was known as Last Acts began in March 1996. Last Acts developed in response to "the disturbing findings" of the SUPPORT study. It brought together a coalition of 72 prominent consumer and healthcare organizations intent on promoting improvements in caring for persons at the end of life.[141] Last Acts was only one of the RWJF's sophisticated and well-funded programs designed to make palliative care accessible to all Americans.[142]

An initiative sponsored by the Milbank Memorial Fund broke new ground. Knowing that modern medicine is specialty based, Christine Cassel and Kathleen Foley, supported by Milbank, convened representatives of medical societies to draft a set of "Core Principles for End-of-Life Care" that ideally would be widely adopted as practice imperatives by a wide spectrum of specialties. Eleven core principles were adopted, beginning with "Respect the dignity of both patient and caregivers," and including alleviating pain and other physical symptoms; attending to psychological, social, and spiritual/religious problems; and providing access to palliative and hospice care.

Medical organizations and societies were asked to deliberate upon and respond to these principles with policy statements. The American Medical Association, the Academy of Hospice and Palliative Medicine, and other groups formally adopted all the "Core Principles" as written. Other groups drafted their own statements that embodied these principles—among them the American Academy of Neurology, American Society of Clinical Oncology, and the Joint Commission on the Accreditation of Healthcare Organizations. Still others adopted the principles with modifications and/or added other principles befitting their specialties—such as the American College of Surgeons, Society of Internal Medicine, the Society of Bioethics and Humanities, and others. Influential groups were now commonly engaged and challenged to follow through with the policies they adopted.[143]

Expanding Responsibilities of Palliative Medicine and Care

Historic proponents of palliative care emphasized attention to the physical, emotional, spiritual, and social dimensions of care for dying persons. Beginning in the 1960s, that comprehensive understanding of comfort care became institutionalized as hospice care in hospitals and various out-of-hospital settings. It became increasingly professionalized and internationalized after the early 1980s.

From the mid–1990s to the present time, the terminology associated with palliative care began to change. Before the 1990s palliative end-of-life care was generally called hospice care in both hospital and out-of-hospital settings. After that time, *hospice care* increasingly denoted comfort-focused care in out-of-hospital settings, while comprehensive end-of-life care for hospitalized patients was typically called *palliative care*. In hospitals and throughout the world, palliative care was often used interchangeably with *palliative medicine*. Both terms were often construed as care for terminally ill patients that integrated the philosophy of hospice into clinical practice.[144] Many physicians who devoted years of attention to hospice care and became palliative care or palliative medicine specialists in hospitals in the 1990s continued to identify palliative care with end-of-life care.[145]

Also by the mid–1990s, the terms *palliative care* and *palliative medicine* increasingly embraced more than terminal care.[146] Palliative care progressives believed that their care and expertise should be extended early on and continually to patients with chronic and relapsing medical problems that warranted potentially life-prolonging treatments up to the time of death.[147] Palliative care thus embraced both end-of-life care and palliation for patients continuing with cure-intended procedures.[148] This historic change continues to be misunderstood and under-appreciated.[149]

The new emphasis on palliative medicine as embracing more than end-of-life care was, in fact, centuries old. As early as 1708, famous and influential physicians such as the world-renowned Hermann Boerhaave (1668–1738) spoke of "palliative cures" or the "*Treatment of* Symptoms"—pain, thirst, sleeplessness, fainting, and weakness—for sick persons generally.[150]

Hospital-based palliative care and palliative medicine programs rapidly increased during the 1990s, sometimes against the grain of ignorance. In 1992, when an expert in home hospice care sought to establish an affiliation with an academic hospital, he was rebuffed by the hospital administer with the angry words, "Dr. Weissman, this is an acute care hospital, our patients do not die." Needless to say, Weissman added, "we were not successful in negotiating a contract ... but oh, how the times have changed!"[151] By the turn of the century, 30 percent of the hospital respondents to a first-ever national survey reported having a palliative care program in place, and another 20 percent had plans to establish such a program.[152]

These hospital programs varied from in-patient consultation services to physician-led palliative care teams that intervened throughout the institution, to special in-patient units for intense symptom control, to hospital-based hospice care, to pain services, to outpatient services.[153] One hospital model was nurse-directed, existed as a separate hospital unit, and relied on the expertise of physician specialists in neurology, oncology, internal medicine, and intensive care.[154] Some hospitals developed models of continuing care for patients with particularly difficult diseases, such as congestive heart failure and COPD.[155] One author praised the development of palliative care units in hospitals as the next frontier of end-of-life care, which "can have a ripple effect within the hospital culture by educating the next generation of doctors and nurses."[156]

Concerning palliative care as a medical specialty, the Institute of Medicine's *Approaching Death* discussed at length its pros and cons and recognized that palliative caregivers already had their own medical society, established journals, organized conferences, and research initiatives. After months of deliberation, the IOM committee concluded that the needs of patients were so great that palliative care should become established, if not as a recognized medical specialty, at least as a "defined and accepted area of teaching, research, and patient care expertise."[157]

Momentously, three weeks after *Approaching Death* was published, the U.S. Supreme Court ruled against the legality of physician-assisted suicide, but in favor of a constitutional right to palliative care and treatment. States should not impose barriers on the availability of palliation for terminally ill patients, including drug laws that interfere with pain relief even if those drugs would hasten death.[158]

The professionalization and internationalization of palliative, comfort-directed care proceeded until the end of the century. A month before the SUPPORT study was published, Linda Blank listed and discussed the "core competencies" required for professionalized palliative care and urged that these should be taught and assessed in board-certified training in family medicine, internal medicine, and surgery. She noted, "Palliative medicine and hospice and home care are gaining recognition as separate distinguished disciplines through increasing research, specialty organizations, federal legislation, quest for certification, and public demand."[159]

The listings of research articles and conferences in *Index Medicus* further attest to the internationalization of palliative care and palliative medicine.[160] In addition to the recognition of palliative care as a medical sub-specialty in Great Britain, Ireland, and New Zealand by 1998, the International Association for Hospice and Palliative Care was formed in 1999, and the Latin American Association was founded in 2000.

Hospice Care

The number of out-of-hospital, Medicare-certified hospices and the number of persons cared for in these hospices greatly increased after 1995. Hospice care for persons diagnosed with terminal illnesses included pain relief, symptom control for sleeplessness and other concerns, emotional and spiritual counseling, and active participation by family and friends.

By 1999 the Medicare Hospice Benefit was widely recognized as an extraordinary and unprecedented benefit that allowed an unusual amount of autonomy for hospice providers in spite of its regulatory limitations.[161] In 1997 there were about 3,000 hospices in the United States, with more than 2,200 of these Medicare certified. Approximately 495,000 terminally ill patients were then receiving hospice care—about 20 percent of the annual deaths in the United States. Some 75–80 percent of these persons were covered by the Medicare benefit program, which greatly contributed to the estimated 16 percent per year growth of hospice coverage between 1985 and 1997. Hospice use expanded another 30 percent from 1998 to 1999—from 540,000 to 700,000 persons. Hospice care occurred most commonly as home care. The explosive growth was fueled by financial reality—the impoverishment of families responsible for terminal care without Medicare support and the fact that most private insurance plans covered high-tech and high-cost hospital care but not the services necessary for best-quality end-of-life care.[162]

While hospice growth was outstanding, the regulatory limits of the Medicare benefits restricted far greater utilization. As predicted, many patients were unwilling to enroll in hospice coverage on the condition that they would no longer seek curative treatment. Due to the entry requirement of a six-month or less terminal prognosis, late physician referrals to hospice continued. On average, patients died within about a month of entering hospice care, and some 15 percent died within 7 days of admission.[163]

Discussions of Good Death

During the 1990s new discussions of good death ensued. Previous chapters of this story reveal that the ideal of enabling persons to experience good deaths began when Francis Bacon coined the term *euthanasia* in 1605. But beginning in the last decades of the 19th century, euthanasia became equated with physician-induced and physician-assisted death for terminally ill patients who want to die.[164] Almost exclusively opposed to euthanasia in its modern sense, proponents of palliative care turned to other terms after the 1880s—natural dying, dying well, dying with dignity, and/or peaceful, gentle, easy deaths. Throughout the long history of palliative care, these terms refer to good dying without rendering death itself as good.

In her 1984 essay titled "On Dying Well," Dame Cicely Saunders concluded that the ways of speaking about a good death were enshrined in the hospice movement to which she was so deeply devoted.[165] Squarely grappling with the changed meaning of *euthanasia*, Kathryn A. Koch contrasted Francis Bacon's definition of euthanasia (a gentle and natural dying) with its modern meaning. The term "good death" should therefore be used as a way to recover Bacon's ideal. She equated good death with "as gentle a death as possible," which involves discontinuing futile treatments, utilizing expert palliative medicine, communicating effectively with patients, respecting patient choices, and offering emotional and spiritual counseling.[166]

Having been trained under and inspired by Dr. Saunders, Porter Storey wrote in 1990 that one of the central goals of hospice care was "to make possible a good death ... one that is as peaceful and comfortable as possible." Because death is inevitably a part of the pilgrimage of every human life, to accept its coming is "neither resignation on the part of patients nor defeatism or neglect on the part of doctors."[167] To be sure, when persons are fatally ill, life's limits are inescapable, yet positive achievements can still be realized. Life-extending treatments can delay death at the cost of detracting from, or nullifying, these achievements.[168] With the assistance of palliative care, terminal illness "can be a time for reconciliation and fulfillment for the patient and his family, and it may well be the most important period that they spend together."[169] Endorsing Storey's perspective, Andrew A. Skolnick added that death can be regarded as good by healthcare professionals who, having done all they can to cure, utilize palliation to "make the dying as comfortable as possible."[170]

In 1993, the philosopher and bioethicist Daniel Callahan advanced the ideal of peaceful death as a corrective to American society's failure to come to terms with the reality of death and to modern medicine's role in fostering that failure. Displaying no awareness of the centuries-old palliative care tradition, Callahan assumed that what he called "a peaceful death" was both innovative and a partial recovery of past understandings of death. He rightly knew his advocacy of peaceful death deeply challenged the underlying assumptions of American society and of modern medicine as the shaping force behind those assumptions.[171] He listed components of a peaceful death as conveying personal meaning, being treated with respect and sympathy, mattering to others, not being unduly burdensome, taking place in societies in which death is not dreaded, preserving conscious awareness, and occurring quickly.[172] Peaceful death opposes violations caused by implementing aggressive, sometimes futile, medical treatments to the very end; by dying after long periods of extreme frailty, disability, and little or no cognitive awareness; by dying anxious and terrified; and by ruinously consuming family and social resources.[173]

As she was finding her true calling in palliative medicine, Diane E. Meier reviewed Callahan's book for the *New England Journal of Medicine*. She noted that medicine's technological imperative, which equates "any acceptance of death as tantamount to rejecting the sanctity of life," had "painted us into a corner." Doctors who pursued the maximum possible prolongation of life were in the mainstream. "Their efforts are not questioned; the tide of the hospital culture is with them." While she criticized Callahan for rejecting the usefulness of medical education to promote a greater acceptance of death, she believed that his book should become required reading for medical students who seldom discussed such topics.[174]

Another breakthrough in discussions of good versus bad deaths was made by the framers of the Institute of Medicine's 1997 report *Approaching Death* (discussed above). That report lists the characteristics of good versus bad deaths and holds that its "expansive vision of a good death is intended to encourage a sensitive regard for dying patients" but should nevertheless not be imposed on dying patients and their families.[175]

Drawing upon that report, Ezekiel J. and Linda L. Emanuel published an extensive "framework for a good death" in 1998. Their framework highlighted the following: assuaging physical and psychological symptoms, attending to caregiver needs and economic realities, providing meaning and purpose through spiritual and existential counseling, withdrawing life-sustaining treatments, and attending to advance-care planning. The authors viewed this framework as a model for the care of dying patients. It would also serve as a guide, "a systematic mechanism" for further research, training, design of healthcare systems, and determinations of the costs of that care. The ideal of good dying thereby became a guiding star for reform of the healthcare system.[176]

Physician-Assisted Suicide (PAS)

The centuries of opposition to doctor-administered death[177] by palliative care proponents continues. But beginning in the late 1980s, several notable palliative caregivers, with the support of like-minded physicians and bioethicists, endorsed the moral permissibility of physician-assisted suicide—that is, enabling terminally ill patients to take their own lives with the assistance of a doctor. They began to accept PAS for several reasons. First, adherents believed PAS should be permissible when medicine's pain-relieving drugs and interventions are unable to ease dire physical and emotional suffering. PAS will thus keep patients from terrible dying.[178] Second, to allow such patients to continue to suffer constitutes an abandonment of the care of patients during the period of their profoundest need. PAS should thereby be viewed as *extending* fundamental aims of palliative care by enabling hopelessly sick and suffering patients to die with as much control as possible.[179] Third, the autonomy of patients extends to their rights to make rational choices about how they prefer to die when dying is inescapable. This accords with patients' right to escape from having their lives prolonged by medical measures over which they have no control.[180] And fourth, additional arguments in favor of PAS rested on refutations of traditional arguments against euthanasia and doctor-assisted death.[181]

The approval of PAS by a select number of notable palliative caregivers began tentatively and gradually because they knew they were disagreeing with traditional medical ethics and with many well-known and respected palliative care colleagues.[182] They also had to distance themselves from Dr. Jack Kevorkian's reckless use of his mobile "suicide machine" to enable some persons who were not yet dying to end their lives, and they had to shun "do-it-to-yourself" guidebooks from members of the Hemlock and other pro-suicide societies.[183]

One of the first articles that spoke openly about PAS and forthrightly identified 10 of its 12 co-authors as believing PAS was not immoral was published in the *New England*

Journal of Medicine in 1989. The authors recognized that assisted suicide posed complex issues that departed from previously accepted norms of personalized, multi-dimensional palliative care. They pointed to recent polls indicating that 58 percent of the American population believed a physician should be able lawfully to end the life of a terminally ill patient at the patient's request. They also emphasized that guidelines—such as proof that the patient's condition is terminal—should be followed, and they called for wide discussion.[184]

In 1990, two prominent palliative care physicians—Christine K. Cassel and Diane E. Meier—called for a shift in medical thinking about the values and needs of patients when medicine is ineffective and death is inevitable. They assert,

> Human support and comfort, adequate control of pain, and true respect for patients' treatment wishes will go a long way toward reducing the demand for assisted suicide or euthanasia. In circumscribed and carefully defined circumstances, however, it may be right to recognize the inevitability of death in a life of unbearable suffering and to help ease this passage.[185]

In 1992 Timothy E. Quill, whose influential article about his participating in the suicide of his patient Diane had been published in 1991,[186] joined Cassel and Meier for the purpose of carefully defining clinical criteria for acceptable—indeed, compelling—PAS. They noted that they supported the legalization of assisted suicide, but not active euthanasia, and, of course, they supported comprehensive palliative, supportive care for the great majority of patients who would benefit from it. Their clinical criteria for PAS included the following: PAS should never be used as a substitute for inclusive palliative care; PAS should be confined to patients with incurable diseases that cause unrelenting suffering; the patient's prognosis should be confirmed by a second medical opinion; patients must clearly, repeatedly, and without distortions from psychiatric illnesses request to die, rather than continue suffering; PAS should be carried out in the context of a meaningful doctor-patient relationship; no physician should be forced to assist a patient in suicide against her or his conscience; clear documentation should be required; the patient should determine whether family members should be told; the lethal medication should be proven to be humane and effective; and the physicians should ideally be present when the lethal medication is taken by the patient.[187]

The physician-ethicist Howard Brody explicated the connections between good death and PAS in 1992. Brody wrote that the aim of palliative care and treatment should be a good death, defined by all the elements of "the highest quality of hospice-style terminal care." But a few patients face bad death in spite of efforts to provide the best terminal care possible. In those instances, PAS should be employed as a last resort that enables patients to exercise final control over their time of death.[188] That same good-versus-bad-death connection was made by Timothy Quill in his 1996 book, which contained haunting stories of his attending to terminally ill patients, several of whom, with Quill's assistance, chose to end their lives. He held that "any intervention that results in a patient's death should be offered only as a last resort, after all reasonable comfort-oriented options have been exhausted." But once all other acceptable alternative measures are tried, "doctors should have the freedom to assist the patient to die as a last resort if it is consistent with their values[s]."[189]

During the 1990s, bills to decriminalize PAS were introduced to 9 states in the

United States. Only one of these bills passed. In 1994 voters of the state of Oregon passed the Death with Dignity Act, legalizing physician-assisted death. Judicial attempts to repeal or limit this act finally ended in 2006. Pressure to pass such legislation continued. In reply to an extensive national survey, 18.3 percent of the reporting physicians indicated they had received a patient's request for assistance with suicide. Six percent replied they had complied with such requests at least once.[190]

Limitations of Aggressive Treatments

The routine use of cardiopulmonary resuscitation changed radically during the 1990s. Whereas in 1987 CPR was being performed on all patients suffering cardiac arrest regardless of their medical conditions, in 1998 it became routine to stop or refrain from starting life-sustaining treatments for terminally ill patients. In the United States and the Netherlands, 90 percent of patients in intensive care units died without resuscitation.[191] In 1996 an empirical study of the care of dying patients in 4 hospitals in Minnesota and Missouri found that 83 percent of patients died without attempted resuscitation, while another 16 percent died during attempted CPR. Another study found that in 1997 65 percent of patients receiving mechanical ventilation had the ventilation withdrawn, in contrast to 10 percent of patients in 1986.[192]

The reasons for this historic change are multifaceted: increasing awareness of the harms and futility of CPR for patients with fatal illnesses; heart-rending stories of overtreatment; the acclaimed but modestly utilized influence of advance directives; the influence of ethical, legal, and medical guidelines for DNR (no–CPR) orders, ventilator support, artificial nutrition and hydration, and other treatments; medical literature on ways to withdraw mechanical ventilation[193]; and increasing awareness that the preconditions for persons experiencing decent, if not good, deaths include the withdrawal of life-sustaining treatments, followed by excellence in end-of-life care.[194]

A fascinating factor that may also have contributed to less CPR use involved the 1996 exposé of the frequency of "miracles" of CPR on television. In a special article in the *New England Journal of Medicine*, Susan J. Diem and others reported what they found after watching and analyzing all the episodes of the television programs *ER* and *Chicago Hope* for a year, as well as 18 episodes of *Rescue 911*. As background, they referenced studies that showed 92 percent of patients over 62 years of age reported obtaining information about CPR from television, and also that patients overestimated their likelihood of survival after CPR—this at a time when end-of-life care was constantly covered in the news media.[195]

Television misinformation abounded. On TV 75 percent of patients survived immediate cardiac arrest and 67 percent appeared to have survived until they were discharged from the hospital. In contrast, the medical literature indicated that between 6.5 percent and 15 percent of hospitalized patients with arrests experienced longer-term survival. On TV only one of the 60 patients depicted suffered a moderate disability from CPR, as opposed to accounts of prolonged suffering, severe neurological damage, and undignified deaths in the medical literature. On *Rescue 911* the term "miracle" was used 56 percent of the time to describe patient survival. As a takeaway message, Diem and her colleagues said,

> To help patients and families make informed decisions, doctors should encourage patients to discuss their impressions of CPR and its chances of success. We should clarify misperceptions, provide actual data on outcomes, and address specifically the differences between CPR as seen on television and CPR as it is experienced by real patients.[196]

A study published a year later found that 90 percent of critically ill patients and/or their surrogate decision makers were accepting physicians' recommendations to limit life-sustaining treatment—an indication that reality could overcome misrepresentation.[197]

Efforts to limit treatments based on doctors' judgments that they would be futile continued on two fronts—medical ethics and policy guidelines. Defending ethical justifications for futility-of-treatment decisions, Timothy Quill and Howard Brody distinguished between two "models" of patient autonomy and defended the second: (1) the independent choice model, wherein the doctor serves as a passive conveyor of medical information to patients about their options and the odds of success for each option and withholds a recommendation that might bias the patient's autonomous decision, versus (2) the "enhanced autonomy option," wherein the physician serves as an active guide in dialogue with patients by informing them about their options and their odds of success, exploring the patient's values, and making recommendations based on the physician's expertise and the patient's values. The central philosophical basis for autonomy is respect for the patient as a person:

> It is not respectful to spare persons from advice or counsel just to maintain neutrality.... Respecting a person means taking the time to listen to that person's unique story and ensuring that medical decisions are integrated into the current chapter of the patient's biography.... Although the final decisions belong to patients, the decisions that result from the intense exchange of medical information, values, and experiences between physician and patient are generally more informed and autonomous than are those made simply on the basis of patient requests.[198]

Further exchanges should occur if patients disagree with physician recommendations. Because the final choice belongs to fully informed patients, if the patient's choice violates the physician's professional integrity, patients should be so informed and attempts should be made to transfer the patient to the care of another physician.

Similar to Quill and Brody, others favored shared patient-doctor decision making over what they termed a "medical cafeteria" approach, in which physicians describe all the therapeutic options and patients choose one.[199] The Scottish authors of a widely sold textbook on palliative care ethics opposed U.S. and U.K. ethicists who advanced "consumer autonomy" that required physicians to continue with patient-requested futile treatments. That view, they argued, forces medicine to cease being a profession upon becoming a service industry. As opposed to an ethics of consumerism, medicine requires professional consultation, "with the patient retaining the right to veto unwarranted treatments and the doctor retaining the right to veto treatments professionally considered useless or harmful."[200] In addition to the United States and Scotland, discussions and debates over futility were occurring in Western Europe, Mediterranean countries, and parts of the Far East.[201]

In the late 1990s, guidelines regarding medical futility began to focus on how to deal with futility *disputes* between doctors and patients and/or family members—often called "futility cases." These guidelines shifted away from earlier ethical justifications for medical futility negotiations between patients and their physicians to *procedures* that should be followed in order to resolve futility disputes—that is, disputes between patients who request continued treatment(s) and physicians who regard the requested treatment(s) as futile. Texas became the first state to adopt a law regulating disputes over medical futility. The Texas Advance Directives Act of 1999 set forth a series of rules for physicians to follow in disputed cases. These included mediation by hospital ethics committees, attempts to transfer the patient to another physician or facility if mediation failed, withholding treatment if no such physician or facility was found within 10 days, and immunity from civil and criminal liability for cessation of treatment by physicians who followed the rules.[202]

Also in 1999, the Council on Ethical and Judicial Affairs of the American Medical Association (AMA) published its report on medical futility disputes in end-of-life care. The council proposed a step-by-step approach to futility disputes: first, earnest attempts by the physician, patient and/or patient's proxy to agree on which treatments are futile; second, attempts to resolve disagreements at the bedside of the critically ill person based on medical outcome data, patient and proxy goals, and informed consent; third, assistance from a medical consultant and patient representative; fourth, involvement by a institutional ethics committee; fifth, attempts to transfer the patient to another physician if resolution seems impossible; and, finally, if transfer is not possible and the patient's and/or proxy's wishes are "considered offensive to medical ethics and professional standards," the medical intervention(s) sought by the patient and/or proxy can be refused.[203] The AMA's approach became a model set of guidelines for years to come.[204]

Education, Training, Textbooks, and Journals

Professional education and training in palliative care from 1995 through 1999 merit a mixed review. In 1997 the Institute of Medicine's *Approaching Death* gave this education and training a failing grade, declaring that they were one of the "very serious" deficiencies in end-of-life care because they failed to provide physicians and other healthcare professionals with "the attitudes, knowledge, and skills required to care well for the dying patient." If that wasn't harsh enough, the IOM committee added that "a curriculum in which death is conspicuous" was mainly notable by its relative absence. Clinical experiences for students and residents largely ignored dying patients and those close to them. In the eyes of the committee, nursing education fared no better: "nursing education also can be faulted for insufficiently preparing nurses to understand the physical, emotional and spiritual needs of dying patients and their families."[205]

Similar low marks were given by others. J. Andrew Billings and Susan Block noted that curricular offerings in palliative end-of-life care were not being integrated into medical teaching and lacked clear standards. T. Patrick Hill held that "by any standard one chooses, medical schools in the United States fail to provide even adequate education in the care of the dying."[206] In 1996 Pam Malloy and others stated that their research on nursing education "demonstrated major deficiencies in palliative care education," revealed that only 2 percent of leading nursing textbooks dealt with end-of-life issues, and proved that nurses were not prepared to provide optimal end-of-life care.[207] Furthermore, reports published in 1995 and 1997 indicated that most U.S. medical schools still only taught death, dying, and terminal care as part of a larger required course—often within a medical ethics course. Approximately 21 percent of the schools polled taught these topics in elective courses.[208]

Yet changes were beginning to occur in post-undergraduate residency programs. Surveys of palliative care teaching in family medicine, internal medicine and other medical residency programs indicated that 60 percent of medical specialty programs had a structured curriculum on end-of-life care—92 percent of family practice and internal medicine residency programs and 65 percent of general surgery programs. An extensive survey of oncology nurses in 1999 found that 26 percent believed they had an excellent level of preparation for effective end-of-life care, and 54 percent felt they had good preparation. Seventy-four percent had received between 1 and 4 hours of continuing education in palliative care over the previous two years. Some educators believed that significant gains and improvements were under way with respect to outlines of basic principles of palliative care in the cure-focused culture of academic medicine, to the design of training initiatives, and to other initiatives.[209] Better education in palliative care was being provided in Canada and the United Kingdom. All of Canada's medical schools required between 5 and 20 hours of education and training, and an average of 7 hours of curriculum time was required in the United Kingdom.[210]

Beyond actual changes in education and training lay ardent hopes that far better palliative care education and training were in the making. Viewing the times as "ripe for changing," Linda Blank proposed ways to define and evaluate competence in end-of-life care. In spite of its initial harsh criticisms, *Approaching Death* spent the better part of a chapter on the core components of professional training and on 11 proven-effective educational strategies for improving end-of-life care. It concluded that most of its goals could be achieved and the initiatives already under way should be encouraged and monitored. In their survey of medical and nursing end-of-life education in the United States, Felicity Audino and Kathleen Foley identified many of the new initiatives, including those sponsored by the American Board of Internal Medicine, fellowship training programs, faculty development programs, the Compassionate Competent Care Initiative of the AMA, and the national initiative of the End-of-Life Nursing Education Consortium.[211]

Textbooks and journals on palliative care up to the end of the 20th century also deserve mixed reviews. With respect to standard nursing and clinical textbooks that served as cornerstones in the training of nurses, medical students, and medical residents, a 1998 critique of the literature found that death was rarely mentioned in these texts, "and the physician's imperative to fight the disease to the bitter end by all means possible, including the latest experimental therapy, is overwhelmingly reinforced." For example, the 1998 edition of *Harrison's Principles of Internal Medicine* gave less than a page to end-of-life issues in its introductory chapter on medicine's mission and gave no index references to the topics of palliative care, comfort care, or hospice.[212] A multi-authored article in 1999 gave the end-of-life content in a top-of-the-line medical and nursing textbook a failing grade in terms of both content areas and indexing.[213]

That was the bad news. The good news was that a number of national medical and nursing organizations at the end of the century were undertaking reviews of nursing and medical texts, identifying experts to write in these texts, persuading publishers that chapters on end-of-life issues were financially worthwhile, rewarding the best of the earliest authors of these chapters, and inserting palliative care questions on licensing examinations.[214]

More good news was that in the 1990s textbooks entirely focused on palliative care "came of age."[215] In Great Britain, where palliative medicine had long been recognized as a medical specialty, the *Oxford Textbook of Palliative Medicine* was first published in 1993, and then revised as a second edition in 1998. That practice-oriented text contained informative chapters on pain management, treatment of common physical symptoms, communication skills, psychological and religious issues, and an overview of palliative care ethics based on patient self-determination. Later editions included internationally known editors and writers.

Additional textbooks published in the United States, Great Britain, and Australia quickly followed. In the United Kingdom, Robert Twycross's continually updated editions of *Introducing Palliative Care* were published in 1995, 1997, 1999, and 2002. Beginning his career as a clinical research fellow at St. Christopher's Hospice with Cicely Saunders in 1971, and renowned for his leadership and additional publications, Twycross developed a training program that served as the foundation for his *Introducing* text, which became used in many nations around the world. Textbooks in the United States included A. Waller and N. L. Caroline's *Handbook of Palliative Care in Cancer* (1996), A. Berger and others' *Principles and Practice of Supportive Oncology* (1997), *Palliative Medicine: A Case-Based Manual* (edited by N. MacDonald in 1998), and the ongoing editions of *Primer of Palliative Care*.[216] Expert information on all aspects of palliative care became available in texts as well as in hundreds of journal articles.

Finally, 1998 witnessed the birth of a pivotal journal that became a flagship in its field: the *Journal of Palliative Medicine* (*JPM*). Recognizing that "never before has medical care near life's end had so much attention in the medical and popular press," the editor of the new *JPM* outlined the need for a peer-reviewed journal devoted entirely to care near the end of life. The new journal would disseminate accurate and timely information to a wide readership, including scientifically rigorous clinical research studies, innovative education methods, and health policy discussions.[217] It began as a quarterly publication but moved to six issues per year in 2002, and then to monthly issues beginning in 2009.

Concluding Perspectives

The journey of palliative care over the 18-year period from 1982 through 1999 is absorbing and multi-themed. Talented, well-trained, and devoted leaders and organizations enabled hospices to experience great growth and to model ideals of good dying. With great efforts on many fronts, overused and onerous practices to stave off inevitable death were significantly curtailed. Greater measures of palliation were now occurring in hospitals, while textbooks and journals were coming of age.

Endurance after the deeply disturbing findings of the SUPPORT study in 1995 reflected a remarkable change in orientation: programmatic and socially powerful commitments to bring palliative, comfort-focused care to greater fruition.

But obstacles remained. Communication between caregivers and fatally ill persons remained poor. And the lack of professional education and training in palliative care and treatment that had been recognized since the time of John Ferriar in 1798 remained deeply problematic. Whether that caring and expertise would become a standard component in medical and nursing education—from its basic science and humanities beginnings to initial clinical training, and then on to post-graduate specialty training—was, in fact, utterly critical.

Thoughtful writers knew that. They knew the SUPPORT study proved that the existing dynamics of the medical system were inhospitable to the essence and aims of palliative medical care. Mirrored in standard medical textbooks, in continually amazing medical discoveries, and in Sherwin Nuland's *How We Die*, the culture of the academic health center remained committed to the curative model of medical care. Diseases—including terminal diseases—were still being treated aggressively until death became inevitable. That goal constituted medicine's "hidden curriculum."[218]

The dominance of cure-oriented diagnosis and treatment created an aversion to (and avoidance of) the care and treatment of terminal patients on the part of many young medical and nurse trainees.[219] Medical and nursing education in palliative care for dying patients faced the uphill challenge of enabling medical and nursing students, resident physicians, and faculty mentors to find meaning and fulfillment in end-of-life care.

For almost 400 years, advocates of palliative care did not equate death with defeat, but rather with the natural and inevitable conclusion of life in patterned and manifold ways. That, they held, becomes a wellspring of motivation for the nurturing of human relationships, for the attainment of worthy ends during life, and for enabling caregivers to ensure that the last chapter of life is as meaningful and peaceful as possible. This quest for peaceful death led a number of palliative caregivers during and after the late 1980s to endorse physician-assisted suicide.

By the end of the 20th century, prominent leaders in palliative care were saying, "By any measure, efforts to improve care for the incurably ill and dying has never been more alive and well."[220] Speaking about the care of dying patients near the end of the 20th century, Jordan Cohen, the president of the Association of American Medical Colleges, exclaimed, "We may be on the verge of a real breakthrough—a 'teachable moment'—in our thinking about an area too long kept in the nether regions of our profession's agenda."[221] To what degrees would the teachable moment of the 20th century become an informed agenda in the 21st century?

9

Choices

2000 to the Present

The chronological brevity of this final era in the story of palliative care disguises the enormity of its significance. It is filled with personal meaning for all readers. As the historical capstone, it describes pivotal developments in contemporary palliative care. At the same time, these developments are laden with personal, existential meaning for seriously ill patients and their family members, for patients-to-be, and for healthcare providers. This is true because several topics in this chapter pertain to *choices* that are being, and will eventually need to be, made.

For centuries, only limited numbers of incurably ill patients could make their own choices regarding aggressive, cure-directed treatment or palliative care. For years physicians made paternalistic life-and-death decisions without the patient's knowledge or input. If patients and their family members were fortunate enough to be cared for by physicians like Alfred Worcester, Walter Alvarez, Edward Rynearson or Porter Storey, they could express their wishes and have them carried out. But with the advent of scientific medicine in the 1880s, hospitalized patients were usually not allowed to choose how they would spend their last months, weeks, and days of life. By the 1960s patients became isolated and virtually powerless in hospitals. Countless persons were subjected to CPR without having any say in the matter. Even after patients' rights of free choice were championed and increasingly upheld by law during and after the 1970s, patients' choices were far more imagined than real—as the SUPPORT study of 1995 proved. This chapter will explore how choices regarding further treatment or palliative care are now far more secure.

Beyond the issue of deciding whether to receive either curative treatment or comfort-directed care, the word *choices* denotes three additional issues. First, it pertains to an expansion of available options—in particular, the option of being able to choose *both* curative and comfort care in hospitals and hospice programs, such that even patients opting for hospice care might be able to continue receiving various types of cure-oriented treatments. Second, to make these choices meaningful, readers, patients, and healthcare givers must clearly understand what contemporary palliative care is—how it is defined and what its components and advantages are. If contemporary palliative care is poorly understood, palliative care is, at best, a secondary, fallback option, not a genuinely informed choice. The historical developments charted in this chapter accent how these choices must be informed. And third, the word *choice* should not be misconstrued as denoting decisions that are easily or lightly made. The choices discussed here often involve arduously and reluctantly made decisions: *Should I continue to pursue further aggressive medical treatments in hopes of prolonging my life? Should I, or when should I, opt for non-aggressive palliative hospital or hospice care? Might I have the option of pursuing **both** curative and palliative care in hospital and even hospice programs? Are the last options real or imagined? What assurances do I have that they are real? What assurances do I have that my choices will be respected?*

It takes no stunning act of the imagination to recognize how these choices are fraught with enormous emotional weight. They encompass ultimate questions surrounding each severely or terminally ill person's life, personality, relationships, and accomplishments in the face of inescapable mortality. Decisions about them are made against the backdrop of the historic successes and continuing promises of modern disease-targeted medicine. Knowingly or not, they are infused by centuries of tension between physicians who sought to soothe the pangs of approaching death and physicians intent on extending patients' lives.

Here is the outline of the main topics that follow: the momentum and magnetism of modern curative medicine; a primer on contemporary palliative care; the remarkable expansion of hospital and hospice programs; enhanced professional status of palliative medicine; physician-assisted suicide; obstacles to, and permissible limitations on, patient choices; ensuring choices; and exploring good death.

The Momentum and Magnetism of Modern Curative Medicine

The remarkable advances in modern medicine's cure-directed and life-prolonging interventions continue without pause. The story of palliative care highlights how it intersects with the history of medical advances and the power of medical institutions. The cascade of medical progress over more than 130 years has saved countless lives. It also accounts for the enduring momentum and institutionalized dynamics of the multi-trillion-dollar edifice of modern medicine.

Medicine's magnetism and mystique attracts constant attention from the media. Like the votive tablets found at the Greek sanctuaries of Asclepius at Epidaurus and Titane, accounts of seemingly miraculous cures have been chiseled into the minds and hearts of healers and the public.[1] Stories like the recovery of renowned paleontologist Stephen Jay Gould from "incurable" abdominal cancer inspire the practices of 21st-century physicians, and they inform decisions of persons who read about cures of patients with seemingly terminal diseases.[2]

No person present at the monthly morbidity and mortality conference at the Dartmouth-Hitchcock Medical Center in New Hampshire will forget the case of a twenty-seven-year-old patient with HIV-AIDS. The patient was diagnosed with acute respiratory distress syndrome (ARDS) due to pneumonia in both lungs. As the audience awaited the answer to the final cause of his death, the former patient and his family entered the conference hall. The audience gasped, and then erupted into applause and a standing ovation. The patient had been hospitalized for 139 days. He'd spent over 50 percent of that time in the intensive care unit at the cost of over a million dollars. That he was now alive seemed "utterly sublime."[3]

Medical breakthroughs in the 21st century include the following:

- The dramatic release of the blueprint of the entire human genome (genetic makeup) in 2000, reissued in even greater detail in 2003 and 2009. This project became extremely important for disease prevention and the promise of medical cures for cancers, cardiovascular disease, and other maladies.
- The development and worldwide use of a far more effective class of "clot busting" drugs for persons suffering from heart disease and acute heart attacks from artery blockage in which angioplasty (opening blockages within the arteries) and the insertion of artery-expanding stents are not readily available.[4]
- New cancer drugs genetically targeted to stop cancer cell growth and prevent breast and other cancers from reoccurring, including the discovery of imatinib—first marketed as Gleevec, approved by the FDA in May 2001 and pictured on the cover of *TIME* as the "magic bullet" to cure cancer.[5]
- A variety of remarkable developments for patients requiring intensive care for heart and respiratory failure, including advances in extracorporeal membrane oxygenation for patients whose hearts and/or lungs are so severely diseased or damaged that they no longer effectively function, and, amazingly, a number of sophisticated artificial heart pumps that promise to "supplant heart transplantation as the ultimate therapy for severe heart failure."[6]
- Minimally invasive and more precise techniques with robotic surgery, as well as numerous other areas of discovery, including breakthroughs based on stem cell research, magnetic resonance images (MRI) to track the workings of the brain, cameras taken as pills, bionic hands and limbs, and face transplant surgery.

These and many other advances enable modern practitioners to believe that "there's almost always something else we could offer" as treatment for patients.[7]

Patients and Doctors Fight for Life

Present-day medicine often inspires patients and their doctors to fight for continued life up to the threshold of death. These fights are mirrored in cancer treatment and research. Consider, for example, efforts to triumph over cancer by patients, on the one hand, and efforts to eradicate cancers by physician oncologists, on the other.

In their study of the use of chemotherapy in 2008, Sarah Elizabeth Harrington and Thomas J. Smith point out how critical it is to understand the perspective of many cancer patients who are "looking death in the eye." Studies from the United States, England, Canada, Japan, Norway, and Italy consistently show that patients with cancer are generally willing to undergo aggressive treatment with major adverse side effects in exchange for minimal benefit. Some patients with previously treated non–small cell lung cancer will accept chemotherapy for a survival benefit as short as one week. Highly educated patients say they are willing to enroll in the initial phase of cancer research with an experimental drug even if the drug will cause the deaths of 10 percent of the enrollees. In 2008 the medical director of a large insurance company reported that 16 percent of its cancer patients receive chemotherapy within 14 days of death, even though chemotherapy produces adverse effects, leads to hospitalization and emergency room visits, excludes patients from enrolling in most hospices, is expensive, and contributes little to the patient's overall quality of life.[8]

Part of Ronald Lands's poem about a patient who battles death to his life's end applies to numerous cancer patients. The patient is "a fighter" in a boxing ring against death. He's looking for the chance to deal a crushing body blow, followed by a mighty uppercut "to death's square jaw."[9]

Patients' expectations and determined efforts to rage against disease are due in part to continued media coverage of new cancer cures. Billboards announced in 2005: "We're closing in on a killer! The killer is leukemia and the cure is at hand!"[10]

Cancer patients' fights for continued life often go hand-in-hand with doctors' determination to keep them alive. A 2007 study found that the very late referrals of cancer patients to hospice care were largely due to oncologists' routinely overestimating patients' remaining life spans.[11] In the mid- to late 1990s various efforts were made to limit the use of anti-cancer drugs to two courses of chemotherapy, but many oncologists refused to stop until up to five different regimens were attempted. By the late 1990s this piece of gallows humor was making the rounds:

> MEDICAL INTERN 1: Why do they put nails in the coffin?
> INTERN 2: I give up.
> INTERN 1: To keep the oncologists from giving one last round of chemo![12]

Serious concerns lie behind the counter-phobic humor. A 2008 study found that only some 30 percent of terminally ill patients with cancer were told they were terminally ill by their oncologists.[13] Equally, if not more troubling, a 2012 empirical study of the relationship between patient preferences and patients' continuing to receive chemotherapy found that, regardless of whether patients personally preferred comfort or palliative care only, they still opted to receive chemotherapy. They also chose to receive additional chemotherapy even if they believed that further treatments would not affect their cancers. The authors offered several possible reasons for these findings: patients feeling that their doubts about additional chemotherapy would undermine their physicians' commitment to cure, inadequate shared decision making by doctors and patients, and physicians' reluctance to engage in painful end-of-life discussions.[14] In May 2014, a palliative care specialist, Diane E. Meier, observed that some oncologists persist in recommending questionable chemotherapy because to do otherwise conveys the idea that they are abandoning their patients.[15] Falsely equating palliative care with surrendering to death, other physicians paternalistically prevent patients from receiving such care throughout the course of serious and fatal illness.[16]

When I was making oncology ward rounds with a research fellow in oncology, we visited a patient whom I will call Willie. Knowing that Willie's metastatic bone cancer was responsible for his suffering from broken bones during the night before our scheduled visit, the head of oncology said he wanted to meet us in Willie's room. When the three of us entered, the chief of oncology gave Willie a pep talk: "I know, Willie, that you had a very bad night. But don't give up! There's always hope! We still have experimental cancer drugs that we're excited about." After the impressive-looking, ever-optimistic chief left, I asked, "Willie, what did you think of what the doctor just said?" Willie paused, then drawled, "I don't believe a word he said, but I sure did like to hear it."

For Willie's doctor and for many other oncologists, "The enemy is cancer, and we want it defeated and destroyed."[17] By 2008 a unifying refrain among palliative caregivers in the United States and around the world voiced the belief that oncologists were the most difficult group to deal with in the provision of palliative care near the end of life. In a second breath, those caregivers recognized that some oncologists are "fabulous" in attending to the emotional needs of their patients, in clearly communicating about end-of-life care, and in helping patients and families cope with death.[18]

The story of Willie raises the topic of experimental chemotherapy, which illustrates the extent to which patients and physician researchers fight to extend life.[19] Phase I cancer research protocols test for the safety and toxicity of drugs proven to have anti-cancer effects in prior animal and laboratory studies. They are *not* designed to measure new drugs' therapeutic effects and benefits, but rather to take the first step that will enable the extent of these benefits to be determined in the next two phases of research.[20] Phase II research investigates approved Phase I drugs on one type of cancer to find if they may be promising treatments.[21] Phase III compares drugs that are shown to work in Phase II with standard, presently approved treatments. The chances of being cured of one's cancer are thus significantly higher in Phase III protocols.[22]

Typically, only patients with metastatic cancers who have already exhausted standard cancer treatment options can enroll in Phase I trials. Their chances of benefiting from Phase I cancer trials, not to speak of being cured, are low.[23] Patients with advanced cancers that have not yet responded to treatments nevertheless readily enter Phase I trials. However small the chance of a cure may be, patients often opt to fight for that chance.[24] Among the 2.5 percent of research subjects whose cancers "respond" to Phase I drugs—usually by not growing or by shrinking—are those who joyfully announce, "A ... Phase I trial saved my life!"[25]

The eight-month journey of Sara Thomas Monopoli depicts the path taken by many cancer patients. Diagnosed with inoperable non–small cell lung cancer that had spread to multiple lymph nodes in her chest and its lining, Sara endured four rounds of four types of approved cancer drugs and five days of radiation treatment. None of these worked, and all contributed to shortness of breath, dry heaves, coughing up blood, and severe fatigue. Her lung cancer had spread through her spine, liver, and brain. But Sara, her family, and her medical team still "remained in a battle mode," which led her to be scheduled for a Phase I drug trial. Telling about Sara's battle, the surgeon and well-known writer Atul Gawande says,

> Our every impulse is to fight, to die with chemo in our veins or a tube in our throats or fresh sutures in our flesh. The fact that we may be shortening or worsening the time we have left hardly seems to register. We imagine that we can wait until the doctors tell us that there is nothing more they can do. But rarely is there **nothing** more that doctors can do.... We want those choices. We don't want anyone ... to limit them.[26]

With her husband's and family's consent, Sara's primary care physician took charge of her care a day and a half before she died. He called in a palliative care team that prescribed a dose of morphine. Her suffering eased. No more inserted catheters, no lab tests, no finger sticks were allowed. "At least she was spared at the very end."[27]

Between Hopeful Determination and Uncertainty

Sara's struggle exemplifies the journeys of many who fight for life with fierce determination and hope. They answer "YES" to the first question posed at the beginning of this chapter: *Should I continue to pursue further aggressive medical treatments in hopes of prolonging my life?* They also illustrate how not death, but rather continued resistance against death, becomes the root cause of physical, emotional, and spiritual suffering.[28] Ira Byock, a well-known author and expert in palliative care, observes that "sometimes families interpret any greater-than-zero prognosis as good news."[29]

The emotional tensions between fighting for further medically prolonged life and accepting one's inevitable death beset numerous critically ill patients and their families with uncertainty, with vacillations between hope for recovery and a final acceptance of dying as peacefully as possible. That was what Robert Arnold found when he entered the ranks of palliative care consultants in 2000: "Ambiguity, ambivalence, and uncertainty rather than acceptance or planning for death dominates ... discussions [with] these patients and their families." While the minds and hearts of patients and families are often filled with double-mindedness, inconsistency, and puzzlement, many of their physicians are action-oriented and focused on the promises of cures. "While 'do no harm' may be the ancient Hippocratic oath, 'do something' is the American way." Over time, Arnold no longer became confused "when a patient who has decided to go to hospice tells me about her interest in a new experimental therapy," and he understood why a doctor at the last minute offers a therapy to a patient he knows to be dying. He found that ambiguity and ambivalence are central to the dying process in contemporary culture.[30] In 2012 Byock described how the uncertainty of "letting a loved one die" on the part of family members sometimes continues until the patient dies with no family members present.[31] A recent survey found that a growing minority of polled patients— 15 percent in 1990 and 31 percent in 2013—believed that physicians should always do everything possible to extend patients' lives.[32]

Costs

Seriously ill patients and patients with multiple chronic conditions and function impairments constitute 10 percent of patients in U.S. hospitals and consume over 50 percent of the nation's healthcare costs. These costs are especially great for patients receiving life-prolonging and life-sustaining treatments during their final year of life. During that time 5 percent of patients consume 25–30 percent of all U.S. Medicare spending, which amounts to more than $150 billion annually. Each day in an ICU can cost at least $10,000, and nearly one in five Americans spend their last days in an ICU. The "sickest patients"—the 5–10 percent of patients with five or more chronic conditions—drive over two-thirds of total healthcare costs, including Medicare and commercial insurance-covered costs.[33]

Medical costs continue to rise exponentially for understandable reasons. They reflect continued advancements in sophisticated ways of prolonging life, as well as the fact that many persons facing death are beset with grave and complex illnesses. They also reflect unresolved problems within the healthcare system. For example, many persons living at home who are not eligible for Medicare hospice coverage experience a series of medical crises that require ambulance services, emergency room treatment, and hospitalization, after which they return home to wait, as it were, for the next emergency to occur. Once patients are hospitalized, they are given numerous diagnostic tests and sophisticated interventions, some of which are unwanted.[34] Underutilization of palliative hospital and hospice care also contributes to these rising costs.[35]

A Primer on Contemporary Palliative (Supportive) Care

Given the prestige, power, and promises of contemporary medical science and life-extending practices, why should patients ever opt for palliative care? Why would supportive care expand in growth and influence? Why wouldn't, why *shouldn't*, this care for severely ill and dying patients languish at the edges of hospital practice? Why, instead, did the provision of palliative care in hospitals, hospices, homes, and nursing homes greatly expand and strengthen in the 21st century and provide many patients with more choices?

The pursuit of answers to these questions acquaints readers with the content, spirit, and driving forces behind contemporary palliative/supportive care, thereby enabling persons to make informed choices with respect to the treatment and care they want to receive during the last phases of life.

The spirit underlying all particular answers is the classic, often-quoted ethical truism articulated in a lecture by Francis Weld Peabody, who, knowing that he was dying, reminded his medical school audience that "the secret of the care of the patient is caring for the patient."[36] That conviction undergirds the moral imperative of caring for increasing numbers of patients with chronic, debilitating, life-threatening, and life-ending illnesses.[37]

Definitions of Palliative Care

The previous chapter shows that beginning in the 1990s palliative care began to extend beyond comfort-directed care at the end of life. Often referred to as palliative medicine, this care includes symptom relief and person-centered attention for patients with life-threatening medical conditions who continue to receive disease-targeted therapies. This expanded understanding characterizes the scope of palliative care in the 21st century. Hospice care, now regarded as a *component* of palliative care/palliative medicine, also includes palliative measures for hospitalized and out-patients whose conditions may be potentially curable, chronic, life-threatening, or life-ending.[38]

The updated 2002 version of the definition of palliative care by the World Health Organization (WHO) serves as the flagship definition worldwide. WHO defines palliative care as "an approach that improves the quality of life of patients and their families facing the problems associated with life-threatening illness" that is "applicable early in the course of illness, in conjunction with other therapies that are intended to prolong life."[39] Translated into many languages, WHO's principles are being promoted beyond the confines of the United Kingdom, Canada, the United States, and Western Europe to Eastern Europe, Central Asia, Africa, India and Latin America.[40]

To ensure consistently high-quality palliative care in existing and developing programs in the United States, in 2002 the National Consensus Project (NCP) carefully defined this care and set forth an extensive set of clinical practice guidelines for all of its components. These guidelines were refined and expanded in 2009. They were formulated after intense debate and discussion by representatives of five major organizations in the United States, including the American Academy of Hospice and Palliative Medicine (AAHPM), the Hospice and Palliative Nurses Association (HPNA), the Center to Advance Palliative Care (CAPC—a palliative care advocacy organization), and the National Hospice and Palliative Care Organization (NHPCO). The NCP blueprint became normative for palliative caregivers and was adopted by the U.S. Center for Medicare and Medicaid Services (CMA).[41] In her impressive autobiographical overview of palliative care in the United States beginning in the 1990s, Diane E. Meier says these guidelines became "a major impetus toward improving access to palliative and hospice care in this country."[42]

Here is the NCP's definition of palliative care and treatment for hospitals and hospices, as well as out-patient, nursing home, and other programs:

> The goal of palliative care is to prevent and relieve suffering and to support the best possible quality of life for patients and their families, regardless of the stage of the disease or the need for other therapies. Palliative care is both a philosophy of care and an organized, highly structured system of delivering care. Palliative care expands traditional disease-model medical treatments to include the goals of enhancing quality of life for patient and family, optimizing function, helping with decision making, and providing opportunities for personal growth. As such, it can be delivered concurrently with life-prolonging cure or as the main focus of care.[43]

Efforts to palliate earlier stages of disease expression and progression have been reinforced by extensive clinical research and have increasingly brought palliative care to the "hard" side of mainline medicine.[44]

Core Elements of Modern Comfort-Focused Care

Many of the essential features of palliative care were described in the writings of notable physicians beginning with John Ferriar at the end of the 18th century. But the modern necessity of defining the purview of all medical specializations led palliative care practitioners to outline the core elements of their work.[45] This is reflected in the work of the NCP. These elements encompass expert relief of physical, bodily symptoms and suffering; communication enabling patients to identify their goals, learn about their options, and choose their preferences; attention to and due care for other dimensions of patient meaning (emotional, social, spiritual, and cultural); continuity of care between hospitals, hospices, homes and nursing homes; bereavement counseling for relatives, partners, and close friends; and responsibility with respect to ethical and legal issues embedded in palliative care.[46] These dimensions of palliative care are presented here as six categories.

First, palliative care providers must become experts in symptom relief for pain, shortness of breath, fatigue, anorexia, nausea, and many other disease sequelae, the details of which are extensively researched and utilized.[47] Foregoing chapters in this book describe how easing the physical symptoms of dying persons became historic concerns for caregivers. As palliative care expanded, palliative measures were discovered and used to ease the symptoms of populations of patients with chronic illnesses, as well as patients undergoing arduous curative and life-saving treatments. Twenty-first-century palliative medicine professionals essentially say to hospitalized and out-patients, "If you opt for ongoing aggressive treatments that have the chance of being successful, we will do all that we can to enable you to receive them as painlessly as possible."

Second, palliative care specialists are trained to assist patients in identifying their personal goals, learning about their treatment options, and choosing which they prefer. This requires expert skills in communication and an awareness of patients' cultural backgrounds. Patients' options may include choosing further aggressive treatment, choosing disease-directed treatment concurrently with palliative care, choosing nonaggressive hospice care, and knowingly and freely choosing to allow the doctor to decide what care seems best.

Decisions regarding these choices are crucial and often challenging. They must be based on each patient's values and preferences insofar as chosen courses of action are compatible with acceptable medical practices. Patients' treatment goals must be aligned with their characteristic approaches to life. Enabling patients to harmonize their life goals with treatment decisions often requires detailed and accurate information sharing provided in a timely manner by caregivers.

Expertise in effective *interpersonal communication* is essential, all the more so because failures in communication became unmistakably apparent after the mid–1990s. The driving forces behind the necessity of effective communication include cultural values, philosophical ethics, the law, and the professional relationships of doctors, nurses, hospital chaplains, and counselors with the patients they serve. Ethically and legally, health professionals are obligated to respect the rights and autonomy of patients and to ensure that patients are benefited rather than harmed. Professionals undermine patient autonomy if they do not share their expertise and knowledge concerning each patient's diagnosis and prognosis and enable patients or their surrogates to make informed decisions.[48]

Representing palliative care specialists, Laura C. Hanson asserted in 2011,

> Communication is our procedure and core skill. Good communication is not sufficient to improve quality of life for a patient living with serious illness, but it is a necessary prerequisite to all of our effective interventions.... When we do this job well, we spend far more time than other clinicians simply listening and communicating with patients and families.[49]

Effective communication is itself palliative, and communication failures can contribute to unnecessary pain and suffering.[50]

Barriers to efficacious physician-patient discussions include physicians' fears of causing emotional suffering, their views of death as an enemy and a sign of medical defeat, their lack of interpersonal skills, and their reluctance to convey bad news.[51] Importantly, however, studies have found that communication over end-of-life issues was not stressful to the great majority of providers and patients[52] and was desired by patients who wanted straightforward, compassionate, and realistic discussions with their doctors.[53] A 2008 study disclosed that patients who had such discussions were more likely to prefer symptom-control treatments and less likely to undergo resuscitation.[54]

Sensitive and workable guidelines for interpersonal communication have been set forth by experienced palliative care professionals. They involve do's and don'ts, steps to follow, tried and true techniques, questions used to initiate discussions and elicit the patient's own questions, and topics to be discussed. In 2000 Timothy E. Quill wrote an outstanding article about initiating discussions with seriously ill patients. Ten years later, with Quill as its lead editor, the 5th edition of *Primer of Palliative Care* succinctly outlined and added to Quill's initial themes that enable patients to make their own choices.[55] R. Sean Morrison, Diane E. Meier, and others added to the wisdom and depth of these discussions.[56] The importance of timely and effective discussions concerning future or near-term enrollment in hospice care have also been thoughtfully analyzed and outlined.[57]

Effective communication inescapably depends upon providers' understanding the cultural backgrounds of patients and their families—their economic circumstances, their educations and preoccupations, and their ethnic and religious worlds of meaning. At times providers must become familiar with patients' cultures—become "culturally competent"—so that patients will be understood and respected. The literature on these matters is extensive.[58] Studies explore the differing cultural perspectives of African Americans, Muslims, and Hindus, as well as the clashes between medical specialists, nurses, and chaplains.[59] Knowing about these perspectives includes, but far exceeds, cultural sensitivity. A recent survey, for example, found that 26 percent of Anglo-Americans report that they want their doctors to do everything possible to prolong their lives, in contrast to 61 percent of African Americans and 55 percent of Hispanic Americans.[60]

Regrettably, studies of physicians in a variety of specializations other than palliative care showed that their communication often falls short of this second core element of palliative care. An innovative study of physician-patient pairs compared what physicians reported they said with what patients reported they heard. The concordances between them varied from very good to very poor: 92 percent agreement on diagnosis, 70 percent agreement on the need for and referral to spiritual counseling, 69 percent on whether hospice was discussed, 49 percent on whether emergency care should be sought, and only 14 percent on whether the physician knew their patients' preferences for pain management and place of death.[61]

Third, palliative care includes attention to the psychological, social, and spiritual dimensions of patients' suffering.[62] This underlines the necessity of collaboration and teamwork. Teams of caregivers should include a core group of professionals from medicine, nursing, social work, clergy, pharmacy, and other areas.[63] Christopher A. Gibson and others give an excellent overview of psychiatrists' and psychologists' roles in palliative care with respect to psychotherapy and medications for anxiety, depression, suicide, delirium, pain, fatigue, and other concerns.[64]

Too often the social dimensions of patients' needs are listed in pro-forma fashion. The National Consensus Project's *Clinical Practice Guidelines*, for example, call for a comprehensive and documented social assessment of everything from social networks to finances, living arrangements, access to transportation, and community resources.[65] Such listings easily overlook the bottom-line importance of family and friendship relationships, communication, forgiveness, gratitude, recollections, and love, which are universal sources of meaning and reasons to live for sick and dying patients.[66]

Maryjo Prince-Paul rightly points out that these dimensions of human life too often remain "untapped" even though they should characterize the care of nurse professionals.[67] Historically, nurses often recognized the value of healing relationships with patients and family members.[68] These relationships were fostered by historic figures in palliative care. In a study published in 2009, Anthony L. Back and colleagues indicated that patients and family members sometimes feel abandoned when their primary care physicians fail to stay in contact after they refer patients to hospice care, not to speak of what patients feel when some doctors tell those who try to stay in contact, "I don't need to see you."[69]

The importance of patients' and family members' religious, spiritual, and existential concerns as sources of meaning and coping has been increasingly recognized and investigated since the 1990s.[70] In the United States, courses on spirituality for medical and nursing students have greatly expanded. They often begin with data about the importance of religion in patients' lives—for example, how over 90 percent of Americans say they believe in God or a universal spirit, and how 40 percent of elderly patients say faith is the most important factor enabling them to cope with illness. Courses then turn to interactive topics, such as how to take a non-intrusive, clinically relevant "spiritual history": Is faith important to you? Are you part of a religious or spiritual community? How would you like me to address these issues in your care? These and many other topics, including when to call for certified chaplain consultations, are discussed as essential dimensions of comfort care, because severe illness can lead patients to question their worth and meaning.[71]

In their practical, well-researched article, Karen E. Steinhauser and others indicated why and how one question can be used to initiate and probe patients' spiritual concerns: "Are you at peace?" Three years later Christina Puchalski and others published a complex report and analysis based on the work of a Consensus Conference that summarized "Quality of Spiritual Care as a Dimension of Palliative Care."[72]

Fourth, palliative care includes providing continuity of care across settings—within hospitals and between hospitals, hospices, homes, and nursing homes.[73] The guidelines of the National Consensus Project outline the duties of palliative caregivers to ensure continuity of care, which is viewed as imperative in order for patients to receive the highest-quality care throughout their illnesses. This requires informing patients with incurable illnesses about available hospice and other community resources. It also presupposes accurate knowledge on the part of caregivers about the differences between hospital-based and hospice palliative care, as well as which hospice programs offer first-rate end-of-life care.[74] Continuity of care also calls for partnerships between hospitals and out-of-hospital palliative care programs, and it requires routine meetings between hospital-based and hospice team members.

Many, if not most, patients and families have problems when they try to negotiate within the healthcare system.[75] The complexities and variety of these systems are daunting—all the more so when patients do not know how to match their respective medical conditions with the best healthcare setting. Expert palliative care includes assisting patients with these matches.

Fifth, expertise in palliative care recognizes and attends to the needs of family members with the recognition that families are multifaceted—relatives, spouses and their relatives, partners, and close friends. Those needs were recognized by William Munk in 1887, Alfred Worcester in 1928, Walter Alvarez in 1952, and, of course, Cicely Saunders throughout her career. The World Health Organization includes family care as an essential component of palliative care.[76] Family support should be provided by physicians, nurses, palliative care teams, trained counselors, and clergy.[77]

Family care includes counsel, emotional support, and regular meetings between family members and palliative care professionals. Discussion topics include how their loved one's condition has changed, what the family's concerns and wishes are, and how they are dealing with grief and loss.[78] Expert family care needs to be thoroughly considered and learned. Its complexities include guidelines for family meetings, communication skills, cultural awareness, and knowledge about varieties of family responses. These responses vary from openness and clarity about hopes, fears, and doubts to masked feelings or strained and conflicting relationships that inhibit communication.[79]

Family members experience the dying and death of loved ones in a variety of ways. John Hardwig poignantly describes the impact of death on many family members: "A death in the family is often ... a *spiritual* crisis ... a crisis *for the family,* not [only] for the patient." Family members need to be helped in finding new hopes—"that Mom will be granted a peaceful and pain-free death, that she knew she was loved, and that the unraveled fabric of the family can be reknit without the pivotal role Mom always played."[80]

The first-hand stories told by Ira Byock confirm and supplement the wisdom of Hardwig's counsel. Families must be encouraged not to postpone making difficult decisions for mentally compromised loved ones. They may need help distinguishing between withdrawal of life-prolonging treatments and abandonment. They may need advice with respect to understanding that transferring a loved one to an ICU or persisting in high-tech rescue efforts can be a form of abandonment. A guilty spouse or child or other relative who demands that everything possible be done for the patient should not be vilified, but rather counseled that he or she is voicing very human emotions, but that his or her demands will possibly add to suffering.[81]

And, *sixth,* palliative care professionals must be acquainted with and responsive to the many ethical issues embedded in the treatment and care they provide—a study in itself.[82] These issues include aligning clinical actions with the fundamental principles of medical ethics inherent in discussions throughout this and foregoing chapters. They include duties of beneficence, prevention of harm, truth telling, respect for patients' rights to make their own choices, and adherence to these moral principles over other values such as cost savings. This history displays the inevitable roles of ethical issues in comfort-directed care. These issues surround advance directives for patients and/ or their surrogate decision makers; withholding or withdrawing life-sustaining ventilation, dialysis, antibiotics, and intravenous nutrition and hydration; judgments regarding medical futility; palliative sedation even if it causes unconsciousness or earlier death, which is widely regarded as morally acceptable[83]; and euthanasia and physician-assisted suicide (the first consistently opposed, the second considered morally acceptable by several palliative care specialists beginning in the last decades of the 20th century).[84]

Generalists' Roles and Education

In accordance with the tradition of expertise in palliative care that dates back to John Gregory in 1772, many physician and nurse generalists offer basic levels of palliative care in the routine course of their provision of health care. In the 20th and 21st centuries, this care continued for hospitalized patients, for ambulatory patients seeking clinical care, and for persons in hospices and nursing homes.

In harmony with the long tradition of palliative care advocacy, Richard A. Parker wrote about his twelve years of experience with 95 patients at the end of life. Some died as in-patients in hospitals, while others passed away in their homes. Parker says,

> To perform end-of-life care, I have had to explore my feelings about death so that I could be open to patients' anxieties, ideas, and questions. In my world view, I accept dying and death as part of the "package deal" of living. This acceptance of the inevitability of death shapes the construct from which I listen to my patients.

He describes the last journeys of several of his patients and exclaims, "Our society awards to physicians the authority and privilege of caring for people at the end of life. I have learned that caring for patients in the last chapter of their lives is the most important part of my job."[85]

The discussion at the end of Chapter 8 showed that palliative care was not a standard component in American medical and nursing education and training at the end of the 20th century. Will that education and training become more extensive in the 21st century? To reach the bedsides of a far greater number of severely ill and dying patients, the basic elements of end-of-life care must become a routine part of the provision of health care by general practitioners, as well as those with specialized training in other medical and nursing disciplines.

The United Kingdom continues to be a model for other nations. The UK General Medical Counsel identified palliative care as one of the core content areas for undergraduate medical education in 2002. The palliative care educational component increased to a mean number of 20 hours per medical school across the United Kingdom by 2005. The objectives of that component included sensitive and sufficient communication; education concerning drugs, signs and symptoms of dying, and ethical issues; and knowledge about when to call for the services of a palliative care team. Training was required for general practitioners and specialists in many medical subspecialties.[86]

A turning point in palliative care education occurred in Germany when a 2013 law called for integration of palliative medicine training in undergraduate medical education.[87] Other nations, including Canada, the Netherlands, Korea, Argentina, Spain, and

Italy, have less extensive requirements, even though students in the last three of these nations widely agree that such training should be included in their curricula.[88]

Due to inadequate levels of palliative teaching and training in the United States up to the end of the 20th century, major national organizations called for standard curricula and required training in end-of-life care. In 2003 the Liaison Committee of Medical Education announced that teaching and training in palliative care should be mandated for all U.S. medical schools. A number of curriculum guides for undergraduate (MD) and graduate physician education were published by several organizations between 1994 and 2000. A two-year initiative supported by the Robert Wood Johnson Foundation and the Department of Veterans Affairs successfully developed a benchmark curriculum for resident physicians in end-of-life care.[89]

These aspirations found measures of fruition in the United States in the first years of the 21st century. A 2001 survey of medical students in six U.S. medical schools found that 49 percent felt prepared to manage common symptoms arising at the end of life. A majority of the students polled said they had been explicitly taught most aspects of terminal care in their formal curricula: 61 percent were taught about discussions of treatment withdrawal, 65 percent about assessing and managing patients' psychological depression, and 71 percent on when to refer patients to hospice. Seventy-three percent reported that they were prepared moderately or very well to manage pain and discuss end-of-life care decisions with patients. Naturally, students from medical schools with a formal curriculum in palliative care reported greater preparation—34 percent better prepared to deal with technical aspects of end-of-life care, and 21 percent better prepared to address psycho-social issues. The 2001 survey should have put an end to the often-voiced view that most doctors view the deaths of patients as medical failures. Asked whether they held that view, 79 percent of the fourth-year medical students responded "Not at all" or "A little."[90]

A 2008 survey of end-of-life care curricula in U.S. medical schools showed progress was occurring, but palliative caregivers' hopes that training in palliative care would become required in medical education had not yet occurred. Thirty percent of the responding medical schools required a course in "Palliative and Hospice Care"— as opposed to only 5 percent in 1998. Another 19 percent required palliative medicine as a clinical rotation, 15 percent offered an elective course, 29 percent an elective rotation, and 53 percent were integrating topics in palliative care in other required courses.[91]

The nursing profession fared far better. A national project titled End-of-Life Nursing Education Consortium (ELNEC) was launched in February 2000 to enable nurses to reduce the physical, psycho-social, and spiritual burdens and distresses of persons facing severe illness and death. The ELNEC project developed a nine-module train-the-trainer program that included a thousand-page curriculum, PowerPoint slides, talking points for each slide, case studies, and other teaching strategies. Modules included pain and other symptom management, communication, and ethical issues. Within three years, 277 nurse practitioners and educators had been trained and were teaching the ELNEC program within and outside their own clinical and hospice settings in the United States and Canada. By 2008 over 4,500 nurses from all 50 U.S. states and the District of Columbia had attended train-the-trainer courses. During these years programs in graduate nursing increased their curriculum coverage of palliative care from a mean of 12 hours to a mean of 34 hours.

Participants found their ELNEC training to be extremely useful, and it inspired them to share what they had learned with multi-disciplinary palliative care teams. Knowing that nurses spend more time at the bedsides and in the homes of persons facing the end of life than any other providers, many nurses regarded their post-training work as a privilege. They could now provide "the most excellent care available" and offer essential levels of education to peers and students.[92]

A number of innovative medical courses and programs added to these developments. They include a team-taught six-seminar education initiative for resident physicians in internal medicine, surgery, neurology, and psychiatry at the New York Presbyterian Hospital and Weill Medical College of Cornell University in 2000; a 20-hour training program for medical students taught by a multi-disciplinary team at the University of Maryland School of Medicine (the instructors of which describe how they secured their curriculum committee's approval of the course as a requirement in 2000); and an education program for physicians in practice (similar to the train-the-trainer ELNEC program for nurses) that by 2004 had 184 trainers who had presented one or more of the program's 16 curriculum modules to approximately 120,000 doctors. These and additional innovative programs were highly, if not enthusiastically, evaluated by their participants.[93]

Specialists

Clinician and nurse specialists in palliative care receive formal training in the field in order to consistently or entirely focus on that care. Many clinician specialists identify their discipline as palliative medicine, which they view as an area of specialization within the larger field of palliative care. Palliative care professionals complement the work of other physicians by providing treatment and care for patients with serious, complex, and terminal illnesses.[94]

By 2005 in the United Kingdom, there were 310 palliative care consultants and sub-specialty recognition in oncology, anesthesiology, radiology and other disciplines. The Royal College of Physicians found that there were some 100 vacancies for full-time palliative medicine consultants in England.[95]

The United States Accreditation Council for Graduate Medical Education (ACGME) Board of Directors finally approved a new sub-specialty in hospice and palliative medicine in 2006. Palliative medicine sub-specialty certification became available to physicians trained in ten primary medical specialties, including internal medicine, family medicine, general surgery, emergency medicine, psychiatry and neurology. A year prior to that approval, over 2,000 physicians were certified by the American Board of Hospices and Palliative Care (ABHPC), and more than 50 fellowship training programs existed nationwide. More than 10,000 nurses and nurse assistants had also been certified by the ABHPC.[96] Clinical nurse specialists now acquire certification through the Advanced Certified Hospice and Palliative Care programs.[97]

Certification of professional expertise in palliative medicine became more formal and extensive over time. The tradition of apprenticeship under an experienced palliative care professional transmogrified into fellowship programs. The professional rigor of these programs soon increased to at least twelve months of mandatory training and required satisfactory or superior ratings in all the core components of palliative care clinical competence, as well as successful completion of a certification examination.[98] Yet a serious shortage of well-trained palliative medicine specialists continues.[99]

Many palliative medicine professionals view themselves as "leaders and facilitators of cultural change" in the hospital-dominated medical system that was found to be so lacking in sensitive terminal care in the 1995 SUPPORT study.

Remarkable Expansion of Hospital and Hospice Programs

The foregoing developments proceeded hand in hand with the amazing expansion of hospital-based palliative care consultants, units, teams, and out-patient services. In 2000 most full-time supportive care professionals worked in hospices, but by 2010 43 percent of certified hospice and palliative medicine (HPM) specialists practiced in academic medical centers and large community hospitals, while 30 percent devoted themselves to hospice, and 15 percent were employed in private practice settings. In 2010 the estimated workforce of certified hospice and palliative medicine specialists—71 percent of whom held full-time palliative care positions—included 4,400 U.S. physicians.[100]

The invasiveness of surgery, the effects of chemotherapy and other treatments, and active interventions for many previously untreatable life-threatening diseases and conditions all require sophisticated forms of symptom relief and complex decisions on the part of patients. The fact that sub-specialization in HPM was approved for specialists in internal medicine, surgery, emergency medicine, anesthesiology, and other areas reflects the extent to which palliative care is needed.

Consider the new emphasis on palliative care in surgery and intensive care units in the United States. Perhaps surprising to some readers, surgeons began to promote palliative medicine beginning in the late 1990s. The dormant state of end-of-life care teaching and research in the field of surgery began to change in 1997—two years after the publishing of the SUPPORT study. A breakthrough occurred in 2001 when the American Board of Surgery included palliative care as a critical area of expertise in post-graduate surgical training. The Surgeons Palliative Care Workgroup created by the Robert Wood Johnson Foundation in conjunction with the American College of Surgeons concluded, "The practice of surgical palliative care is a fundamental component of good surgical clinical care." Surgeons must become competent in providing comfort-directed care along with curative care. Core competencies in surgical palliation include management of pain and other symptoms, effective communication that includes compassionately conveyed bad news about poor prognoses, and knowledge about advance directives. Increasing research in these areas contributed to these developments.[101]

Long active in palliative medicine initiatives, Geoffrey Dunn, a surgeon with hospice training, wrote in 2011, "The surgical world has too many seriously ill people in its care and has too much to offer the seriously ill with all diagnoses to not assume a leadership role for the continued growth and development of palliative care. Recent developments in the field of surgery give reason for optimism that this will occur."[102]

In 2000 Kathy Faber-Langendoen and Paul N. Lanken outlined the reasons why clinicians in intensive care units (ICUs) should be skilled in palliative care. Critically ill and dying patients and their family members must make decisions about withdrawing ventilator support, dialysis, intravenous fluids, and antibiotics. They are often beset with anxiety, an overwhelming sense of loss, and spiritual distress. Patients' symptoms of sleeplessness, nausea, and pain also require expertise in the use of opiates and other drugs. Their care, therefore, "often requires a dramatic shift from the 'rescue' mode to approaches that recognize death's inevitability and focuses on patient and family comfort." Requisite palliative care skills must be learned and mastered, not assumed.[103]

Others added to the ICU literature. Because 1 of every 5 Americans dies in ICUs, the core competencies of those working in such units should include quality end-of-life care in addition to life-sustaining care. The difficulties inherent in transforming ICUs into suitable places for sensitive terminal care call for special measures such as turning off as many monitors as possible, liberalizing visitation times, and enabling clergy visits if desired. ICUs contain the sickest patients with high risks of dying and with problems that deeply affect their quality of life. These units require the combined attention of intensive care specialists and palliative care consultation teams of physicians, nurses, pastoral caregivers, and social workers.[104]

By 1999 hospital programs in palliative care were expanding rapidly, such that these units in hospitals were praised as the "next frontier" in end-of-life care.[105] Dramatic changes occurred after 2000. A reported 24.5 percent of hospitals had palliative care programs in 2000, 40.4 percent in 2003, 52.8 percent in 2006, and 63 percent in 2009. As trendsetters, 84.5 percent of U.S. medical schools were affiliated with at least one hospital with a palliative care service by 2008.[106]

In 2010 palliative care teams in U.S. hospitals increased for the tenth consecutive year. That year there were 1,635 teams in hospitals—an increase of 4.3 percent over 2009. In 2010 nearly all Veteran Administration hospitals contained palliative care teams; 88 percent of large hospitals with 300 or more in-patient beds housed palliative programs; and 57 percent of small hospitals with 50–299 beds had such programs. By 2010 program directors spoke of how the steady and continuous growth had forged expansions of their own programs, overwhelmed existing staff members, and called for more palliative care specialists than were being trained.[107]

Unfortunately, studies indicated that access to palliative care programs in the United States varied significantly according to geographical location. Regionally, the American South had fewer hospitals with palliative care teams (53 percent) than the Northeast (76 percent), the Midwest (75 percent), and the West (71 percent).[108] Programs in individual states varied still more significantly: the lowest number of programs were in Mississippi (10 percent) and Alabama (16 percent), while the highest were in New Hampshire (85 percent), Montana (88 percent), and Vermont (100 percent).[109] Nevertheless, the Center to Advance Palliative Care estimated that by 2014 these care programs would be available in 84 percent of U.S. hospitals with 50 or more beds for patients.[110]

Geographical and other disparities characterized palliative care in other nations. In 2005 the United Kingdom had 3,195 palliative medicine hospital beds—one bed for every 18,370 citizens; Italy had one bed for 26,974 of its citizens, while on a descending scale Germany, France, Hungary, and Lithuania had far fewer beds per number of citizens.[111] A world-wide survey of palliative care services in 2007 pointed to the creation of new regional associations: the Latin American association in 2000, the Asia Pacific Hospice Palliative Care Network in 2001, and the African Association for Palliative Care in 2003. Eighty in-patient palliative care units existed in Japan in 2000; 250 designated programs existed in Australia by 2002; 113 programs in India by 2006; and a total of 467 palliative care programs in Poland, Romania, and Hungary in 2002.[112]

A majority of large Canadian hospitals and almost 90 percent of the medical facilities in rural areas offer palliative care services, even though, somewhat similar to the United States, general medical staff tend to have inadequate training and more specialized palliative medicine staff are needed. More than 60 percent of Canadians die as hospitalized patients who receive varying degrees of supportive care from generalists and specialists. Patients who experience severe suffering are treated by pain control specialists or by palliative caregivers who have unique access to methadone.[113]

In 2012 most European hospitals did not have mobile teams of palliative care professionals. Patients in ICUs were not permitted to die in more peaceful hospital settings. So within hospitals, ICU physician "specialists of life" were also becoming specialists in end-of-life care who would occasionally be called to provide help with palliative care in other medical wards.[114]

Hospice Care: Growth and Calls for Reform

In contrast to the United Kingdom, the United States, and Canada, most nations have not developed separate hospice care institutions for persons facing the end of life, so those who investigate the status and spread of palliative care across the world speak broadly about the availability of palliative services.[115] In 2003 some 200 hospices existed in the United Kingdom. One hundred fifteen of the world's 234 countries had one or more hospice-palliative care services by 2007, but only 35 of these nations had integrated these services into mainstream medicine. Progress was being made, but, globally speaking, "unrelieved suffering" continued on a massive scale.[116]

In the United States the more than 4,500 hospice programs that existed in 2007 increased to almost 5,000 by 2010. In 2000 513,000 Americans were enrolled in hospice. This expanded to 1.2 million persons in 2005, and to 1.56 million in 2010. Of the total number of Americans dying each year, 5.5 percent died with Medicare hospice coverage in 1990, 22.9 percent in 2000, and 44 percent in 2010.[117] What a correction these figures are to the assertion made in 2005 that only a "lucky few" die in hospices![118]

The stunning levels of growth reflect the highly positive dimensions of the U.S. Medicare benefit program. That program provides alternative settings from traditional hospital care and consistently attends to patients' and family caregivers' emotional and spiritual needs through interdisciplinary teams. Expert pain management is generally available, and patients who continue to live beyond the original 180-day coverage period can be recertified for continued care. (Recertification required face-to-face physician or nurse practitioner visits with patients after January 2011.[119]) High levels of patient and family satisfaction with hospice continues.[120]

Nevertheless, criticisms of the Medicare hospice benefit program intensified in the 21st century. The surging number of *hospital-based* palliative programs offered symptom relief and personalized care for severely and chronically ill patients, as well as care for patients judged to be terminally ill. Because Medicare coverage was limited to the last group, the coverage began to be viewed as overly restrictive.

The majority of U.S. hospices only enrolled patients with certified six-months-or-less prognoses of continued life and did not offer continuing cure-directed treatments. Hospice programs also labored under severe per-day financial restrictions that, for example, discouraged or forbade newer and more expensive pain-relieving medications, as well as continuity-of-care visits by oncologists and other physician specialists.[121] These limitations led many patients and providers to equate hospice with giving up attempted cures and accepting oncoming death. They also resulted in patient referrals to hospice care when some patients were only days or hours away from dying.[122]

So hospice coverage remained largely off limits or unavailable to three groups of patients: those desirous of fighting for life via curative-oriented care regardless of six-months-or-less prognoses; patients with end-stage diseases who were likely to live longer—perhaps much longer—than 6 months; and patients who might well opt for hospice enrollment, but whose physicians did not effectively explain the benefits of hospice to them.[123]

Efforts have been made to break down barriers to hospice use. Several life insurance companies developed programs that paid for cure-directed treatment along with hospice care. UnitedHealth offered open access coverage for patients who chose continued curative treatments along with hospice care.[124] The Aetna Insurance Company developed a program that offered disease-targeted treatments along with comfort-focused hospice care for patients with prognoses of 12 months of continued life instead of the standard 6 months. A study found that patients were twice as likely to enter the expanded-coverage program, stayed in the new program 73 percent longer than patients receiving standard hospice care, and required fewer numbers of acute care hospital visits.[125] Only very large hospices that serve more than 400 patients per day over time can afford these open access policies. Unfortunately, only 2.5 percent of the United States' 4,100 hospices in 2007 were that large.[126]

These limitations and pilot programs led to calls for systematic reform. Writing in the *New England Journal of Medicine* in 2012, David G. Stevenson renewed criticisms that the 6-month Medicare prognosis requirement made it extremely difficult to give timely hospice care, especially for patients with terminal non-cancer conditions. It also required patients to disavow curative therapy, which impedes enrollment into hospice and, by extension, patients' receiving better quality-of-life care. To overcome disconnects between hospital-based palliative care and hospice care, Stevenson called for reform of Medicare hospice coverage into a coordinated system of care with a continuum of high-quality care ranging from hospital-based palliative medicine to end-of-life hospice care.[127]

Enhanced Professional Status of Palliative Medicine

As major medical institutions increasingly engaged specialists in palliative medicine after 2003, the standing of these physicians improved, along with their career satisfaction and their sense of meaning and purpose.[128] A variety of developments contributed to that status and sense of satisfaction.

Specialists in palliative care acutely realized how the softness of their discipline must become hardened and specific like other medical specializations. To become fully respected, it must develop an expanded body of literature, including sophisticated peer-reviewed empirical research. That imperative is now being realized. In the 21st century the journal literature on all aspects of palliative medicine and care expanded exponentially. A window into this growing literature can be found in this chapter's references (with their numerous annotations), the references in the 2009 edition of National Consensus Project's *Clinical Practice Guidelines*, and the ever-expanding number of journal articles found in medical indexes.[129] These examples attest to the expansion of clinical and observational research on all aspects of palliative medicine from pain assessment and management in clinical specialties to studies of anxiety, grief, delirium, depression, emotional and psychiatric issues, and all the other core elements of modern palliative care.

In his impressive overview of advances made in the United Kingdom, D. Doyle wrote, "The knowledge base continues to grow, good research is being published, [and] more than 50 reference books and textbooks on the subject are now published in the UK alone." These advances accounted for a continuing number of excellent recruits into the sub-specialty and the fact that colleagues in many other specialties increasingly requested the expertise of palliative care specialists.[130]

Similar developments were occurring in the United States. A virtual drumbeat of summons by palliative medical specialists called for increasing research in the field, enhanced funding from the National Institutes of Health (NIH), greater representation on NIH committees appointed to approve research, and more evidence-based studies that measure the effectiveness of supportive care interventions. Such measures would enable these specialists to speak with greater authority and conviction to their medical colleagues and the public.[131]

Conferences, Foundation Support, and the Public Media

International and national conferences and the impressive support of funding agencies contributed to the status of palliative care in medical and nursing institutions and in the eyes of the public. International conferences included comprehensive sets of topics on the world-wide growth of supportive care; the roles of respective team members and family caregivers; the roles of culture, ethnicity, and spirituality; and many other subjects.[132] One national conference was the 2004 NIH State-of-the-Science on Improving End of Life Care sponsored by the NIH Office of Medical Applications of Research, the National Institute of Nursing Research, and other organizations. Annual assemblies of the American Academy of Hospice and Palliative Medicine (AAHPM)—primarily a physician organization—are both national and international. Beginning in 2004, the AAHPM met jointly with the Hospice and Palliative Nurses Association

(HPNA). These state-of-the-art, relationship-building assemblies are attended by over 2,000 medical and nursing professionals from North America, along with representatives from India, Korea, Vietnam, Uganda, and other nations.

No foundation has contributed more to the improvement, expansion, and professionalism of palliative medicine and care than the Robert Wood Johnson Foundation (RWJF). Several of its funded initiatives have already been noted. The RWJF's multiyear, multi-million-dollar Last Acts program, designed to promote improvements in end-of-life care, began in response to the alarming negative findings of the RWJF-funded SUPPORT study of 1995. Last Acts involved a coalition of more than 800 national health and consumer groups and six task forces designed to improve patient-provider communication, change the culture of healthcare institutions, and alter American attitudes toward death. Also critically important was the Soros Foundation's Project on Death in America, which funded $14 million of faculty fellowship programs in palliative care between 1995 and 2004.[133]

Numerous television programs and films, and an almost countless number of websites, offer important and accessible information about end-of-life care. The inspiring and intimate four-part PBS television series *On Our Own Terms: [Bill] Moyers on Dying in America* was first aired in September 2000 and became widely used in undergraduate medical ethics courses. *Consider the Conversation: A Documentary on a Taboo Subject* premiered in 2011 and has been viewed and discussed across the world.

Two Surprises

Surprising findings increased the status of palliative care. The first disclosed how comfort-focused care lowers the enormous costs of medical treatments for persons in their last years, months, and days of life. A 2008 study analyzed data on 25,459 patients, 4,908 of whom received palliative care consult services, while the rest received none. Palliative team consultation saved $2,642 per patient admission for those who were discharged from the hospital alive and $6,896 per admission for those who died in the hospital. For a 400-bed hospital, the addition of a palliative medicine program that made 500 consults per year would save that hospital $1.3 million each year. Later studies found that patients receiving care from palliative consults were 43 percent less likely to be admitted to ICUs during hospitalization, were less likely to die in ICUs, received fewer numbers of treatments, experienced shorter hospital stays, and were more likely to be referred to hospice care. These factors accounted for impressive savings. A March 2013 study showed that the U.S. Medicare hospice benefit program both lowered hospitalizations and resulted in significant cost savings even for patients who were enrolled in hospice from 30 to only 1–7 days.[134]

The second surprise revealed that palliative care extends rather than shortens life. A study published in 2007 validated what palliative care providers in hospices had long suspected—that hospice patients with several types of serious illnesses lived longer than their non-hospice counterparts. The length of survival was highest for patients with congestive heart failure (on average 81 days longer), lung cancer (39 days longer), and pancreatic cancer (21 days longer). None of the 6 groups studied experienced shorter life spans in hospice.[135]

Another study in 2010 randomly assigned newly diagnosed patients with metastatic non–small cell lung cancer, the leading cause of death from cancer world-wide, into two groups. The first received palliative care along with standard oncologic care, and the second only standard care. The researchers found that those receiving palliative care integrated with standard care lived 30 percent longer—an average of 11.6 months versus 8.9 months for those receiving standard care alone. Patients receiving palliative care experienced fewer depressive symptoms, better clinically measured quality of life, reduced levels of chemotherapy, less aggressive end-of-life treatment, and longer periods of hospice care.[136]

Control of pain and other symptoms enables persons to sleep and eat better and talk more with friends and loved ones. Psychological support and the comforts of meaningful social relationships contribute to desires for continued living. The interplay between these treasured elements of comfort care and the quality and length of patients' lives calls for additional, methodologically rigorous research.[137]

Not as surprising, but still remarkable, palliative hospital programs greatly affected the number of patients discharged from hospitals to hospices. Discharges from hospitals to hospice increased fifteen-fold between 2000 (27,912) and 2009 (430,882). These discharges greatly increased the number of patients entering hospices with diseases other than cancer, including patients with heart failure, chronic obstructive lung disease, and other conditions. They also lowered the cost of hospital care for these patients.[138]

Physician-Assisted Suicide (PAS)

The section on PAS in Chapter 8 discussed why physician-assisted death became an important topic in the story of palliative care in the last decades of the 20th century. Several leading palliative care providers recognized that the unbearable and unrelenting suffering of a small number of terminally ill patients could not be eased by comfort-assuaging measures. As a last resort, they believed that mentally competent patients with fatal illnesses who want to end their lives by taking lethal drugs should be provided with the means of doing so as long as a series of safeguards are followed.[139] Arguably, PAS in such cases is an extension of palliative care because it ensures a serene death.

Physician-assisted suicide in the 21st century has been surrounded by heated controversy. To focus on developments in the United States,[140] voters in the state of Oregon approved physician-assisted death in 1994 under the rhetoric of its Death with Dignity Act. Legally challenged for years on several fronts, that act, which included safeguards against abuse, was upheld by the U.S. Supreme Court in 2006. Acts similar to Oregon's were passed by voters in the state of Washington in 2008, by the Montana Supreme Court in 2009 and by legislators in Vermont in 2013. Most official medical associations strongly oppose these measures, including the American Medical Association, the World Health Association, the American College of Physicians–American Society of Internal Medicine, the Vermont and Massachusetts Medical Societies, and many other entities.[141]

Polls of American citizens display mixed results. Proponents of PAS cite a 2005 poll indicating that 70 percent of U.S. adults favor laws allowing doctors to comply with the wishes of a dying patient in severe distress who asks to have her or his life ended.[142] Opponents point to waning support, with 2010 polls showing 55 percent of adults in favor and 45 percent opposed to PAS. Even fewer would vote to legalize PAS.[143] Polls in 2013 indicate 50 percent of Americans believe PAS should be legal, 29 percent say it should be illegal, and 45–49 percent think it's morally wrong.[144]

Palliative care physicians are divided over the morality of physician-assisted suicide. Some experienced and notable palliative caregivers believe that PAS should be opposed, feared, and loathed, as it makes physicians complicit in putting persons to death. It harms, rather than protects, vulnerable persons who may feel that they are shameful and burdensome. It is disguised by phrases like "death with dignity" and "aid-in-dying." It betrays medicine's historic devotion to healing and to life. It is subject to abuse. It directly conflicts with the Hippocratic Oath's principle, "I will give no deadly medicine to anyone if asked nor suggest any such counsel."[145]

In a 2003 article, Timothy E. Quill and Christine K. Cassel contend that medical associations opposed to PAS should shift to positions of neutrality. They believe these associations "generally understate" how often palliative drugs "fail to alleviate some end-of-life suffering," and they present data suggesting that up to 17 percent of suffering patients would have wanted PAS. These associations fail to provide their members with guidelines for dealing with terminally ill patients whose suffering is severe and intolerable. Quill and Cassel also review findings indicating that the legalization of PAS in the state of Oregon has not been abused, since it only accounts for .1 percent of the deaths in Oregon. And they list medical, nursing, and bioethics organizations that have assumed positions of neutrality toward PAS, including the American Academy of Hospice and Palliative Medicine and the Society for Health and Human Values.[146]

The most fervent and lengthy physician defense of PAS was published in 2008 in a book titled *To Die Well* by Sidney Wanzer and Joseph Glenmullen. At the time, Wanzer was the president of the Boston chapter of Compassion and Choices, formerly known as the Hemlock Society.[147] He had been the lead author of the innovative 1989 article that forthrightly, and for the first time in a U.S. medical journal, identified physician proponents of PAS.[148] *To Die Well* highlights stories of Wanzer's dying patients and includes chapters on patients' rights, pain control, palliative or comfort care for persons who are no longer receiving cure-directed treatments, irreversible dementia, and advance directives. He refers to PAS as merciful death, aid-in-dying, "a progressive approach to hastening death in intolerable situations," and deliverance.[149] The emphasis on PAS is embedded in the book's framework, which sets forth two critical turning points in palliative care—the first turning from active treatment to comfort care, the second turning to hastened death when it is imminent, suffering is intolerable, and all comfort measures have failed. The authors observe that a majority of persons will experience the first turning point, and only a very few will reach the second.[150]

Wanzer and Glenmullen surround acceptable PAS with an impressive list of 15 safeguards. These include assurances that all acceptable forms of up-to-date palliative care have been exhausted, that clinical depression has been ruled out, that relevant expert consultants have been called in, that the suffering person has been fully informed about all treatment alternatives, that the patient is mentally competent, that the patient's request is voluntary, and that suffering is intolerably severe.[151] They also appeal to State of Oregon data that shows how PAS has not led to abusive overuse, and they hold that patients' rights of free choice are decisive.[152]

Obstacles to, and Permissible Limitations on, Patient Choices

In 2012 Robert Y. Lin and colleagues accurately observed, "The past decade has been a dynamic period for hospice and palliative care."[153] Palliative medicine became professionally defined, broadened its scholarly base, greatly expanded as a field of medical specialization in hospitals, and dramatically increased patient referrals to hospices.

Yet obstacles stood in the way of palliative care as a truly available choice for many patients. First, the science and art of palliative care are still poorly understood by an apparently large number of medical practitioners. In his powerful article in the *New Yorker* in 2010, the surgeon and writer Atul Gawande castigates the failure of cure-directed medicine to improve the lives of patients with end-stage disease. Yet even Gawande knew very little about palliative and hospice care before he wrote the article. He admits, "I didn't know much about hospice." He proves how little he knew by observing that hospice is trying to offer "a *new* ideal for how we die," but that many have not embraced its "rituals." He confesses he once believed that hospice care hastens death. Upon working closely with expert nurse and physician palliative care professionals in his own hospital, however, his appreciation of their work dramatically changed.[154] In 2012, Porter Storey, a pioneer palliative care professional since 1983, commented that hospice and palliative medicine "is one of the fastest-growing, but least understood [medical] specialties."[155] And in 2014 an oncology nurse described how some physicians still equate palliative care with only hospice care.[156]

The central aims and components of palliative medicine also appear to be misunderstood by many non-physicians and politicians. Ignorance about the contributions of palliative care fueled the turmoil over death panels in the United States beginning in 2009. Palliative caregivers and those who championed what they were doing widely believed that communication with patients about end-of-life choices would increase if caregivers were paid for the time required for truly effective communication. Payments to practitioners with proven communication training were added to House Bill 3200 (the Affordable Care Act), Section 1233, titled "Advance Care Planning Consultation." However, the ensuing uproar led to the removal of Section 1233 from the bill that was finally passed. Politicians and editorialists, backed by outcries from American citizens, turned the intent of that section on its head. Advanced planning discussions were labeled as the work of grisly "death panels" intent on coaxing patients away from expensive life-sustaining treatments.[157] Some palliative care professionals felt that they'd become dangerously "radioactive." They were being stereotyped as physicians who wanted to get severely ill and dying patients out of the way in order to save money via rationing. Paying them to do what they had long been advocating—promote choice through expert and extended conversations with patients—had been distorted as taking choice away.[158] This controversy over payments to palliative caregivers for time-intensive conversations with patients continues.

Permissible limitations on patient choices by physicians continued with respect to performing futile treatments. The 20th-century limitations on patient rights to receive non-beneficial and often harmful treatments persist in the 21st century. A review of the literature in 2005 noted that the developing medical and ethical consensus against futile treatments in the 1990s remained in place in 2000 and 2001. The author urged legislative action beyond the established guidelines of Texas and California and advocated further development of futility-of-treatment guidelines in ICUs.[159]

Other authors between 2004 and 2011 argued that doctors have ethical and fiduciary duties *not* to undertake non-beneficial interventions.[160] Doctors should initiate sensitive, honest, thorough, and nonconfrontational discussions that explain why further attempts to prolong life will be ineffective and harmful. Patients and family members should be given time to adjust to a lack of curative options. If needed, medical consultants and ethics committee members should become involved as counselors. Those who conduct these discussions should convey that palliative *care* is never futile.[161]

Little is known about the extent to which doctors limit patient choices in accordance with futility-of-treatment guidelines. A survey of the responses of 10,000 physicians in 2010 asked, "Would you ever recommend or give life-sustaining therapy when you judged that it was futile?" showed that 37 percent replied "No," 39.4 percent responded "It depends," and 23.6 percent said "Yes."[162]

Ensuring Choices

The rights of and opportunities for patients to make informed choices respecting critical and end-of-life care are pivotal for all patients. Advance directives as living wills and durable healthcare powers of attorney were signed into law by state legislatures during the 1970s and 1980s. To seek to ensure the effectiveness of these laws, hospitals established guidelines for DNR orders and other life-sustaining treatments. The U.S. Congress's passage of Patient Self-Determination Act (PSDA) in 1991 required all hospitals and other patient care facilities to provide patients with information about these directives. Yet the 1995 SUPPORT study proved that these choices were far more theoretical than real.

In spite of their apparently *decreasing* utilization after the PSDA was instituted, living wills and durable powers of attorney ascended to the status of conventional wisdom and medical ethics orthodoxy. In 2012, the surgeon and senator Bill Frist wrote that all persons should have signed living wills and durable healthcare powers of attorney. Yet he lamented that 4 out of 5 persons had not done that, even though these directives, he asserted, "provide an essential roadmap of your preferences" and also relieve family members and doctors "from having to guess what you would really have wanted."[163]

Problems with Living Wills

But the effectiveness of living wills has been profoundly questioned in the 21st century. In 2002 Mark D. Sullivan gave cogent reasons for why they offered the illusion of patient choice, rather than actually securing patient autonomy. They fail to provide meaningful instructions about end-of-life care because half of them are not relevant to or predictive of patients' actual situations.[164]

Angela Fagerlin and Carl E. Schneider crafted a devastating critique of living wills in 2004. Even though they were being advanced by the "grandees of law and medicine," no degree of "tinkering" will ever "make the living will an effective instrument of social policy." The conditions upon which they are written are "unmet and largely unmeetable." For them to work, people would have to predict their preferences accurately—preferences regarding unidentifiable maladies and unpredictable treatments. Numerous studies indicate that patient preferences change over time. Even if living wills happen to correctly predict patient preferences, those who interpret them may not do so accurately. Durable powers of attorney are far more preferable, but the PSDA should be repealed because of "arrogant indifference to its effectiveness" and administrative costs.[165]

Writing from the perspective of ICU physicians in 2007, James E. Szalados describes why the wording in written advanced directives is "inherently ambiguous" in settings filled with complex and powerful technologies. Hence, the values and judgments of specific ICU teams often "drive the actions that are taken, with or without advance directives."[166]

Studies have also indicated that surrogate decision maker perceptions of patients' preferences are often inaccurate[167] and that numerous problems beset DNR orders.[168] To be effective, legally binding designations of a family member or friend as a substitute decision maker must include full and updated conversations about one's preferences. When that occurs, durable powers of attorney are far more reliable than living wills. This points to the greatest value of living wills: their helpfulness as a means to enable surrogates to understand the types of choices their appointees would make.

Two New Initiatives: POLST Programs and Right to Know Laws

Fortunately, the disenchantment with living wills and the far better, but still imperfect, durable healthcare powers of attorney have given rise to two innovative 21st-century initiatives designed to secure the rights of patients to make their own choices.

The first of these initiatives is the POLST Paradigm Program. POLST stands for Physician Orders for Life-Sustaining Treatment. Like a small cloud on the horizon in the waning years of the 20th century, POLST programs became a frontal system of fundamental change in ensuring terminal patient rights of choice in the 21st century. The cloud formed at the Oregon Health Sciences University between 1991 and 1996. The frontal system consisted of the development of the National POLST Paradigm Task Force in 2004, which was recommended for nation-wide adoption in 2006. By 2012 the program had been adopted by 13 U.S. states and in-state regions, and programs were developing in 28 states and regions and in a number of nations.[169]

The National Paradigm Task Force requires a careful set of conditions to be met before POLST programs are approved. Approval includes compliance with existing state laws, ongoing training of healthcare professionals across the continuum of care facilities, education in communication skills, and commitments to improve end-of-life care.[170]

POLST programs apply to persons with advanced, life-threatening illness whose life expectancies are within the range of one or two years. Patient care must begin with honest and detailed conversations between physicians and patients and/or patients' families that will enable doctors to fill out the one-page, clearly organized POLST form. The form contains a simple list of checkboxes regarding four patient preferences: first, whether to attempt CPR; second, what medical interventions are (or are not) wanted with respect to one of three options—"Comfort Measures Only," "Limited Additional Interventions," or "Full Treatment"; third, whether antibiotics are rejected, limited to when infection occurs, or used when medically indicated; and, fourth, whether artificially administered nutrition through tubes is refused, accepted for a trial period, or wanted long term.

After the chosen boxes are checked, the form must be signed by both the doctor and the patient or the patient's surrogate. The form thereby explicitly registers choices *and* rises to the status of a *medical order* regarding all four sets of options. These forms—readily found on the web—are printed on brightly colored paper and expressly designed to be visible in medical charts, as well as transferable when patients are moved from a hospice or nursing home to a hospital or moved within the hospital.

Filling out the POLST form requires consultation between patients and providers to ensure that patients receive the treatment they desire. The POLST form itself can serve as an important conversation starter, even though at first some palliative care specialists were concerned that the "very fluid and changeable" nature of patient choices requires updated forms, and that filling them out should not replace time-consuming and emotionally complex conversations.[171]

POLST far exceeds the limited effectiveness of previous advance directives for the following reasons: They extend to greater numbers of patients than those who become mentally incompetent. They improve communication over end-of-life issues. They result in *actionable* medical orders that square with the real world of medical practice. They pertain to patients' current medical conditions and balance the authority of doctors with the rights and decisions of patients. They transfer care between different settings, which eases the worries of hospital-based palliative care professionals who are concerned that their careful planning will evaporate shortly after hospital discharge. They have inspired the development of other types of workable programs.[172]

Studies prove the superior effectiveness of POLST programs in ensuring that choices are respected. One found that 98 percent of patients' preferences for treatment limitations were respected and found that no patient with a POLST form received unwanted CPR, ventilator support, ICU admission, or feeding tubes. Another study of 400 patients found that these forms not only limited treatment but also guaranteed that patients wanting more aggressive levels of treatment received them.[173]

A second set of 21st-century initiatives could prove to be important for patients and families, even though they have been resisted by a number of physicians. These initiatives, which began in 2008, turned again to the force of law and legislation that originally instituted advance directives. They are "right to know" laws designed to ensure that patients are told about their prognoses and treatment options and are empowered with the legal and moral rights to make their own decisions. These new laws require physicians to offer information about patients' full range of options upon request. Recognizing that too many patients were not being informed about end-of-life options, the laws aimed to further change the medical system.[174] Most of them sought to impose by law what POLST programs were accomplishing for patients nearing the end of life.

The first of these laws, the Right to Know End of Life Options Act, was signed into law in California in 2008. The act requires information and counseling for patients with diagnoses of terminal illness that must include the following: the right to refuse or discontinue mechanical ventilation, chemotherapy, antibiotics, and artificial nutrition and hydration; the right to pursue disease-target therapy with or without concurrent palliative care; the right to comprehensive pain and symptom management; the right to enroll in hospice; and the right to execute advance directives. A similar law was passed in Michigan in 2011 under the title "The Michigan Dignified Death Act." The impact of these acts is presently unknown.

Three acts have been signed into law in New York State: the Family Health Care Decisions Act (FHCDA) in 2010; the Palliative Care Information Act (PCIA), which took effect in February 2011; and the Palliative Care Access Act (PCAA), which became effective in September 2011.

The FHCDA focuses on mentally incompetent patients and only applies to general hospitals and nursing homes. It tells doctors when life-sustaining treatment should stop, and it expressly gives legal rights to family members or friends who had not been designated as decision makers in advance directives. "Now at last," the director of a hospital fund exclaimed, "the law has been changed." The change was needed because New York State "lagged behind nearly every other state" with respect to giving decision-making power to non–legally designated persons.[175] The law sets forth in priority order the persons who are legally empowered to make end-of-life decisions for incompetent patients.[176]

The PCIA law is similar to, but extends beyond, the right-to-know acts of California in 2008 and in Michigan in 2011. The PCIA requires physician and nurse practitioners to *offer* information and counseling regarding palliative care and end-of-life options— in contrast to California's law, which mandates that information and counseling should be provided for patients who *request* them. Furthermore, violations of PCIA are punishable by fines up to $5,000 for repeated offenses and jail terms up to one year long for willful violators.[177]

The New York Palliative Care Access Act (PCAA) became law seven months after PCIA. It expanded upon the preceding act in four ways: First, beyond the information and counseling required by the PCIA, the PCAA requires providers to ensure patient *access* to specialist-level palliative and pain care consultation and services. Second, beyond hospitals, it applies to home care agencies, assisted living residences, and individual practitioners. Third, it applies to patients or residents with advanced life-limiting illnesses, not just those who are terminally ill. And fourth, it includes the penalties outlined in the PCIA, but adds additional penalties for failures to comply with the PCAA, including the possibility of medical misconduct action for those who negligently fail to comply.[178]

Both the PCIA and the PCAA are designed to make sure patients are empowered to make choices "consistent with their goals for care, and wishes and beliefs, and to optimize their quality of life."[179] If legislative law can implant palliative care within the culture of medical practice and in other institutional settings, these laws should do it. They make extensive demands on healthcare providers and administrators—requirements backed by penalties for noncompliance. They are also worded as deeply expressed concerns for the travails of many severely ill and dying persons.

Yet worries remained. Some doctors recognized that many of their colleagues were falling short of effective communication, sensitive quality-of-life care, and full discussions of patients' treatment options. But they questioned the adequacy of correcting these failures by law. A pioneer in hospice care wrote that the PCIA "gives impetus to begin to meet crying needs" but is an unfunded mandate that defines neither what compliance is nor how it will be monitored.[180]

To be carried out, these laws will require additional levels of palliative care training in medical and nursing schools, institutional changes, increased funding, initiatives in compliance oversight, explicit and workable standards of care, and further expansions of palliative care workforces. Will these laws forge change? Might they be resisted more than welcomed? Will other states and nations enact similar laws? These questions await answers.

Expanded Choices

Even as the enduring momentum of modern medicine's curative capabilities builds, the overarching story in the 21st century emphasizes how palliative care is achieving its rightful status in hospital-based medical practice, as well as in hospice programs. Palliative care at the present time is an increasingly available alternative for patients with life-threatening and life-ending diseases. In numerous hospitals, life-prolonging and aggressive treatments with or without comfort care interventions vie for the hearts and minds of patients, their families, and healthcare professionals. In an ever-increasing number of hospice programs, persons can receive expert comfort-focused care that is sometimes supplemented by curative treatments. These developments have taken center stage in 21st-century dramas of life and death.

The coexistence of cure-directed interventions and palliative care forges a third choice. Previously existing choices included opting for cure-directed treatments or non-curative hospice care. Now a third option is increasingly available—continuing disease-targeted treatments along with palliative care.

Exploring Good Death: "The Debate of the Age"

As in previous eras, the term *good death* in the 21st century was used synonymously with the terms *peaceful/gentle dying*, *dying well*, and *dying with a sense of worth*—all opposed to bad deaths.[181] Those terms call into play actions and emotional responses that will enable end-of-life care to be good—actions and emotions that should serve as guideposts for caregivers in numerous settings.

Over time remarkable similarities existed between advocates of palliative care with regard to the fundamental elements of good dying. Cicely Saunders evoked the writings of Francis Bacon in the 17th century, William Munk in the 19th century, and Albert Worcester in the 1930s. In her 1984 essay "On Dying Well," Dame Saunders spoke of the elements of good death that resonated with those of the Institute of Medicine's discussion of "decent or good death" versus "bad death" in 1997, and with Ezekiel and Linda Emanuel's "The Promise of a Good Death" in 1998.[182] Discussions of good death mushroomed in the 21st century.

Explorations of good death assume that dying persons should be freed from isolation, neglect, pain, pointless prolongation, and disregard for one's values and wishes. With sensitive and expert care, many persons can experience good death—that is, meaningful and even new levels of insight, reconciliation, and peace to the point of death. But given the way some persons are struck with life-draining and painful end-stage conditions, it seems wise and accurate to augment "good" with "as good as possible" or "decent" or "acceptable."[183]

Richard Smith, the editor of the *British Medical Journal*, began discussions of good death in the 21st century with his January 2000 article on "A Good Death." He contends that insofar as death is viewed as a failure by physicians, medicine is diverted from giving due attention to helping persons experience good deaths. "How to reinstate that attention into medical practice and the fabric of culture," Smith says, is "the debate of the age." He lists the "principles of a good death," which should be incorporated into professional codes, the plans of individuals, and healthcare systems. These principles include "knowing when death is coming and understanding what can be expected"; having control over pain and other symptom relief; having "access to information and expertise of whatever kind is necessary"; having "access to any spiritual and emotional support"; controlling "who is present and who shares the end"; having access "to hospice care in any location, not only in hospitals"; and being able to die "when it is time to go and not have life prolonged pointlessly."[184]

Respondents to Smith's article spoke of ways these principles exemplify hospice care in Great Britain.[185] One offered "one further ingredient" to his list: having an *amicus mortis*—a chosen "friend at death" present during one's last months, weeks, and days of life.[186] Other authors re-emphasized Smith's principles, often discussed them in greater detail, and sometimes, informed by social scientific research, added to the listing. In keeping with the long-standing emphasis on patient autonomy, a study based on interviews of 75 patient participants by Karen Steinhauser and her colleagues noted that having a choice is contingent on patients' clearly understanding their treatment options and having their preferences honored. Participants valued the principles listed by Smith and wanted to be recognized as unique persons by caregivers. Surprising to these authors, several participants also wanted to continue contributing to the well-being of others.[187]

The social scientific study by Elizabeth Tong and her colleagues in 2003 summarized data derived from 13 focus groups of non-minority and minority persons. Their study confirmed the value of the core components of palliative and hospice care. The ten domains they found to be characteristics of good death included physical comfort, emotional well-being, a home-like environment, non–medically-invasive care, recognition of cultural concerns, respect for autonomous choices, and attentive care and counseling for family members.[188]

Reviews of the literature on good death in the United Kingdom, the United States, and other nations in 2006 and 2008 spoke of the burgeoning interest in the topic. Almost all the dimensions of good dying were those just listed. Two additional themes emphasized trust in one's caregivers and a sense of completion of important life tasks on the part of dying patients who want to feel they are leaving a memorable legacy. One review mistakenly claimed that the first attempt to define a good death was made in 1983.[189]

Under the controversial rubric of "dying with dignity,"[190] the Canadian psychiatrist Harvey Max Chochinov developed what he termed a "dignity model" of palliative care.[191] He maintained that it was "A New Model for Palliative Care" that surpasses the "mechanistic" and narrowly "technological paradigms" of other palliative caregivers.[192] He equated his model with holistic, compassionate, medically savvy, and novel end-of-life care.[193] "Dignity-conserving care needs to become part of the palliative care lexicon and an overarching therapeutic aim and standard of care for *all patients* close to death."[194]

Chochinov's model, however, rests upon commonly used terms for the overall purpose of palliative care,[195] and it reflects all the previously discussed core principles of that care.[196] Ironically, Chochinov and his colleagues' survey of 213 patients in palliative care hospital units found that only "a small group of patients reported that loss of dignity was a problem."[197]

Nevertheless, Chochinov and his fellow researchers offer two contributions to the meaning of good, or at least better, death. Both are informed by the tradition of meaning-centered group psychotherapy in the logo therapy of Victor Frankl and in the work of William Breitbart, an American psychiatrist and palliative care consultant. Breitbart's interests turned from treating the psychiatric disorders of dying persons to enabling them to find greater meaning in life when struggling with terminal illnesses. Chochinov began working with Breitbart in 2004.[198]

Chochinov's first contribution highlights specific things caregivers can do to maintain and enhance dying persons' hopefulness, sense of self-worth, and peaceful well-being. He and his colleagues developed a repertoire based on easily used "interventions" that would enable persons to feel valued. These include displaying interest in terminally ill patients' treasured roles in life, encouraging them to participate as much as possible in purposeful activities—such as listening to music, light exercise, outings, prayer, and meditation—and enabling them to begin or continue life projects that will be remembered, such as writing letters, making audio and/or video recordings, and keeping journals.[199]

Calling these "interventions" may secure the attention of caregivers, and they identify specific things caregivers can do to maintain and bolster dying persons' sense of meaning and purpose. Yet they reflect broader aspects of care emphasized by numerous palliative caregivers. They also reflect values of devoted clinicians. Many palliative care specialists, including Chochinov, quote Francis Weld Peabody's famous words that equate patient care with "caring for the patient."[200] Yet within Peabody's most-cited article in the medical literature lies this unforgettable precept: "What is spoken of as a 'clinical picture' is not just a photograph of a sick man in bed; it is an impressionistic painting of the patient surrounded by his home, his work, his relations, his friends, his joys, sorrows, hopes and fears."[201] Clinicians, medical students, nurses, counselors, and clergy who become skilled impressionists in Peabody's sense will bring greater meaning, hope, and comfort to those approaching death.

Chochinov's second contribution involves terminally ill persons who are experiencing depression, meaninglessness, and a loss of worth. He designed a "Dignity Psychotherapy Question Protocol" consisting of a step-by-step procedure that psychiatrists and other palliative caregivers can use to sustain and enhance dying persons' uniqueness and worth. The protocol includes answering a series of questions. Patient answers are recorded, shaped into a narrative by a caregiver, and returned to the patient and family. The questions pertain to their most important roles in life, the accomplishments they are most proud of, and words they want to say to loved ones and friends.[202]

Most incurably ill patients who participate in this protocol feel they are helping their families. It assures them that they are passing on a legacy that will endure beyond the grave.[203] Family members confirmed that the Dignity Protocol heightened their loved ones' sense of purpose and enabled them to prepare for death. They also said the document would continue to be a source of comfort.[204] Caregivers who conduct this life review display personalized attention and sensitivity. This approach would also contribute to the well-being of numerous persons who are not terminally ill, but whose thoughts and stories for any number of reasons are never invited, not listened to when uttered, or overtly silenced.

This story from a fourth-year medical student conveys the value of this protocol:

> I tried to write THE NEXT GREAT NOVEL. As part of my ambulatory care clerkship, however, I was given the opportunity to help write the story of a patient's life. I was the first medical student at NYU to participate in dignity therapy. I was nervous. Recording a patient's life history and thoughts seemed daunting.
>
> As soon as I met my patient, "Sarah," all my worries dissipated. Like me, she had always wanted to write a novel or a memoir; she was delighted to tell her story. Sarah was almost blind and spent her time listening to the TV in a nursing home, but she had been a teacher who loved to read and write. She wanted her children to know about her many experiences throughout the years and to communicate her hopes for them.... She was a natural story teller.
>
> I recorded everything Sarah told me, then transcribed and edited our 2-hour conversation. The document was both touching and insightful. It was twice as real and powerful as any of my discarded novels. When I read Sarah the final document we created, she cried and said she had no idea that she was so interesting.
>
> Perhaps one day I will write that novel, but for now, I am happy to have written something that will have a positive impact on the lives of Sarah and her children.[205]

Concluding Perspectives

Palliative care has achieved remarkable gains in the 21st century. It became more thoroughly defined and spelled out as a multifaceted medical discipline. Its successes have been secured through great effort, sophistication, and leadership by caregivers who gave themselves to their callings.

To be sure, further challenges remain, the most important of which include rectifying poor communication on the part of many healthcare providers, providing more education and training for undergraduate medical students, overcoming geographical disparities and the worrisome shortage of palliative care specialists, and enabling persons enrolled in U.S. hospice coverage to gain access to needed and effective cure-directed treatments. Furthermore, too many persons—including physicians—still misunderstand what palliative care is,[206] the meaning of which appears to be more readily conveyed by terms such as comfort-directed, quality-of-life, and supportive care.[207]

Given the power and prestige of contemporary curative medicine, the recent gains in palliative care are stunning. Within *hospitals*, the sanctuaries of curative medicine, palliative medicine now makes numerous life-extending medical treatments less painful by bringing greater measures of symptom relief to persons suffering from complex illnesses. Palliative care generalists and specialists attend to patients with end-stage diseases by easing their symptoms, enabling them to clarify their choices, and providing emotional, social, and spiritual support and counsel. This care also extends the lives of patients and decreases healthcare costs.

So, in the first years of the 21st century, palliative medical treatment and care began to take a rightful place both alongside and within major medicine disciplines, including surgery, internal medicine, anesthesiology, and other specializations. Palliative care teams are increasingly being called in as consultants for practitioners in a variety of medical disciplines, even as many of these practitioners are becoming more skilled in the essential components of palliation.

The widespread coexistence of palliative and cure-directed care in increasing numbers of hospitals is very good news for severely and fatally ill patients. Coexistence gives patients choices with respect to their preferred treatment options. POLST programs secure these choices much more effectively than living wills. They are invaluable supplements to patient-appointed durable powers of medical attorney, and they merit expansion across the United States and in other parts of the world.

Comfort-focused end-of-life care also expanded impressively in hospices, and hospice care continues to serve as a model for fundamental components of palliative care and treatment. Even though hospice is now recognized as a coexisting and essential part of palliative care/palliative medicine, it is an indescribably valuable choice for countless persons.

While the rights, protections, and number of patient choices at the present time are fully deserving of celebration, the choices themselves are often replete with emotional struggle and pain. Patients and family members deserve sensitive and expert counseling as they struggle with inner ambiguities and choose their preferred courses of action. Fully understanding the nature of contemporary palliative care is imperative for making good choices.

Epilogue

This 400-year history of palliative care has explored stories and traditions situated in time and place and bound together by ribbons of legacy. The centuries-old quest for peaceful dying with the aid of healthcare professionals embodies elemental features of life: growth, dreams, expectations, times of testing, dedication, elation, disappointments, unexpected surprises, and hard-won successes.

From the time of Francis Bacon to the inauguration of palliative medical care by 1772, and up to the present time, healthcare professionals devoted to comfort-centered care have held that death is natural and inevitable. Richard A. Parker reaffirmed this fundamental premise when he said in 2002 that dying and death are part of "the 'package deal' of living."[1]

With this premise as its starting point, palliative care practitioners defined their unique specialty: physicians and other caregivers should use medical knowledge and skills to enable persons to die peacefully. They created a new type of package deal, one that paired dying with physical, emotional, and spiritual peacefulness. Parker affirmed that with the steadfast assistance of the doctor, patients usually experience a good death.[2] Others concurred. Expert palliative care enables patients to experience peaceful death as "a natural last step in the progression of aging and disease."[3]

The search for a good death with the help of medical measures began in 1605 with the challenge Bacon made to the physicians of his time. He reasoned that in addition to correcting other deficiencies, physicians should acquire the skill to enable persons to "pass more easily and quietly out of life."[4] He set forth reasons why death should be accepted as a natural, non-feared fixture in human life. Wisely, he recognized that the fruition of his challenge to physicians would require "a succession of ages ... not within the hour-glass of a man's life."[5]

At the same time, Bacon championed science as the foundation for improvements of the human condition. This history has shown how the search for a good death and the advancement of medical science played off one another over the centuries that followed. Bacon presented medical palliation and medical science as fully compatible with and supportive of each other. He could not, of course, have foreseen how the medical science he championed would for many decades marginalize and threaten to undermine peaceful and natural dying.

Beginning in the 1890s, scientific medicine within modern hospitals steadfastly focused on saving and prolonging human life with ever-increasing technological sophistication and invasiveness. Medicine's focus on healing and rescue led practitioners in hospitals to isolate and neglect persons sick unto death, as well as seek to prolong the lives of many others to the point of death.

Rather than viewing death as a natural end to life, numerous practitioners fought against it as a dreadful, evil enemy. The idea of death as enemy accords with the beliefs of the vast majority of physicians and non-physicians alike, religious or not. In Jewish and Christian scripture and its legal legacies, life is sacred and death is its ultimate foe. Secularists agree that death is their enemy. Upon castigating religion as a "vast moth-eaten musical brocade," the English poet Philip Larkin speaks of death as sure and total extinction, compared to which nothing is more terrible.[6]

So physicians equating death with evil accorded with common conviction. On the one hand, that equation profoundly motivated modern medical scientists to create amazing forms of healing and life extension from the 1890s to the present time. On the other, it has repressed acknowledgment of death's inevitability and delayed recognition that dying can be a time of peace, reconciliation, and newfound meaning.

Modern scientific medicine's war against death began to betray Bacon's palliative care legacy. Beyond viewing death as their enemy, many doctors regarded the deaths of their patients as manifestations of personal ineffectiveness and failure. Enmeshed in the dynamics of modern hospitals, they identified themselves as the rightful guardians of human life. So they assumed the roles of authoritarian paternalists who, without the knowledge and consent of those who came to hospitals for healing, turned the bodies of dying patients into medical battlefields. For some 90 years—roughly between 1895 and 1985—many doctors aggressively treated non-consenting, fatally ill patients up to the moment of death, and sometimes even after the body manifested signs of death. With far greater restraint after the late 1980s, most physicians ceased battles to prolong life when restitution became clearly hopeless.

However small their numbers became, defenders of palliative care and treatment opposed these and earlier excessive attempts to prolong life. The voices of these defenders resonate throughout the eras of this history—John Ferrier in 1798, William Munk in 1887, Walter Alvarez in 1952, Cicely Saunders from 1958 to 2004, Paul Ramsey in 1970, and a great chorus of others. At critical times in this story, nurses shouldered most of the care and spoke eloquently about their convictions for doing so. Together these persons speak to and for the women and men of our times.

Physicians without special expertise in the care of dying persons joined the ranks of these defenders insofar as they opposed the paternalism of their peers. "Do you want to continue that [chest messaging until] his pupils are fixed and dilated?" a doctor asked his colleague in the 1960s.[7] "When will **mercy** enter into the aggressive protocols and permit the ravaged patient to die peacefully?" another physician asked in 1983 after describing his daughter's ghastly ordeal.[8] "Must we always use the desperate measure of CPR regardless of the underlying illness?" still another asked in 1987.[9]

Physicians, along with nurses, ethicists, theologians, lawyers, commissions, and palliative care organizations, condemned physician paternalism as exceeding the boundaries of moral conscience. Programmatic guidelines and policies were developed to rein in such paternalism. The numbers of palliative care professionals expanded and became far more influential. They turned unremitting medical treatment into a choice, not a necessity. They also enabled patients, along with their family members, to choose medically sophisticated palliative care and treatment in lieu of (and, later, along with) medical efforts to sustain life. These momentous efforts and contributions have moved organized medicine far beyond past neglect, stonewalling, isolation, and abuse of dying patients.

This history is the legacy of practitioners of palliative care and treatment. It has persisted for hundreds of years. The voices, personalities, experiences, passions, firsthand stories, sacrifices, and exemplary expertise of the past are still insightful and inspiring. They have not gone with the winds of time. They remain sources of wisdom and instruction. They capture the ideals of palliative care and identify the moral and philosophical pillars upon which it stands. They account for the nature of contemporary hospice and hospital-based palliative care and treatment, and they will continue to inspire and enrich this care. Present-day practitioners are challenged to add new chapters to this legacy, to tell about that which is not told here.

Unfortunately, the good news about what palliative medicine includes is not as well known as it should be both in the minds of many medical professionals and in the eyes and minds of the public. This history informs readers about the nature of palliative care, past and present.

The legacies of patients, families, and friends are also portrayed in this history. Thankfully, at the present time increasing numbers of patients are respected with the right to make their own choices—exceedingly hard-won choices over centuries. Up to the point of manifest medical futility, many patients and their surrogates can choose aggressive medical treatment and choose to have the effects of those treatments relieved by palliation. They can also opt for only comfort care in various settings—most notably in hospice settings. Hospice care attends to the physical, emotional, spiritual, and social needs of patients and includes bereavement counseling for family members.

Persons who choose to continue with aggressive life-extending treatments should learn about their downsides. The surgeon and Jesuit priest, Myles Sheehan, counsels that "a good death, regardless of the circumstances, means putting medical care in proper perspective and not allowing it to dominate." That takes planning and wise choices.[10] Atul Gawande puts the matter memorably:

> Death is the enemy. But the enemy has superior forces. Eventually, it wins. And, in a war that you cannot win, you don't want a general who fights to the point of total annihilation. You don't want Custer. You want Robert E. Lee, someone who knew how to fight for territory when he could and how to surrender when he couldn't, someone who understood that the damage is greatest if all you do is fight to the bitter end.[11]

Persons faced with fatal illness and those who are legally empowered to make decisions for them will do well to identify their bottom-line beliefs. Gawande describes the story told to him by the nationally and internationally known palliative care expert, Susan Block. Catching herself after visiting with her severely ill father, she realized, "Oh, my God, I don't know what he really wants." Going back, she talked with him about what he would be willing to go through "to have a shot at being alive." In the midst of their agonizing conversation, he shocked her with the words, "Well, if I'm able to eat chocolate ice cream and watch football on TV then I'm willing to stay alive." Three minutes before his surgery she asked the surgeons whether he would still be able to eat chocolate ice cream and watch football on TV if the operation was successful.

Yes, they said. So she gave them the OK, and her father lived for another ten years. The outcome might have been different, but the honoring of his choice symbolized a bottom line.[12]

Present levels of choice for persons with life-threatening and life-ending illnesses represent the ultimate, crowning achievement of modern advocates of palliative, comforting care. The journey detailed in this book accounts for why these choices are increasingly accessible at the present time. Knowing about the core elements of present-day palliative medicine and care described in this work's final chapter enables patients and their families to make informed choices with respect to treatment options. Their decision to receive continued cure-directed medical treatments should hinge on health-care professionals' enabling them to become truly informed about the nature, promises, limits, harms, and costs of these treatments—namely, their effects on meaningful life and consciousness.

The central challenge faced by patients with catastrophic and terminal illnesses now involves wrestling over, and then making, decisions regarding their available options within the unalterable constraints of human mortality. Studies explored at the beginning of the last chapter show that these decisions often involve great ambivalence and anxiety. No patient and no family should feel guilt for those natural responses. Patients should, however, carefully weigh the burdens of their choices on themselves and their families.

During the times when heroic treatments were forced on patients, medical paternalism and authoritarianism ruled. Those tables should not be overturned, such that palliative care becomes a new form of paternalism. Patients should not be censured for not choosing comfort-focused end-of-life care. They should not be denied the right to opt for proven and promising curative treatments that may slow down or possibly reverse their present conditions and delay the visitation of death. Persons with severe and terminal illness have the right to say, "Thank you for expert symptom-easing care during the course of my illness, but with hopes still tied to yet-untried medical treatments, I choose to fight for life until I die." Alternatively, having undergone cure-intended treatments, persons with terminal illnesses can also say, "Thank you for the availability of expert palliative care that will ease my symptoms, add meaning to the last days of my life, and enable me to experience a good death."

Chapter Notes

Preface

1. The comprehensiveness of this history nevertheless focuses on palliative care for adult patients. Expansive histories of palliative medical care for infants and children, and for many of the other particular topics in this story—for example, the care for poorer patients and minorities, surgical palliative care, types of palliative sedation, and the biographies of numerous care professionals over time—have not yet been fully explored. Hopefully, this history will foster complementary studies.

2. Emily K. Abel, *The Inevitable Hour: A History of Caring for Dying Patients in* America (Baltimore: Johns Hopkins University Press, 2013).

3. For example, James L. Hallenbeck, *Palliative Care Perspectives* (Oxford: Oxford University Press, 2003), 3; Bruce Jennings, "Preface," *Improving End of Life Care: Why Has It Been So Difficult? A Hastings Center Special Report* 35, no. 6 (2005): S2–S4; and David Clark, "From Margins to Centre: A Review of the History of Palliative Care in Cancer," *Lancet Oncology* 8 (May 2007): 430–438, esp. 430.

4. Lawrence R. Samuel, *Death, American Style: A Cultural History of Dying in America* (New York: Rowman & Littlefield, 2013).

5. Shai J. Lavi, *The Modern Art of Dying: A History of Euthanasia in the United States* (Princeton, NJ: Princeton University Press, 2005).

6. Milton J. Lewis, *Medicine and Care of the Dying: A Modern History* (Oxford and New York: Oxford University Press, 2007).

7. At points Dr. Saunders herself contributed to the myth that palliative care began in the 1960s with the flourishing of the modern hospice movement she originated. Cicely Saunders, "The Evolution of Palliative Care," *Patient Education and Counseling*, no. 41 (2000): 7–13. For examples of others who take this view, see Hallenbeck, 3; Ian Dowbiggin, *A Concise History of Euthanasia: Life, Death, God, and Medicine* (New York: Rowman & Littlefield, 2005), 112; David Clark, "End-of-Life Care Around the World: Achievements to Date and Challenges Remaining," *OMEGA* 56, no. 1 (2007–2008): 101–110, esp. 101–102; and Lewis, 6–7.

Chapter 1

1. Bacon was promoted to the English peerage (which included several ranks of nobility) in 1618 under the title of Baron (and therefore Lord) Verulam. At the height of his social, legal, and legislative career, Bacon was elevated to the rank of Viscount St. Alban in 1621. His historical title Lord Verulam is indebted to his being the first holder of title Baron Verulam. See Perez Zagorin, *Francis Bacon* (Princeton, NJ: Princeton University Press, 1998), 21ff.

2. Three years before Bacon died in 1626 he published a heavily revised edition of *Advancement* in Latin for the purposes of reaching an international audience and registering his own intellectual growth. Bacon's revision of *Advancement* was titled *De Dignitate and Augmentis Scientiarum Libri IX—The Dignity and Advancement of Learning in Nine Books*, first published in 1623. Bacon's admonitions with respect to palliative care by and large remained the same in both works and, therefore, reflect his thinking between 1605 and 1623.

3. Francis Bacon, *The Major Works: Oxford World's Classics*, edited with introduction and notes by Brian Vickers (Oxford: Oxford University Press, 2002), 299. This work contains the translation of Bacon's original 1605 version of Bacon's *The Advancement of Learning*. References to Bacon's works in Vickers will be referred to as Bacon, *The Major Works* (Vickers, 2002).

4. Bacon, *The Major Works* (Vickers, 2002), 20–21 and 512–513.

5. Bacon, *The Major Works* (Vickers, 2002), 147–148.

6. Bacon, *The Major Works* (Vickers, 2002), 174.

7. Bacon, *The Major Works* (Vickers, 2002), 175 and 612. The quote is from Proverbs 22:13 and 26:13.

8. Francis Bacon, *The Great Instauration in New Atlantis and the Great Instauration*, ed. Jerry Weinberger (Wheeling, IL: Harlan Davidson, 1989), 15–16. In his preface to the greatly expanded version of *The Advancement of Learning* first published in 1623, Bacon says that he is writing not for pleasure, profit, fame, self-promotion, or out of contentiousness, but for the purposes of propagating "Varity in Charity." Francis Bacon, *Of the Advancement and Proficiencie of Learning: Or the Partitions of the Sciences, Nine Books*, translated (from Latin) by Gilbert Wats (London: Thomas Williams, 1674), 13–14. Wats's translation will be referred to as Bacon, *Of the Advancement* (Wats, 1674).

9. Bacon, *The Major Works* (Vickers, 2002), 174.

10. This quote is from Bacon's expanded *Advancement of Learning* published in 1623 as translated in Lord Bacon, *Advancement of Learning*, ed. Joseph Devey (New York: P.F. Collier and Son, 1902), 184–184–185. Devey's translation will be referred to as Lord Bacon, *Advancement of Learning* (Devey, 1902). Wats translates the phrase "impatience of diseases" more graphically as "the vexations of sickness." Bacon, *Of the Advancement* (Wats, 1674), 121.

11. Lord Bacon, *Advancement of Learning* (Devey, 1902), 186.

12. Lord Bacon, *Advancement of Learning* (Devey, 1902), 186, on the three "offices" of medicine, and 186–

187, on the first office or preservation of health.

13. Francis Bacon, *The Historie of Life and Death* (New York: Arno Press, 1977 [1638 edition]).

14. Lord Bacon, *Advancement of Learning* (Devey, 1902), 193–195.

15. Bacon, *Of the Advancement* (Wats, 1674), 123.

16. Lord Bacon, *Advancement of Learning* (Devey, 1902), 187–193.

17. Lord Bacon, *Advancement of Learning* (Devey, 1902), 192–193.

18. This text is taken from the translation of Bacon's expanded 1623 *Advancement* by Spedding, Ellis, and Heath because it precisely reflects Bacon's language regarding "attention" to the dying, as well as rightly translates the term "euthanasia exteriori" as "outward euthanasia." Bacon's 1623 text differs only slightly from his original text of 1605. Francis Bacon, *The Works of Francis Bacon*, edited by James Speeding, Robert Leslie Ellis, and Douglas Demon Heath, vol. IX (Boston: Taggard and Thompson, 1864), 34–35. For the Latin text, see Francisci Baconi Boronis De Verulamic, *Dignitate et Augmentis Scientiarum* (Londini: Edwardi Griffini, 1638). The translation by Speeding and others will be referenced as *The Works of Francis Bacon*, IX (Speeding et al., 1864).

19. Antoninus Pius was the fifteenth Roman emperor, who reigned from 138 to 161 CE. His famous final word was "aecquanimitus" (equanimity). See E. E. Bryant, *The Reign of Antoninus Pius* (Cambridge: Cambridge University Press, 1895), 91.

20. The Stygian water refers to the bitterness of death. In Greek mythology the river Styx was the boundary between life on earth and habitation in the underworld.

21. That is, set it down as something desired and essential.

22. That physicians were often at the bedsides of dying persons in the 16th century is confirmed by Ian Mortimer in *The Dying and the Doctors: The Medical Revolution in Seventeenth-Century England* (Rochester, NY: Boydell Press, Royal Historical Society, 2009), 73–189 and 204–211. Mortimer focuses on statistical changes regarding the increased number of physician, apothecary, and nursing services, as well as the greater use of medicines, ointments, dietary regimens, and bloodletting. Palliative care is not mentioned, nor is attention given to specific cases of provider-patient interaction.

23. Bacon, *The Major Works* (Vickers, 2002), 213 and 630.

24. The reference to and wording about Augustus Caesar is based on Bacon's reliance on Suetonius's *The Lives of the Caesars: Book II*, which says that Octavius (Augustus) "suddenly passed away as he was kissing Livia, uttering these last words: 'Live mindful of our wedlock, Livia, and Farewell,' thus blessed with an easy death and such a one as he had always longed for. For almost always on hearing that anyone had died swiftly and painlessly, he prayed that he and his might have a like *euthanasia*, for that was the term he was wont to use." Suetonius, *Suetonius in Two Volumes*, trans. J.C. Rolfe (Cambridge, MA: Harvard University Press, 1944), 281. Bacon first mentioned Augustus Caesar's use of "euthanasia" in the essay "On the Praise of Fortitude," probably written in 1592. Bacon, *The Major Works*, 28.

25. Ezekiel J. Emanuel claims that "possibly the first reference to euthanasia in the English literature was made in 1516 [by] Sir Thomas More in … *Utopia*." Against that claim, the term "euthanasia" or any equivalent of that word is never used by More, nor is it found in the English translations of More's *Utopia* beginning with the classic translation by Ralph Robynson in 1556, and including numerous translations thereafter, such as the scholarly side-by-side Latin and newly translated English texts by Logan, Adams and Miller in 1995 and the recent translation by Clarence H. Miller in 2001. After 1975, the indexed texts of More's work typically refer to his famous discussion of the honorable nature of voluntary death under the subject of "euthanasia" in the index. Emanuel, "The History of Euthanasia Debates in the United States and Britain" *Annals of Internal Medicine* 121, no. 10 (November 15, 1994): 793–802, esp. 794; Ralphe Robynson, *More's Utopia*, edited with introduction by J. Rawson Lumby (Cambridge: Cambridge University Press, 1892), 121–123; Thomas More, *Utopia: Latin Text and English Translation*, eds. George M. Logan, Robert M. Adams, and Clarence H. Miller (Cambridge: Cambridge University Press, 1995), 186–187 and 224–227; and Thomas More, *Utopia*, translated with introduction by Clarence H. Miller (New Haven, CT: Yale University Press, 2001), 96–97 and 120–121.

26. Bacon says in his 1605 edition of *Advancement* that "a fair and easy passage" is "that same *Euthanasia*" which "Augustus Caesar was want to wish for." Bacon, *The Major Works* (Vickers, 2002), 212.

27. Some authors say that Bacon promulgated physicians ending the lives of dying patients in pain. See Ezekiel J. Emanuel, "The History of Euthanasia"; Emanuel, "Euthanasia: Historical, Ethical, and Empiric Perspectives," *Archives of Internal Medicine* 154 (September 12, 1994): 1891; and L. Tad Cowley, Ernle Young, and Thomas A. Raffin, "Care of the Dying: An Ethical and Historical Perspective," *Critical Care Medicine* 20, no. 10 (October 1992): 1473–1482, esp. 1479.

28. See Harold Y. Vanderpool, "Doctors and the Dying of Patients in American History," in *Physician-Assisted Suicide*, ed. Robert F. Weir (Bloomington: Indiana University Press, 1997), 33–66; and Harold Y. Vanderpool, "Life-Sustaining Treatment and Euthanasia: III. Historical Aspects of," In *Bioethics*, 4th ed., six vols., ed. Bruce Jennings (Farmington Hills, MI: Macmillan Reference, 2014), vol. 4, 1849–1863.

29. The contents of these craft of dying books from the early 15th century through Jeremy Taylor's Anglican book first published in 1651 and titled *The Rule and Exercises of Holy Dying* are discussed by Nancy Lee Beaty, *The Craft of Dying: A Study of the Literary Tradition of the "Ars Moriendi" in England* (New Haven, CT: Yale University Press, 1970).

30. Beaty, 110.

31. David W. Atkinson, "The English Ars Morendi: Its Protestant Transformation," *Renaissance and Reformation* XVIII (1982): 1–10.

32. Bacon held to the Protestant doctrine of *sola scripture*—the authority and sufficiency of Scripture for Christian belief, practice, and morality. Bacon, *The Major Works* (Vickers, 2002), 1–19, 111–112, 122–126, 191–192, 289–299, and 373–374. See the excellent essay by Johann Mouton, "Reformation and Restoration in Francis Bacon's Early Philosophy," *Modern Schoolman* 60 (1983): 101–120, as well as Stephen A. McKnight, *The Religious Foundations of Francis Bacon's Thought* (Columbia: University of Missouri Press, 2006), esp. 134–159.

33. These quotes are from "Of Earthly Hope," and from *Advancement*. Bacon, *The Major Works* (Vickers, 2002), 94 and 245.

34. Quoted from Vickers in Bacon, *The Major Works* (Vickers, 2002), 565. Vickers discusses the background, themes, and unique ordering of Bacon's confession of faith at length (560–572).

35. The discussion and quotations that follow are from "Of Death" in Bacon, *The Major Works* (Vick-

ers, 2002), 343–344. At points I am indebted to Vicker's excellent footnotes on present-day meanings of some of Bacon's terminology (718–719).

36. A reference to the Romans 6:23 in the New Testament: "For the wages of sin is death."

37. In his essay titled "Of Superstition" Bacon caustically criticizes Roman Catholic scholastic theologians in the Council of Trent (the Ecumenical Council of 1545–1563 that codified Catholic teaching in opposition to the Protestant Reformation) as inventing unfounded and intricate dogmas. His criticism of friars fueling unwarranted fears of death accord with Bacon's Protestant-fueled criticisms of Roman Catholic superstition.

38. Here Bacon quotes from Seneca the philosopher: "Pompa mortis magis terret, quam mors ipsa" ("It is the trappings of death that scare us more than death itself"). Bacon, "Of Death," *The Major Works* (Vickers, 2002), 343.

39. Bacon, "Advice to the Earl of Rutland on His Travels," in Bacon, *The Major Works* (Vickers, 2002), 70.

40. The Roman emperor Marcus Salvius Otho, who died in 69 CE.

41. Bacon, "Of Death" in *The Major Works* (Vickers, 2002), 343.

42. Roman emperor from 31 BCE to 14 CE.

43. Roman Emperor from 69 to 79 CE.

44. Servius Sulpicius Galba, Roman emperor, 68–69 CE.

45. This text is from the New Testament gospel of Luke 2:29.

46. This and previous quotes are from Bacon, "Of Death," in *The Major Works* (Vickers, 2002), 343–344.

47. Laurence McCullough credits this position to the Prussian physician-professor Frederich Hoffman (1660–1745) and calls Hoffman's practices the medical "custom" of the time. Laurence B. McCullough, *John Gregory's Writings on Medical Ethics and Philosophy of Medicine* (Dordrecht/Boston/London: Kluwer Academic Publishers, 1998), 22.

48. Shai J. Lavi, *The Modern Art of Dying: A History of Euthanasia in the United States* (Princeton, NJ: Princeton University Press, 2005), 6.

49. Lavi, 1. In contrast, Cotton Mather's sermon in 1723 that describes Mather's visit with a young minister who died suddenly, happily, and easily with acclamations of "joy unspeakable" was entitled "Euthanasia." Mather, *Euthanasia: A Sudden Death Made Happy and Easy* (Boston: S. Kneeland, 1723), 1–28.

50. Mortimer, 207.

51. William Perkins, *A Salve for a Sicke Man, or a Treatise of … the Right Way to Die Well*, in *The Workes of that Famous and Worthie Divine in the University of Cambridge*, ed. J. Legatt (Cambridge: M. W. Perkins, 1608), vol. 1, 484. Eighteen editions of Perkins's work were published between 1561 and 1632.

52. Richard Baxter, *The Saint's Everlasting Rest* [personal copy with date unknown], 230. First published in 1650, after which over 16 editions were published by 1800, with numerous editions thereafter.

53. John Willison, *The Afflicted Man's Companion* (New York: J. C. Totten, 1806), 106 and 220. Willison's book was first published in 1727 and again in 1737, 1741, and many later editions.

54. David Carlin, "Sir Thomas Browne's *Religio Medici* and the Publishing House of Ticknor and Fields," *Osler Library Newsletter*, no. 89 (October 1998): 1–4.

55. Thomas Brown, *Pseudodoxia Epidemica: or, Enquiries into vary many received Tenants and commonly presumed Truths* (Sixth and Last Edition, 1672), esp. Book I, 17–20.

56. Browne, *Pseudodoxia or Enquiries*, Books I–VII.

57. The famed Greek physicians to whom, traditionally, the "Hippocratic" medical writings are attributed and who lived from c. 460 to 370 BCE.

58. This text is from sirbacon.org, which advances the study of Bacon. See http://www.sirbacon.org/history lifedeath.htm, 68 (accessed July 21, 2010).

59. Thomas Browne, "A Letter to a Friend," http://penelope.uchicago.edu/letter.html (accessed June 10, 2010), 3.

60. Browne, "To a Friend," 11.

61. Browne, "To a Friend," 17.

62. Thomas Browne, *Religio Medici*, edited by Jean-Jacques Denonain (Cambridge: Cambridge University Press, 1955), 57.

63. Browne, *Religio Medici*, 50 and 93, quote from 93.

64. Browne, *Religio Medici*, 92–93.

65. Browne, *Religio Medici*, 93 and 95.

66. Browne, *Religio Medici*, 93 and 53.

67. Browne, *Religio Medici*, 50.

68. Browne, *Religio Medici*, 98–99.

69. The best discussion of Bonet that I have found in English was published more than 70 years ago by Ernest E. Irons, "Theophile Bonet

1620–1689: His Influence on the Science and Practice of Medicine," *Bulletin of the History of Medicine* XII, no. 5 (December 1942): 623–665.

70. Irons, 643–654; John Crellin, "Theophile Bonet (1620–1689)," *American Journal of Pathology* 98 (January 1980): 212; Philip Rieder, "Bonet, Theophile," *Dictionary of Medical Biography*, vol. I (Westport, CT: Greenwood Press, 2007): 238–239.

71. Theophile Bonet, "The Office of a Physician," *A Guide to the Practical Physician*, Book XX (London: Thomas Flesher, 1688), 854–868.

72. Bonet, *A Guide to the Practical Physician*, Book I, 7–8.

73. Bonet, *A Guide to the Practical Physician*, 8.

74. Bonet, "The Office of a Physician," 855.

75. Bonet, "The Office of a Physician," 855.

76. Bonet, "The Office of a Physician," 855.

77. Donald D. McNeil Jr. "Palliative Care Extends Life, Study Finds," *New York Times*, August 19, 2010, A15.

78. Bonet, "Agonia, or Pangs of Death: How Persons at the Point of Death Are to Be Revived," *A Guide to the Practical Physician*, Book I, 7–8.

79. Bonet, "The Office of a Physician," topic 40, 862.

80. Bonet, "The Office of a Physician," topic 35, 861.

81. Samuel Bard, *A Discourse Upon the Duties of a Physician* (Bedford, MA: Applewood Books, 1996 [1769]), 11. Drs. John Morgan and Samuel Bard graduated together from the University of Edinburgh in 1765. Each aspired to establish a medical school in his respective city. Morgan returned to Philadelphia, where he, along with William Shippen, became instrumental in establishing the first medical school in America—the Medical Department of the University of Pennsylvania—three years before the medical school in King's College. See the excellent essay by Fielding H. Garrison, "Samuel Bard and the King's College School," *New York Academy of Medicine* 1 (May 1935), 87.

82. Garrison, 85.

83. Garrison, 88.

84. *Discourse*, 13–23, quote from 16.

85. Garrison, 87.

86. *Discourse*, 20–21.

87. Editorials, "Samuel Bard (1742–1821) Colonial Physician," *JAMA* 205, no. 8 (August 19, 1968): 586–587.

88. McCullough, 33–36; and Robert M. Veatch, *Disrupted Dialogue* (Oxford: Oxford University Press, 2005), 7–16.

89. John Gregory, *Lectures on the Duties and Qualifications of a Physician* (London: W. Strahan and P. Cadell, 1772), 109. These lectures are now available in a copy print book by ECCO Print editions. Bioethicists and historians are indebted to Laurence B. McCullough for highlighting Gregory's philosophical sophistication and contributions to medical ethics The carefully inscribed notes from 1767–1768 are found in McCullough, 71–99. Then Gregory's lectures were published anonymously (London: W. Strahan and T. Cadell, 1770), and definitively by Gregory himself in *Lectures on the Duties*, 1772.

90. These texts are from Gregory, *Lectures on the Duties*, 193 and 220. Gregory displays indebtedness to Bacon far more than any other authority, as evident in 107, 111, 130, 152, 159, and 189–193.

91. Gregory, *Lectures on the Duties*, 1772, introductory pages.

92. McCullough, 14–15. Cullen's mentorship included John Brown (1735–1788) and Benjamin Rush (1736–1808) of Philadelphia. For Cullen's theories of medicine, see Lester King, *The Medical World of the Eighteenth Century* (Huntington, NY: Robert E. Krieger, 1971 [1958]), 139–143 and 214–219.

93. See Erwin H. Ackerknecht, *Therapeutics from the Primitives to the 20th Century* (New York: Hafner Press, 1973), 78–92.

94. Gregory, *Lectures on the Duties*, 1772, 35.

95. See Herman Boerhaave's (1668–1738) discussion of "The Palliative Cure, or Treatment of Symptoms," in *Dr. Boerhaave's Academical Lectures of the Theory of Physic* (London: W. Innys, 1751), 432–440, and Dorothy Porter and Roy Porter, *Patient's Progress: Doctors and Doctoring in Eighteenth-century England* (Stanford, CA: Stanford University Press, 1989), 149–151.

96. Gregory, *Letters on the Duties*, 1772, 35.

97. Ministers and others viewed as displaying unbridled religious doctrinal and emotional excesses were labeled and opposed as "enthusiasts" by Enlightenment Protestants. The 1744 broadside against the "Enthusiasm" of the itinerate evangelist, George Whitefield, by the president and fellows of Harvard College displays that opposition. H. Shelton Smith, Robert T. Handy, and Lefferts A. Loetscher, *American Christianity: An Historical Interpretation with Representative Documents*, vol. I (New York: Scribner's, 1960), 330–330.

98. Gregory, *Letters on the Duties*, 1772, 36.

99. Gregory, *Lectures on the Duties*, 1772, 69–70.

100. Gregory, *Lectures on the Duties*, 1772, 35.

101. Gregory, *Lectures on the Duties*, 1772, 34–35.

102. On presaging the signs of death, see the discussion above about the Hippocratic signs of death and the discussion of the renowned physician Herman Boerhaave in *Academical Lectures on the Theory of Physic* (London: W. Innvs, 1751), 59.

103. Gregory, *Lectures on the Duties*, 1772, 22. Gregory did, however, credit patients with certain "rights," including, for example, patients and family members recommending a remedy to the physician without being criticized (33).

104. This phrase was used to summarize the description of Gregory's death published in 1788. Quoted in McCullough, 17.

105. Porter and Porter, 144–152, quote from 151.

Chapter 2

1. John Ferriar, *Medical Histories and Reflections*, 4 vols. (Philadelphia: Thomas Dobson, 1816), 392. The "little book" of Ferriar's essays published in 1796 became volume I of his 4-volume work, first published in 1809. Ferriar dedicated his little book to his older colleague and friend, Thomas Percival. Ferriar, *Medical Histories and Reflections* (London: Printed by W. Eyres for T. Cadell, 1792), iii and iv.

2. Thomas Percival, *Medical Ethics; or, A Code of Institutes and Precepts, Adapted to the Professional Conduct of Physicians and Surgeons* in *Percival's Medical Ethics*, ed. Chauncey D. Leake (Huntington, NY: Robert E. Krieger, 1975), appendix IV, 243. Percival's book will be referenced in this chapter as *Percival's Medical Ethics*, the pages of which refer to the pages in Leake's edition.

3. *Percival's Medical Ethics*, 91.

4. See the remarkable, profoundly appreciative review of Rush's life by Meredith Clymer in an annual oration to the society of graduates of the Medical Department of the University of Pennsylvania: Clymer, *Dr. Benjamin Rush: The Annual Oration* (Philadelphia: Collins Printer, 1876).

5. William G. Rothstein, *American Physicians in the Nineteenth Century: From Sects to Science* (Baltimore and London: Johns Hopkins University Press, 1972), 34–36.

6. Rothstein, 34; and Rush, "Duties of a Physician," in *The Selected Writings of Benjamin Rush*, ed. Gagobert D. Runes (New York: Philosophical Library, 1947), 308–309.

7. Rush, "Vices and Virtues," 298, in *The Selected Writings*.

8. Rush, "Vices and Virtues," 294 and 296.

9. Rush, "Duties of a Physician," 315, in *The Selected Writings*.

10. Rush, "Duties of a Physician," 313.

11. Rush, "Duties of a Physician," 313.

12. J. V. Pickstone and S. V. F. Butler, "The Politics of Medicine in Manchester, 1788–1792: Hospital Reform and Public Health Services in the Early Industrial City," *Medical History* 28 (1984): 227–249.

13. John M.T. Ford, "John Ferriar," Wellcome Institute for the History of Medicine, 1987, found at http://www.thornber.net/cheshire/ideasmen/ferriar.html (accessed October 29, 2009).

14. Corey E. Andrews, "'Ev'ry Heart can Feel': Scottish Poetic Responses to Slavery in the West Indies, from Blair to Burns," *International Journal of Scottish Literature* 4 (Spring/Summer 2008).

15. Ferriar, *Medical Histories and Reflections* (1816). In his preface (9–10), Ferrier describes the history of his publications and his "professional duty" to base all his "discussion" on "a convincing display of facts." The dates when his 4 volumes were first published are found in W. Bruce Fye, "Profiles in Cardiology: John Ferriar," *Clinical Cardiology* 21 (1998): 533–534.

16. Ferriar, *Medical Histories and Reflections* (1816), 9.

17. Ferriar, "Of the Treatment of the Dying," in *Medical Histories* (1816), 392.

18. Ferriar, "Of the Treatment of the Dying," 393.

19. Ferriar, "Of the Treatment of the Dying," 392.

20. Ferriar, "Of the Treatment of the Dying," 392.

21. Ferriar, "Of the Treatment of the Dying," 393.

22. Erwin H. Ackerknecht, *Therapeutics from the Primitives to the 20th Century* (New York: Hafner Press, 1973), 78–92, esp. 82–85.

23. "Opium in Medical Practice," at http://www.drugtext.org/library/books/opiumpeople/opiummedprac.html (accessed September 19, 2010).

24. P. N. Bennett, "Alexander Gordon (1752–99) and His Writing: In-

sights into Medical Thinking in the Late Eighteenth Century," *Journal of the Royal College of Physicians of Edinburgh* 42 (2012): 165–171, quote from 170.

25. Lester S. King, *The Medical World of the Eighteenth Century* (Huntington, NY: Robert E. Krieger, 1971 [1958]), 316–317.

26. Ferriar, "Of the Treatment of the Dying," 392–393.

27. Ferriar, "Of the Treatment of the Dying," 393–395.

28. Ferriar, "Of the Treatment of the Dying," 393.

29. The renowned English poet Edmund Spenser (1552?–1599).

30. Ferriar, "Of the Treatment of the Dying," 394.

31. Ferriar, "Of the Treatment of the Dying," 394.

32. Ferriar, "Of the Treatment of the Dying," 397–398.

33. Ferriar, "Of the Treatment of the Dying," 394–395.

34. The history and ethical bases for these practices have been explored by Michael Stolberg as expressive of popular traditions of actively ending persons' lives. Michael Stolberg, "Active Euthanasia in Pre-Modern Society, 1500–1880: Learned Debates and Popular Practices," *Social History of Medicine* 20 (July 7, 2007): 205–221.

35. Stolberg; Harold Y. Vanderpool, "The Responsibilities of Physicians toward Dying Patients," in *Medical Complications in Cancer Patients*, ed. J. Klastersky and M. J. Staquet (New York: Raven Press, 1981), 117–133.

36. Especially women who took it upon themselves to care for sick and dying persons. Nursing with special training would emerge in the 1840s and reach greater levels of professionalization with the career of Florence Nightingale (1820–1910).

37. Ferriar, "Of the Treatment of the Dying," 396.

38. Ferriar, "Of the Treatment of the Dying," 396.

39. James Mackness, *The Moral Aspects of Medical Life* (London: John Churchill, Princes Street, Solo, 1846), 340–341.

40. Mackness, 340–341.

41. Ferriar, "Of the Treatment of the Dying," 396–398.

42. This topic will be discussed in the later chapters of this book, and a window into its importance is found in Kathleen A. Culhane-Pera et al., *Healing by Heart: Clinical and Ethical Case Stories of Hmong Families and Western Providers* (Nashville: Vanderbilt University Press, 2003).

43. The Rev. Thomas Gisborne, *On the Duties of Physicians, Resulting from Their Profession* (Oxford: John Henry Parker, 1847).

44. "Austenonly: Jane Austen's People: Thomas Gisborne," at http://austenonly.com/2009/12/08/jane-austens-people-thomas-gisborne/ (accessed May 3, 2013).

45. This is a short-hand name for Percival's *Medical Ethics; or, A Code of Institutes and Precepts, Adapted to the Professional Conduct of Physicians and Surgeons* (Manchester: S. Russell, 1803).

46. *Percival's Medical Ethics*, 68.

47. *Percival's Medical Ethics*, 65–67 and 171.

48. Rush, "Duties of a Physician," 313 in *The Selected Writings*.

49. Quoted by Percival in his *Medical Ethics*, 186.

50. Gisborne, *On the Duties of Physicians*, 25.

51. The New Testament's book of Romans (3:8).

52. Ethical reasoning and problem-solving based on the probable consequences of actions is called consequentialism, the most prominent form of which is utilitarianism. Utilitarianism weighs the respective principles of utility (well-being, pleasure, happiness and the like) versus disutility to determine the rightness and/or wrongness of human actions. See the excellent and succinct overview of ethical theories, including utilitarianism, in Tom L. Beauchamp and James F. Childress, *Principles of Biomedical Ethics*, 6th ed. (New York: Oxford University Press, 2009), 333–368.

53. Gisborne, *On the Duties of Physicians*, 26–28.

54. Gisborne, *On the Duties of Physicians*, 27.

55. Gisborne, *On the Duties of Physicians*, 31 and 35–36.

56. *Percival's Medical Ethics*, 189.

57. Daniel K. Sokol, "How the Doctor's Nose Has Shortened over Time: A Historical Overview of the Truth-Telling Debate in the Doctor-Patient Relationship," *Journal of the Royal Society of Medicine* 99 (December 2008): 632–633; and Robert Baker and Laurence McCullough, "Medical Ethics' Appropriation of Moral Philosophy: The Case of the Sympathetic and Unsympathetic Physician," *Kennedy Institute of Ethics Journal* 17, no. 1 (2007): 4.

58. Robert M. Veatch, *Disrupted Dialogue* (Oxford: Oxford University Press, 2005), 4ff; and J. B. Morrell, "The University of Edinburgh in the Late Eighteenth Century: Its Scientific Eminence and Academic Structure," *Isis* 62 (Summer 1971): 158–171.

59. See the biography of Percival by Chauncey Leake in *Percival's Medical Ethics*, 24–34.

60. Preface to *Percival's Medical Ethics*, 65.

61. *Percival's Medical Ethics*, 65.

62. *Percival's Medical Ethics*, 66.

63. *Percival's Medical Ethics*, 120–166.

64. *Percival's Medical Ethics*, 68–69 and 170–172.

65. See Percival's preface in *Percival's Medical Ethics*, 65–69, and the discussion of Veatch, 63–70.

66. *Percival's Medical Ethics*, 67.

67. *Percival's Medical Ethics*, 167–205. In these pages, the editor of *Percival's Medical Ethics*, Chauncey D. Leake, abbreviates Percival's "Notes and Illustrations."

68. *Percival's Medical Ethics*, 74.

69. The phrase "rob the philosopher of fortitude" should probably be construed as "even rob the *philosopher* of fortitude." That interpretation accords with the widely held belief that philosophers (Socrates and others) and other heroic figures of the past embraced fortitude as an essential virtue of character. See the emphasis on "people of courage" in Francis Bacon's text on the naturalness of death in Chapter 1, and also Bacon's discussion of "how men endued with this virtue Fortitude have entertained death" (Bacon, *The Major Works*, 26–29, quote from 26).

70. *Percival's Medical Ethics*, 91.

71. *Percival's Medical Ethics*, 98.

72. Sir William Temple, Baronet, wrote a pioneering history of England and employed Jonathan Swift as his secretary. See http://www.britinnica.com/EBchecked/topic/586878/Sir-William-Temple-Baronet (accessed August 7, 2014).

73. Earlier in his code, Percival noted that "officiating clergymen" with propriety and discrimination were present in hospitals and medical charities (*Percival's Medical Ethics*, 73). He also greatly praised assisting clergy as "*Physicians* of the soul" who aid the skill of medicine with "the supports and comforts, which it is your sacred function to afford." These quotes are found in the original copy of Percival's medical ethics, which were deleted from Leake's edition. Thomas Percival, *Medical Ethics* (Manchester: S. Russell, 1803), 131.

74. Gisborne, *On the Duties of Physicians*, 25.

75. *Percival's Medical Ethics*, 186–194.

76. *Percival's Medical Ethics*, 194–195.

77. *Percival's Medical Ethics*, 194–195.

78. *Percival's Medical Ethics*, 195.

79. That is, during labor.

80. In bed awaiting the delivery of her child.

81. *Percival's Medical Ethics*, 195–196.

82. *Percival's Medical Ethics*, 91 and 194.

83. Leake, *Percival's Medical Ethics*, 35 and 47; and Veatch, 71 and 286–288.

84. Ferriar, "Of the Treatment of the Dying," 392 and 394.

85. See the brilliant essay by William May on the moral and metaphysical foundations of benevolent paternalism: William May, "The Metaphysical Plight of the Family" in *Death Inside Out*, eds. Peter Steinfels and Robert M. Veatch (New York: Harper and Row, 1974), 49–60.

Chapter 3

1. See these stories in the texts quoted from Percival in the last chapter.

2. Worthington Hooker, *Physician and Patient: or, A Practical View of the Mutual Duties, Relations and Interests of the Medical Profession and the Community* (New York: Baker and Scribner, 1849), 357–360. Hooker's quotes and texts are from the reprinted edition of *Physician and Patient* (New York: Arno Press, 1972).

3. Fielding H. Garrison, *An Introduction to the History of Medicine*, 4th ed. (Philadelphia: W. B. Saunders, 1929), 103, 571, 664–665.

4. Carl Friedrich Heinrich Marx, "Medical Euthanasia," 1826, trans. Walter Cane, *Journal of the History of Medicine and Allied Sciences* 7 (1952): 401–416, quotes from 405.

5. Marx, "Medical Euthanasia," 405–406.

6. We have seen how Marx referred to euthanasia (good dying) as a science (405). At the end of his essay, Marx also refers to euthanasia as "this art in medicine" (416).

7. Marx, "Medical Euthanasia," 405.

8. Marx, "Medical Euthanasia," 406

9. Marx, "Medical Euthanasia," 406.

10. Marx, "Medical Euthanasia," 407–408.

11. See the notable biography of Nightingale by Judith Lissauer Cromwell, *Florence Nightingale, Feminist* (Jefferson, NC, and London: McFarland, 2013), 73–83. See also Richard Harrison Shryock,

"Nursing Emerges as a Profession: The American Experience," in *Sickness and Health in America*, eds. Judith Walzer Leavitt and Ronald L. Numbers (Madison: University of Wisconsin Press, 1978), 203–215; and "Florence Nightingale," at http://www-history.mes.st-and.ac.uk/Biographies/Nightingale.html (accessed July 9, 2014).

12. Marx, "Medical Euthanasia," 408.

13. Marx, "Medical Euthanasia," 408–409.

14. Marx, "Medical Euthanasia," 407.

15. For references to the terms "heroic," "heroic treatments," and "heroic practices" in this age, see, for example, Alexis Berman, "The Heroic Approach in 19th-Century Therapeutics," in *Sickness and Health in America*, 77–79; Erwin H. Ackerknecht, *Therapeutics from the Primitives to the 20th Century* (New York: Hafner Press, 1973), 83–84, 119, and 191.

16. Marx, "Medical Euthanasia," 409.

17. Marx, "Medical Euthanasia," 407 and 409–410.

18. See the overview by John Duffy, *The Healers* (New York: McGraw-Hill, 1976), 98–106 and 232–233.

19. William G. Rothstein, *American Physicians in the Nineteenth Century: From Sects to Science* (Baltimore and London: Johns Hopkins University Press, 1972), 49–52; and John S. Haller Jr., *American Medicine in Transition, 1840–1910* (Chicago: University of Illinois Press, 1981), 77–90.

20. Rothstein, 53 and 59.

21. Quoted by Rothstein, 61–62.

22. Martin S. Pernick, *A Calculus of Suffering* (New York: Columbia University Press, 1985), 45.

23. These sects included Thomsonians, homeopaths, and hydropaths. See Ronald L. Numbers, "Do-It-Yourself the Sectarian Way," in *Sickness and Health in America*, 87–95; and Duffy, 107–128.

24. An operation bought relief to Ludwig van Beethoven that enabled him to live for another two days. "History: Liver and Ascites," at http://depts.washington.edu/physdx/liver/history.html (accessed May 20, 2013).

25. For a superb article on the anatomical details about and types of hernia surgeries, see Ira M. Rutkow, "A Selective History of Groin Hernia Surgery in the Early 19th Century," *Surgical Clinics of North America* 78 (December 1998): 921–940.

26. Marx, "Medical Euthanasia," 410.

27. See the still relevant biographies of notable surgeons in the first decade of the 19th century in Garrison (417–512). For a discussion of the surgical innovations of one of the domineering surgeons of the time, see G. Androutsos, M. Karamanou, and A. Kostakis, "Baron Gullaume Dupuytren (1777–1835): One of the Most Outstanding Surgeons of the 19th Century," *Hellenic Journal of Surgery* 83 (2011): 239–243.

28. Matt Soniak, "'Time Me, Gentlemen': The Fastest Surgeon of the 19th Century," at http://www.theatlantic.com/health/archive/2012/10/time-me-gentlemen-the (accessed May 21, 2013).

29. Marx, "Medical Euthanasia," 410.

30. Marx, "Medical Euthanasia," 406 and 413.

31. Marx, "Medical Euthanasia," 410.

32. Marx, "Medical Euthanasia," 411.

33. Marx, "Medical Euthanasia," 410–411 and 416.

34. Marx, "Medical Euthanasia," 412.

35. Marx, "Medical Euthanasia," 412.

36. Marx, "Medical Euthanasia," 413–414.

37. Marx, "Medical Euthanasia," 414.

38. Marx, "Medical Euthanasia," 414–415.

39. Marx, "Medical Euthanasia," 414–415.

40. Marx, "Medical Euthanasia," 415.

41. Marx, "Medical Euthanasia," 415–416.

42. Marx, "Medical Euthanasia," 405 and 406.

43. The quote is from Marx, "Medical Euthanasia," 411.

44. Robley Dunglison, *Address to the Medical Graduates of the Jefferson Medical College* (Philadelphia: Printed by Adam Waldie, 1837), 15–16.

45. Dunglison's discussion of the physiology of death as a corrective to received and popular opinion was emphasized by many others. See the book by A.P. W. Philip, *An Inquiry into the Nature of Sleep and Death* (London: Henry Renshaw, 1834); Anonymous, "Physiological Nature of Death," *Boston Medical and Surgical Journal* 15 (September 21, 1836): 109; and Bennet Dowler, "Researches on the Natural History of Death," *New Orleans Medical and Surgical Journal* 6 (January 1850): 594–615, esp. 607–608. Intense discussion also occurred regarding the many signs of death that surpassed the

classic facial signs of Hippocrates. See, for example, Henry W. Ducachet, "On the Signs of Death, and the Manner of Distinguishing Real from Apparent Death," *American Medical Recorder* 5 (1822): 39–52; and Christopher W. M. Hufeland, *The Art of Prolonging Human Life* (London: Simpkin and Marshall, 1829), 181–182.

46. Dunglison, *Address to the Medical Graduates*, 16.

47. Dunglison published his landmark text, *Human Physiology*, in 1832 and 2 volumes of essays on a comprehensive spectrum of human diseases in 1842. See the brief biography of Dunglison by Caroline Hannaway, "Dunglison, Robley," *Dictionary of Medical Biography*, ed. W. F. Bynum and Helen Bynum, vol. 2 (Westport, CT: Greenwood Press, 2007), 440–441.

48. Dunglison, *Address to the Medical Graduates*, 16.

49. C. W. Hufeland, *Enchiridion Medicum, or The Practice of Medicine*, 2nd ed. (New York and London: William Badde, 1844), iii–iv. The references and quotes that follow refer to this text, which duplicated the first (1842) edition.

50. See the excellent study by Thomas H. Broman, *The Transformation of German Academic Medicine, 1750–1820* (Cambridge and New York: Cambridge University Press, 1996), 104–113 and 122–125. Brief biographies of Hufeland are found in Hufeland, *Enchiridion*, v–vi; and I. A. Abt, "Christopher Wilhelm Hufeland," *Annals of Medical History* (1931): 27–38.

51. "Three Cardinal Means" is paginated separately at the end of *Enchiridion*. Hufeland's reference to them as "heroics" is found on 15.

52. Hufeland, "Three Cardinal Means," 4–15; and Broman, 114–119.

53. Hufeland, *Enchiridion*, quotes from 77. For an excellent discussion of emphases on the qualities of character of German physicians at the time and for the ways these accents increased the social status of the profession, see Broman, 70–72, 97, 104–108, 169–173, and 184–184.

54. Hufeland, *Enchiridion*, 7.

55. Hufeland, *Enchiridion*, 7.

56. Hufeland, *Enchiridion*, 7–9.

57. Hufeland, *Enchiridion*, 7.

58. Hufeland, *Enchiridion*, 7.

59. Hufeland, *Enchiridion*, 7–8.

60. Hufeland, *Enchiridion*, 7.

61. Hufeland, "Three Cardinal Means," 46.

62. Hufeland, "Three Cardinal Means," 47.

63. Hufeland, "Three Cardinal Means," 46–47.

64. Hufeland, "Three Cardinal Means," 47.

65. That is, experienced-based practitioners who magnify the efficacy of their cures—and their earnings—in spite of their lack of formal medical education. Physicians with MDs often over-censored empirics for their lack of formal training and their dependence on "quack" remedies. While an assortment of empirics deserved these criticisms, empirics like John Wesley, who opposed standard heroic remedies, probably benefited patients as much as or more than their medically educated counterparts. The AMA surely included under "empiricism" various assortments of mountebanks and quacks—traveling venders of patent medicines, hucksters of magical curatives for purposes of profit, and not a few "Cheats and Bubbles." Unfortunately, these cheats and bubbles are still around and exposed now and then. See, for example, Lester King, *The Medical World of the 18th Century* (Huntington, NY: Robert E. Krieger, 1971 [1958]), 34–58, quote from 46.

66. *Code of Ethics of the American Medical Association: Adopted May 1847* (San Francisco: Jos. Winterburn, 1867), 4. For Percival's words, see Chapter 2 and Thomas Percival, *Percival's Medical Ethics*, ed. Chauncey D. Leake (Huntington, NY: Robert E. Krieger, 1975), 91 and 98.

67. See, for example, the beliefs of a physician from New Orleans, Bennet Dowler, who briefly discusses the elements of "euthanasia" and adds that the art of enabling patient's to die peacefully, "next to the restoration of health, ought to be the object of every physician." Dowler, 611.

68. The phrase "cordials to the drooping spirit" in Percival and the AMA code very likely include the words of the physician as well as the medicines given.

69. The emphasized words are mine.

70. Hooker, *Physician and Patient*, quote from x.

71. For a discussion of these groups, see Numbers, "Do-It-Yourself the Sectarian Way," in *Sickness and Health in America*, 87–96.

72. Laurence B. McCullough, "Hooker, Worthington," in *Dictionary of Medical Biography*, eds. W. F. Bynum and Helen Bynum, vol. 3 (Westport, CT: Greenwood Press, 2007), 664.

73. Hooker, 345.

74. The quote is from Hooker, 355–356. In 1850 Bennet Dowler says succinctly, "Hope is an excellent medicine." Dowler, 611.

75. Hooker, 345.

76. Hooker, 347.

77. Hooker, 346–353.

78. Hooker, quotes from 348 and 351.

79. Hooker, 347.

80. Hooker, 353.

81. Hooker, 347–348.

82. Hooker, 348–355.

83. Hooker, 346–347.

84. Hooker, quotes from 348.

85. Gisborne's statement was quoted in *Percival's Medical Ethics*, 186. For Rush's position, see Benjamin Rush, "Duties of a Physician" in *The Selected Writings of Benjamin Rush*, ed. Gagobert D. Runes (New York: Philosophical Library, 1947), 313.

86. Hooker, 356–357.

87. Hooker, 357.

88. See the quotes and discussion of Percival in Chapter 2, and Percival's texts in *Percival's Medical Ethics*, 194–196.

89. Hooker, 359–360.

90. Hooker, 360.

91. These three arguments are made by Hooker, 360–363.

92. Hooker, 363.

93. Hooker, 365.

94. Hooker, 365–372, for these injuries.

95. Hooker, 372–373.

96. Hooker, 374–375.

97. Hooker, 375–376.

98. Hooker, 378.

99. Hooker, 380.

100. Hooker, 382.

101. Tom L. Beauchamp, "Worthington Hooker on Ethics in Clinical Medicine," in *The Codification of Medical Morality*, vol. 2, ed. Robert Baker (Dordrecht: Kluwer Academic Publishers, 1995), 106. Beauchamp situates Hooker within the philosophical and theological ethics of his time (105–119).

102. Review: Medical Ethics, "*Physician and Patient*, by Worthington Hooker," *American Journal of Medical Sciences* 23 (January 1852): 149–177, esp. 172–174, with quotes from 174.

103. Clifford Hawkins, "Writing the MD Thesis," *British Medical Journal* (November 6, 1976): 1121–1124.

104. Hugh Noble, *Euthanasia* (University of Edinburgh, 1854), 26 pages. I found Noble's thesis while doing research in library of the Society of Royal Physicians in Edinburgh. It is available in the Centre for Research Collections in the Edinburgh University Library.

105. Noble, 1, 6, 12, and 15.

106. Noble, 2.

107. Noble, 1–5.

108. Noble, 12–13, and 23, quotes from 12 and 13.

109. Anesthetics were discovered in 1842. The germ theory of disease was validated by Louis Pasteur in 1861 and became the basis for the transformative work on antisepsis by Joseph Lister in 1867. In 1847, however, Ignaz Phillip Semmelweis's discovery that the frequency of obstetrical infections could be greatly decreased if obstetricians washed their hands in a chlorinated lime solution was publicized in *The Lancet.* Perhaps that and other aseptic and antiseptic practices were being used in Edinburgh by 1856. See also Rothstein, 250–259.

110. Noble, 16–17.

111. Noble, 5–8 and 12–15.

112. The Scottish physician, James Young Simpson, discovered the anesthetic qualities of chloroform in 1851, the use of which rapidly expanded in surgery thereafter. See J. Wawersik, "History of Chloroform Anesthesia," *Anaesthesiologie und Reanimation* 22 (1997): 144–152.

113. Noble, 2–3, 9–11, and 19–22.

114. Noble, 25.

115. Noble, 24–25.

116. Noble, 16.

117. Noble, 17.

118. Noble, 17.

119. Noble, 17–18. The bold words are mine. The underlined word is in Noble's text.

120. Noble, 26.

121. Noble, 2.

Chapter 4

1. Carl Friedrich Heinrich Marx, "Medical Euthanasia," 1826, trans. Walter Cane, *Journal of the History of Medicine and Allied Sciences* 7 (1952): 406.

2. A Hospital Nurse, "Some Notes on How to Nurse the Dying," *The Trained Nurse* 5 (July–December 1890): 17–21.

3. The identification of exact diagnosis with modern, scientific medicine continued into the first decades of the 20th century. See Alfred Worcester, "Past and Present Methods in the Practice of Medicine," *Boston Medical and Surgical Journal* 166 (February 1, 1912): 162–164.

4. C. J. B. Williams, "On the Success and Failures of Medicine," *The Lancet* 5 (April 5, 1862): 345–347.

5. Alex Berman, "The Heroic Approach in 19th-Century Therapeutics," in *Sickness and Health in America*, eds. Judith Walzer Leavitt and Ronald L. Numbers (Madison: University of Wisconsin Press, 1978), 81–83.

6. Berman, 82–83.

7. William G. Rothstein, *American Physicians in the Nineteenth Century: From Sects to Science* (Baltimore and London: Johns Hopkins University Press, 1972), 183–184, quote from a family member in 1889.

8. Antipyrine, a drug based on coal tar, began to replace quinine as an anti-febrile drug in the late 1880s and was elevated to panacea status by 1893.

9. See the discussion of Hufeland in Chapter 3, as well as Rothstein, 186–195.

10. Simon Flexner and James Thomas Flexner, *William Henry Welch and the Heroic Age of American Medicine* (Baltimore: Johns Hopkins University Press, 1993 [1941]), 181–210, quote from 207.

11. Rothstein, 249–260.

12. Fielding H. Garrison, *An Introduction to the History of Medicine*, 4th ed. (Philadelphia: W. B. Saunders, 1929), 590–616; Gerald Imber, *Genius on the Edge* (New York: Kaplan, 2010), 9–35; John Duffy, *The Healers* (New York: McGraw-Hill, 1976), 255–256; and Erwin H. Ackernecht, *Therapeutics from the Primitives to the 20th Century* (New York: Hafner Press, 1973), 130–136.

13. Florence Nightingale, *Notes on Nursing* (New York: D. Appleton, 1860, first published in 1859); see especially the important biography of Nightingale by Judith Lissauer Cromwell, *Florence Nightingale, Feminist* (Jefferson, NC: McFarland, 2013).

14. The war broke out in 1854 when Russia began fighting the combined armies of England, France, and Turkey.

15. Bernard Cohen, "Florence Nightingale," *Scientific American* 250 (March 1984): 128–137; and Cromwell's biography.

16. Richard Harrison Shryock, "Nursing Emerges as a Profession: The American Experience," in *Sickness and Health in America*, 205.

17. Williams, 346.

18. From Shryock, 207.

19. Nightingale, 17–18. For additional references to death and the care of terminally ill persons, see 46, 130, and 134.

20. For example, Nightingale, 12–16, 17–20, 30–32, and 130.

21. Nightingale, 12.

22. Nightingale, 30.

23. Discoveries that microorganisms or germs caused disease and infection were made by Louis Pasteur (1822–1895), Joseph Lister (1827–1912), Robert Koch (1843–1910) and others in the late 1860s and thereafter. See Rothstein, 253–259, and Imber, 13–19.

24. See the discussion of Harold Y. Vanderpool, "Changing Concepts of Disease and the Shaping of Contemporary Preventive Medicine," in *Preventive Medicine and Community Health*, ed. Anne W. Domeck (Galveston: University of Texas Medical Branch, 1982), 7–34, esp. 10–14. The quote is from Nightingale, 127.

25. Nightingale, 32–33.

26. Nightingale, 28.

27. Nightingale, 28, 30, 35, 78–80, and 85, quotes from 28, 78 and 85.

28. Nightingale, 38–39 and 44–49.

29. Nightingale, 29 and 40–43, quote from 42.

30. S. D. Williams, "Euthanasia," in *Essays by Members of the Birmingham Speculative Club* (London: Williams and Norgate, 1870), 210–237.

31. For the British origins of that debate and its prominence in American medicine, see Harold Y. Vanderpool, "Doctors and the Dying of Patients in American History," *Physician-Assisted Suicide*, ed. Robert F. Weir (Bloomington: Indiana University Press, 1997), 33–66. See also the discussion by Larna Jane Campbell, "Principle and Practice: An Analysis of Nineteenth and Twentieth Century Euthanasia Debates (1854–1969)" (PhD dissertation, University of Edinburgh, 2003), 118–134.

32. For an historical overview of the five major meanings of euthanasia, see Harold Y. Vanderpool, "Life Sustaining Treatment and Euthanasia: II. Historical Aspects of," in *Encyclopedia of Bioethics*, 4th ed., ed. Bruce Jennings (Farmington Hills, MI: Macmillan Reference USA, 2014), Vol. 4, 1849–1863. For books that intertwine doctor-induced death with physicians' attention to palliative care, see, for example, Shai J. Lavi, *The Modern Art of Dying: A History of Euthanasia in the United States* (Princeton, NJ: Princeton University Press, 2005; and Milton J. Lewis, *Medicine and Care of the Dying: A Modern History* (Oxford and New York: Oxford University Press, 2007).

33. S. D. Williams, 212.

34. S. D. Williams, 212–213, quote from 212.

35. S. D. Williams, references to 211, 213, 223–5, 228–229, 231–232, 234, and 237, with quote from 219.

36. S. D. Williams, 212.
37. S. D. Williams, quotes from 236 and 224.
38. S. D. Williams, 230.
39. S. D. Williams, 214–217.
40. S. D. Williams, 215–218.
41. S. D. Williams, 235–237.
42. "Euthanasia," *Spectator Archive* (March 18, 1871), 10ff. For the historic replaying of these opposing positions, see Vanderpool, "Doctors and the Dying of Patients in American History."
43. Paul Starr, *The Social Transformation of American Medicine* (New York: Basic Books, 1982), 85–88.
44. The texts below will be taken from D. W. Cathell, *The Physician Himself* (Baltimore: Cushings and Bailey, 1882), which was reprinted in New York (Arno Press, 1972). Later editions expanded on his 1882 publication but did not change them substantively. See, for example, D. W. Cathell, *Book on the Physician Himself* (Philadelphia: F. A. Davis, 1903).
45. Praise for Cathell's advice has continued for well over a century. See, for example, "Review of Cathell, D. W., *Book on the Physician Himself*," *Journal of Laryngology* 6 (1892): 594–595; Book Notices, *"Book on the Physician Himself,* by D. W. Cathell," *JAMA* 62 (January 24, 1914): 318; and D. Neuhauser, "Public Opinion Is Our Supreme Court: D. W. Cathell MD, *The Physician Himself,*" *Quality and Safe Health Care* 14 (2005): 389–390.
46. Starr, 80–92.
47. Cathell, 87.
48. Cathell, 82–83 and 200–201.
49. Cathell, 87.
50. Cathell, 200.
51. Cathell, 201–202.
52. Cathell, 198–199.
53. Cathell, 202.
54. Cathell, 81, 83, 199–201. See the discussion of Robley Dunglison in Chapter 3.
55. Cathell, 198.
56. Cathell, 81 and 86.
57. Cathell, 86 and 87.
58. Cathell, 82.
59. Cathell, 81–82.
60. Cathell, 82.
61. See Debra Campbell, "Catholicism from Independence to World War I," in *Encyclopedia of the American Religious Experience*, Vol. I, eds. Charles H. Lippy and Peter W. Williams (New York: Scribner's, 1988), 357–374, esp. 362–369.
62. Cathell, 83–86. In these pages he also describes baptism for newborns and says that others besides priests can baptize by using the precise rituals and words he gives to his readers.

63. For example, Daniel W. Foster, "Religion and Medicine: The Physician's Perspective," in *Health/Medicine and the Faith Traditions*, eds. Martin E. Marty and Kenneth L. Vaux (Philadelphia: Fortress Press, 1982), 245–270; Harold Koenig, Michael McCullough, and David Larson, *Handbook of Religion and Health* (New York: Oxford University Press, 2001); and Harold Y. Vanderpool, "The Religious Features of Scientific Medicine," *Kennedy Institute of Ethics Journal* 18 (2008): 203–234.
64. Nic Hughes and David Clark, "'A Thoughtful and Experienced Physician': William Munk and the Care of the Dying in Late Victorian England," *Journal of Palliative Medicine* 7 (2004): 703–710, esp. 705.
65. Reviews and Notices of Books, "*Euthanasia, or Medical Treatment in Aid of an Easy Death*, by William Munk, M.D.," *The Lancet* 7 (January 7, 1888): 21–22.
66. William Munk, *Euthanasia or, Medical Treatment in Aid of an Easy Death* (London and New York: Longmans, Green, 1887). Munk's book was initially published in both London and New York. A facsimile of the original text was republished by the Arno Press (New York, 1977), from which the references and texts in this chapter are taken.
67. Munk, iii, 89, and 100–101.
68. Munk, 3. At this point Munk supplies his readers with Francis Bacon's full text on palliative care in Latin.
69. Munk regularly quotes from William Heberden's (1710–1801) Latin text, *Commentaria de Morborum Historia et Curatione* (first published in 1802), constructed from the careful notes made in his pocketbook at the bedside of patients. His *Commentaries on the History and Cure of Diseases* were published in English in 1802, 1806, and 1818.
70. Munk, 5–6. Known as Henry Vaughn before he became a baronet and changed his name in 1809, Sir Henry Halford (1766–1844) served as a physician to King George III from 1793 to 1830, and he continued to attend to British royalty. William Munk himself published *The Life of Sir Henry Halford* (London: Longmans, Green, 1895). See John S. Morris, "Sir Henry Halford, president of the Royal College of Physicians, with a note on his involvement in the exhumation of King Charles I," *Postgraduate Medical Journal* 83 (June 2007): 431–433.
71. Munk, v–vi. Munk relies on Sir Henry Halford, *Essays and Orations Read and Delivered at the Royal College of Physicians*, 3rd ed.

(London: John Murray, Albemarle Street, 1833).
72. Benjamin Collins Brodie (1783–1862) was one of the great surgeon-philosophers of his time, who entered surgical practice because he had nothing better to do and rose to the recognized rank of "the first surgeon in England." Munk refers to and quotes from Brodie, *The Works of Sir Benjamin Collins Brodie*, ed. Charles Hawkins (London, 1865). The prominent British surgeon William Scovell Savory became highly influential within the London College of Surgeons. Having not earned an MD degree, Savory was referred to as "Mr. Savory" in Munk's treatise (Munk, 10 and 24). Munk refers to Savory's *On Life and Death* (London, 1863), a book consisting of four lectures.
73. Munk, 77–78.
74. Munk, 4.
75. Munk, 4–5.
76. Munk, 7.
77. John Ferriar, "On the Treatment of the Dying," in *Medical Histories and Reflections* (Philadelphia: Thomas Dobson, 1816), 394.
78. For the next 10 pages, Munk offers further proof of this point by referring to published cases of apparent death from drowning, including testimonials of revived sailors.
79. Munk, 20.
80. Munk, 21–22.
81. Munk, 22–23.
82. Muck, 22–23.
83. See Norman Moore, "Munk, William," *Dictionary of National Biography*, 1901 supplement at http://en.wikisource.org/wiki/Munk,_William-(DNB01) (accessed October 26, 2010). See also the valuable discussion of Munk by Larna Jane Campbell, 127–128.
84. Here Munk refers to William Savory's *On Life and Death* (178).
85. Munk, 26–27.
86. Munk, 26–30.
87. Munk, 30.
88. Munk, 31–49, quote from 47.
89. Munk, 7.
90. See the bestselling book by Sherwin B. Nuland, *How We Die* (New York: Vintage Books, 1993), esp. xv–xviii, 264–268, quote from xv. Nuland's book will be discussed in Chapter 8.
91. Munk, 54–55.
92. Munk, 53–56.
93. Munk comments on page 57 that Watson's 5th lecture is impressive and detailed for its time. He focuses on various causes of death—disability, apnea, coma, and so on. Watson (1792–1882) delivered his lectures at King's College in London. Printed and revised in several British

and American editions (first published in 1858), his lectures influenced generations of practitioners. Greatly respected, Watson became a fellow in the Royal College of Physicians and a physician to the English queen.

94. This is the footnote from Munk on 57. It refers to Thomas Watson, *Lectures on the Principles and Practice of Physic*, 5th ed., 2 vols. (London, 1871), 62.

95. Munk, 57–60.

96. Munk, 61–62.

97. Munk, 86–87.

98. Munk, 86.

99. Munk, 97–100, with the quote and reference to Nightingale on 100.

100. Munk, 101.

101. Munk, 85–86.

102. Munk, 105.

103. Munk, 66.

104. Munk, 66–68.

105. Munk, 69–70.

106. Munk, 72–75.

107. Munk, 74–81.

108. Munk, 83–85.

109. Munk, 86.

110. Munk, 65 and 104.

111. Munk, 71–72.

112. Munk, 88 and 103.

113. Munk, 9 and 105.

114. Reviews and Notices of Books, "*Euthanasia*," 21–22.

115. William Osler, "Notes and Comments," *Canada Medical and Surgical Journal* 16 (March 1888): 510–511.

116. Charles B. Williams, "Euthanasia," *Medical and Surgical Reporter* 70 (June 30, 1894): 909.

117. Williams, 909–911.

118. Williams, 911.

119. Munk, 81.

120. A Hospital Nurse, 17.

121. A Hospital Nurse, 17.

122. A Hospital Nurse, 17.

123. A Hospital Nurse, 17.

124. A Hospital Nurse, 17

125. A Hospital Nurse, 18.

126. A Hospital Nurse, 18.

127. A Hospital Nurse, 19–21.

128. A Hospital Nurse, 21.

129. Oswald Browne, *On the Care of the Dying: A Lecture to Nurses* (London: George Allen, 1894), 5.

130. Browne, 10–37, quote from 30.

131. Browne, 22–24. The quotes are from an address by Dr. Matthews Duncan to the Abernethian Society in 1886. This is James Matthews Duncan (1826–1890), a fellow in the Royal College of Physicians in Edinburgh.

132. Browne, 25–26.

133. Browne, 7 and 31.

134. Browne, 29.

135. Munk, 4.

136. C.J.B. Williams, 345–347.

137. Austin Flint, *A Treatise on the Principles and Practice of Medicine*, 3rd ed. (Philadelphia: Henry C. Lea, 1868), 17.

Chapter 5

1. Sir William Osler, "Man's Redemption of Man" in Sir William Osler, *Osler's "A Way of Life" and Other Addresses* (Durham, NC: Duke University Press, 2001), 355–370.

2. Osler, "Mans Redemption," 358, emphasis mine.

3. Osler, "Man's Redemption," 363–370.

4. Osler, "Man's Redemption," 363.

5. "The Doctor," *Medical Review of Reviews* 20 (January 1914): 76–77.

6. George E. Ranney, "Death, a Universal Law," *Transactions of the Michigan State Medical Society* 16 (1892): 9–29, quote from 10. Ranney also calls death "the grim monarch," the "arch enemy," and "the great and invisible conqueror" with a black flag "unfurled over an appalling legion of diseases" (10–13).

7. See the introductory chapter by Austin Flint, *A Treatise on the Principles and Practice of Medicine*, 3rd ed. (Philadelphia: Henry C. Lea, 1868), 17–23; and William Osler, *The Principles and Practice of Medicine* (New York: D. Appleton, 1892). Flint's textbook was first published in 1866, with a 5th edition in 1884. Osler's text was first published in 1892, with its 16th edition published in 1947. Each consumed enormous time and effort.

8. Ira Rutkow, *Seeking the Cure: A History of Medicine in America* (New York: Scribner, 2010), 134–180.

9. Alfred Worcester, "Past and Present Methods in the Practice of Medicine," *Boston Medical and Surgical Journal* 166 (February 1, 1912): 163.

10. Christopher Crenner, *Private Practice* (Baltimore: Johns Hopkins University Press, 2005), 69–81, 214.

11. Creener, 77–78, 208–220.

12. William Osler, "Treatment of Disease," *British Medical Journal* (July 24, 1909): 185–189; and Gerald Imber, *Genius on the Edge: The Bizarre Double Life of Dr. William Steward Halstead* (New York: Kaplan, 2010), 105–110.

13. Edmund D. Pelligrino, "The Sociocultural Impact of Twentieth-Century Therapeutics," in *The Therapeutic Revolution*, eds. Morris J. Vogel and Charles E. Rosenberg (Philadelphia: University of Pennsyl-

vania Press, 1979), 246–253. For the stellar career of William H. Welch at Johns Hopkins in pathology and bacteriology, see Simon Flexner and James Thomas Flexner, *William Henry Welch and the Heroic Age of American Medicine* (Baltimore: Johns Hopkins University Press, 1993 [1941]).

14. For William Welch's devotion and involvement in public health, see Flexner and Flexner, 341–364; see also William G. Rothstein, *American Physicians in the Nineteenth Century: From Sects to Science* (Baltimore and London: Johns Hopkins University Press, 1972), 261–281.

15. Worcester, "Past and Present Methods," 164.

16. Imber, esp. 111–124, 229–245, and 283–286, quote from 139. See also, for example, Michael Bliss, "Cushing, James Harvey," in *Dictionary of Medical Biography*, eds. W. F. Bynum and Helen Bynum (Westport, CT: Greenwood Press, 2007), 388–392; Harvey Cushing, *Consecratio Medici and Other Papers* (Boston: Little, Brown, 1928); and Rutkow, esp. 125–132 and 180–190.

17. Lindsay Granshaw, "The Hospital," *Companion Encyclopedia of the History of Medicine*, vol. 2, eds. W.F. Bynum and Roy Porter (London: Routledge, 1993), 1180–1203, esp. 1189–1891; James Bordley III and A. McGehee Harvey, *Two Centuries of American Medicine* (Philadelphia: W. B. Saunders, 1976), 283–288; and A. J. Oschner, "Hospital Growth Marks Dawn of New Era," *Modern Hospital* 1 (September 1913): 1–5.

18. Flexner and Flexner; and Paul Starr, *The Social Transformation of American Medicine* (New York: Basic Books, 1982), 116.

19. For example, Henry A. Christian, "The Medical Profession's Obligation to the Patient," *Modern Hospital* 7 (1916): 9–12; and S. S. Goldwater, "The Hospital and the Surgeon," *Modern Hospital* 7 (October 1916): 273–277 and (November 1916): 371–377. For the roles of trained nurses, see Starr, 155–156.

20. Hugh Cabot, "Avoiding Psychological Damage in the Care of Hospital Patients," *Modern Hospital* 17 (September 1921): 184.

21. Thomas F. Reilly, "Signs and Symptoms of Impending Death," *JAMA* 66 (January 18, 1916): 161.

22. J. V. DePorte, "Where Do People Die—at Home or in Hospitals?" *Modern Hospital* 33 (August 1929): 73–80.

23. A Hospital Nurse, "Some Notes on How to Nurse the Dying,"

The Trained Nurse 5 (July–December 1890): 17–21; Hermine Kane, "The End," *American Mercury* 19 (April 1930): 458–461; and Alfred Worcester, "The Care of the Dying," in *Physician and Patient*, ed. L. Eugene Emerson (Cambridge, MA: Harvard University Press, 1929), 201.

24. A Hospital Nurse, 17–21.

25. Kane, 458–461. Kane is writing about her work as a "trained nurse" responsible for most of the care of dying persons.

26. See the outstanding analysis of the nature of authority and the growth and consolidation of medicine's professional authority by Paul Starr, 3–29 73–189, esp. 3–17 116–156. Starr shows that medicine as an extraordinary work of reason based on specialized knowledge, technical expertise, and rules of behavior was indelibly linked to the power of its system of organization.

27. Texts of the 1847 Code's articles regarding palliative care are given in this book's Chapter 3; the full text of the 1903 code is found in Chauncey D. Leake, ed., *Percival's Medical Ethics* (Huntington, NY: Robert E. Krieger, 1975), 240–257. The word *"Ordinarily"* is new to the 1903 code, and the italics are mine.

28. Leake gives the full text of the 1912 code on 259–273. The quotes from that code are on 260.

29. William Osler, "Notes and Comments," *Canada Medical and Surgical Journal* 16 (March 1888): 510–511.

30. Osler, "Treatment of Disease," 185.

31. A Hospital Nurse, 17–21. See the discussion of the care of this nurse toward the end of Chapter 4.

32. B. W. Richardson, MD, "Natural Euthanasia," *Popular Science Monthly* 13 (1875): 612–620, quote 618.

33. E. P. Buffett, "Euthanasia: The Pleasures of Dying," *New Englander and Yale Review* 55 (August 1891): 231–242, quotes from 240 and 241.

34. John Ferriar, "Of the Treatment of the Dying," in *Medical Histories and Reflections* (Philadelphia: Thomas Dobson, 1816), 392. The discussion of Ferriar, Marx, and others are found in Chapters 2–4.

35. W. R. Albury, "Ideas of Life and Death," in *Companion Encyclopedia of the History of Medicine*, vol. 1, eds. W. F. Bynum and Roy Porter (New York: Routledge, 1993), 249–280, esp. 266–269. The quote is from Ivan Pavlov in 1900, in Albury, 266.

36. Albury, 268–271.

37. John Anthony Tercier, *The Contemporary Deathbed: The Ulti-* *mate Rush* (New York: Palgrave Macmillan, 2005), 49–94 and 157; Richard V. Lee, "Cardiopulmonary Resuscitation in the Eighteenth Century," *Journal of the History of Medicine and Allied Sciences* 27 (1972): 418–433; and Peter Safar, "On the History of Modern Resuscitation," *Critical Care Medicine* 24 (Supplement, February 1996): 35–115.

38. A. H. P. Leuf, "Resuscitation After Apparent Death," *Medical News* 54 (January 26, 1889): 97–99.

39. L. Pierce Clarke, "The Injection of Stimulants into the Heart-Walls," *Boston Medical and Surgical Journal* 82 (April 18, 1895): 395.

40. Julius Gottesman, "Resuscitation by the Intra-Cardiac Injection of Epinephrin," *JAMA* 79 (October 14, 1922): 1334–1335. For a brief discussion and a description of additional cases in both internal medicine and surgery to attack disease "even in the face of death," see Crenner, 203–204.

41. Kane, 458–461, quotes from 459 and 460–461.

42. Simeon E. Baldwin, "The Natural Right to a Natural Death," *St. Paul Medical Journal* 1 (December 1899): 875–889.

43. Baldwin, 888.

44. Baldwin, 884.

45. Baldwin, 883–884.

46. Baldwin, 888.

47. Baldwin, 877.

48. Baldwin, 878.

49. Baldwin, 878–879.

50. Baldwin, 881.

51. Baldwin, 883.

52. Baldwin, 881.

53. Baldwin, 879.

54. William Munk, *Euthanasia or, Medical Treatment in Aid of an Easy Death* (London and New York: Longmans, Green, 1887), 70.

55. Baldwin, 880.

56. Baldwin, 877, 878 and 888.

57. Baldwin, 888–889.

58. Baldwin, quotes from 876, 877, 878, 882, and 888.

59. Baldwin, 877.

60. Albert R. Jonsen, *The Birth of Bioethics* (New York: Oxford University Press, 1998), 236–281.

61. For the great praise of Sainsbury's work, see Reviews, "*Principia Therapeutica*, by Harrington Sainsbury," *Journal of Mental Sciences* 52 (1906): 788–789; and William Osler, "Treatment of Disease," 187. Osler said that Sainsbury's work "should be in the hands of every practitioner and senior student."

62. Harrington Sainsbury, *Principia Therapeutica* (London: Methuen, 1906), 224–225.

63. Sainsbury, 226–227.

64. Sainsbury, 228–229.

65. Arthur MacDonald, "Death in Man," *Medical Times* 49 (July 1921): 149–180; and MacDonald, "Human Death," *Medical Times* 56 (August and September 1928): 206–216.

66. MacDonald never mentions Munk in the body of his article, but the contents of his sub-section are a rehash of Munk, whom MacDonald lists in his bibliography (180).

67. A brief overview of Glaister's work that mentions his psychiatric practice is found at http://www.braziers.org.uk/research-and-publications/john-norman-glaister/ (accessed August 12, 2013).

68. J. Norman Glaister, "Phantasies of the Dying: Some Remarks on the Management of Death," *The Lancet* (August 6, 1921): 315–317.

69. Glaister, 315.

70. Glaister, 315.

71. Glaister, 315.

72. Glaister, 315–316.

73. Glaister, 316.

74. Glaister, 316.

75. Glaister, 316.

76. Glaister, 316–317.

77. Glaister, 317.

78. The story of Ruth's grappling with cancer, a condition that was never revealed to him, is found in my article drawn from a lecture given to the Philosophical Society of Texas: Harold Y. Vanderpool, "Caring for People with Cancer," *Philosophical Society of Texas Proceedings* 55 (1992): 85–92. That article draws upon the outstanding study by James T. Patterson, *The Dread Disease: Cancer and Modern American Culture* (Cambridge, MA: Harvard University Press, 1987).

79. Alfred Worcester, "The Care of the Dying," in *Physician and Patient*, ed. L. Eugene Emerson (Cambridge, MA: Harvard University Press, 1928), 200–201. This reference will be identified as "The Care of the Dying" (1928).

80. For an overview of Worcester's career, see Derek Kerr, "Alfred Worcester: A Pioneer in Palliative Care," *American Journal of Hospice and Palliative Care* 9 (May/June 1992): 13–14 and 36–38.

81. Kerr, 14.

82. Worcester, "Past and Present Methods," 159, 162, and 164.

83. Worcester, "Past and Present Methods," 152.

84. Worcester, "Past and Present Methods," 164.

85. The influence of Peabody and this quote from Peabody are found in the introduction to the published volume of the Harvard lectures. See also Francis Weld Peabody, "The

Care of the Patient," *JAMA* 88 (1927): 877–882.

86. Alfred Worcester, *The Care of the Aged, the Dying, and the Dead* (Springfield, IL: Charles C. Thomas, 1935). Worcester's chapter on "The Care of the Dying" in this book (33–61) will be referenced as "The Care of the Dying" (1935).

87. Worcester, "The Care of the Dying" (1935), 33.

88. See the discussion of Kerr, 13.

89. Worcester, "The Care of the Dying" (1935), 46.

90. Worcester, "The Care of the Dying" (1935), 33; Ferriar, 392.

91. Worcester, "The Care of the Dying" (1935), 33–34.

92. Worcester, "The Care of the Dying" (1935), 34–36.

93. Worcester, "Past and Present Methods," 164.

94. Worcester, "The Care of the Dying" (1935), 45–47.

95. Worcester, "The Care of the Dying" (1935), 37–41.

96. Worcester, "The Care of the Dying" (1935), 41–49, quotes from 42, 43 and 45–46.

97. Worcester, "The Care of the Dying" (1935), 48–49.

98. Worcester, "The Care of the Dying" (1935), 51–54, quote from 53–54.

99. Worcester, "The Care of the Dying" (1935), 58–59; Kane, quote on 459.

100. Worcester, "The Care of the Dying" (1935), 59.

101. This appears to refer to Worcester's becoming critically ill and being nursed back to health by his medical partner. Derek Kerr comments that the care Worcester received when he was critically ill influenced his views of terminal care. Kerr, 35–36.

102. Worcester, "The Care of the Dying" (1935), 46, 48, and 60.

103. "Physician and Patient, Personal Care," *American Journal of Nursing* 29 (June 1929): 756.

104. Book Notices, "*The Care of the Aged, the Dying, and the Dead*," by Alfred Worcester," *JAMA* 105, no. 3 (July 20, 1935): 225.

105. These quoted words are part of the title of the book by Flexner and Flexner.

Chapter 6

1. See the discussion in the first pages of the last chapter, as well as the informative discussion on the changes and dynamics of teaching hospitals from the 1910s through the 1950s in Kenneth M. Ludmerer, *Time to Heal* (Oxford: Oxford University Press, 1999), 102–113.

2. See, for example, Ira Rutkow, *Seeking the Cure: A History of Medicine in America* (New York: Scribner, 2010), 173–250.

3. A disease of deficiency, pernicious anemia causes unsteady ambulation, shortness of breath, chronic tongue swelling, and numbness and tingling in hands and feet.

4. See Ludmerer, 134–161; and Harold Y. Vanderpool, "Introduction and Overview: Ethics, Historical Case Studies, and the Research Enterprise," in *The Ethics of Research Involving Human Subjects*, ed. Harold Y. Vanderpool (Frederick, MD: University Publishing Group, 1996), 1–30.

5. Claude S. Beck, "Reminiscences of Cardiac Resuscitation," *Review of Surgery* (March–April 1970): 77–86.

6. Thomas L. Petty, "The Modern Evolution of Mechanical Ventilation," *Clinics in Chest Medicine* 9 (March 1988): 1–10.

7. Peter Safar, "History of Cardiopulmonary-Cerebral Resuscitation," in *Cardiopulmonary Resuscitation*, eds. William Kaye and Nicholas G Bircher (New York: Churchill Livingstone, 1989), 1–53.

8. David M. Oshinsky, *Polio: An American Story* (New York: Oxford University Press, 2005).

9. For the years 1936–1951, see, for example, the description of surgeries for cancers found to be "inoperable" in Richard C. Cabot and Russell L. Dicks, *The Art of Ministering to the Sick* (New York: Macmillan, 1936), 298–314 and 331–374 (republished in 1937, 1938, 1942, 1943, and 1944); mention of "the subjection of dying folk to dramatic but indulgent surgery" by Clifford Hoyle in "The Care of the Dying," *Post-Graduate Medical Journal* 20 (April 1944): 120; and the comments of Frank Hebb in 1951 about the "belated attempts at remedial treatment … the subjection of dying people to dramatic but useless surgery or to investigations of no practical value" that "may invite criticism" (Frank Hebb, "The Care of the Dying," *Canadian Medical Association* 65 [1951]: 262). This chapter will indicate how heroic medical interventions for patients with fatal diseases became all the more frequent and technologically complex over the next 10 years.

10. William F. Mengert, "Terminal Care," *Illinois Medical Journal* 122 (September 1957): 100.

11. William B. Bean, "On Death," *Annals of Internal Medicine* 101 (February 1958): 202.

12. Clair Hooker and Hans Pols, "Health, Medicine and the Media," *Health and History* 8 (2006): 1–13.

13. Hooker and Pols, 2–5.

14. Bean, 201.

15. See, for example, C. J. Gavey, *The Management of the "Hopeless" Case* (London: H. K. Lewis, 1952), 39: "In this age of far-reaching scientific discovery when one must be continually prepared for the announcement of new potent remedies (as happened in the case of penicillin for bacterial endocarditus which was formerly always fatal), the term 'hopeless' is applicable to fewer and fewer." David A. Karnofsky, "Why Prolong the Life of a Patient with Advanced Cancer?" *CA: A Cancer Journal for Clinicians* 10 (January–February 1960): 9 and 11.

16. C. S. Cameron, *The Truth About Cancer* (Englewood Cliffs, NJ: Prentice-Hall, 1956), 116.

17. Earle M. Chapman, "He Was in the Prime of Life," *Rhode Island Medical Journal* 39 (September 1956): 494.

18. Worcester's *The Care of the Aged, the Dying, and the Dead* was also republished in 1972. Nine or more articles on palliative care were published in the United States and United Kingdom the 1940s, 25 or more in the 1950s, and, as testimony to the birth of "the death and dying movement," over 72 articles and books on death, dying, and terminal care in the 1960s.

19. W. N. Leak, "The Care of the Dying," *Practitioner* 161 (1948): 80–87, quote from 87.

20. Virginia Kasley, "As Life Ebbs: The Art of Giving Understanding Care and Emotional Tranquility to the Dying Patient," *American Journal of Nursing* 48 (March 1948): 170 and 173. Similar comments were made by the Reverend Rollin J. Fairbanks that same year in "Ministering to the Dying," *Journal of Pastoral Care* 2 (1948): 6–14.

21. Clifford Hoyle, 119 and 123, quote from 119. Hoyle's assertion was repeated by the Canadian physician Frank Hebb in 1951 (261).

22. Hoyle, 120.

23. Hoyle, 121–123. Hoyle comments, "Almost always the nurse's responsibility is greater than the doctor's" in the stages of life. "She is constantly with the patient, and better tells the needs as they arise" (122). See also Leak, 81, 87; Gavey (24–26) discusses how "certain *minor medical operations* may help." The italics are his.

24. A study of 200 terminally ill cancer patients published in 1945 by Abrams and others indicated that in Boston, 35 percent died in hospitals,

45.5 percent in their own homes, and 19.5 percent in nursing homes. Only 15.5 percent said they preferred to stay at home. Ruth Abrams, Gertrude Jameson, Mary Poehlman, and Sylvia Snyder, "Terminal Care in Cancer," *New England Journal of Medicine* 232 (June 21, 1945): 719–724.

25. Hoyle, 122.

26. Gavey, 16.

27. S. Shindell, "Editorials: Home Medical Care—A Pilot Study," *Medical Annals of the District of Columbia* 19 (1950): 89–90; Mildred C. J. Pfeiffer and Eloise M. Lemon, "A Pilot Study of Home Care of Terminal Cancer Patients," *American Journal of Public Health* 43 (1953): 909–914; and Jean Aitken-Swan, "Nursing the Late Cancer Patient at Home," *Practitioner* 183 (1959): 64–69.

28. Cabot and Dicks, 7 and 37.

29. Hoyle, 119. During the 1940s no consensus existed with respect to what patients should be told when their illnesses were considered fatal. Some physicians rejected revealing the patient's prognosis even if asked by the patient; others guardedly told when asked; and a minority believed that patients have a right to know the nature of their conditions. See, for example, Cabot and Dicks, 306–307. Hospital-based clergy spoke about the necessity of conforming to doctor's decisions with respect to what patients were or were not told. Cabot and Dicks, 307–308, and 339.

30. See the present author's discussion of the successful hiding of Babe Ruth's cancer in the late 1940s and the breaking of that taboo with the treatment of the great woman athlete, Babe Didrikson in the early 1950s. Harold Y. Vanderpool, "Caring for People with Cancer," *Philosophical Society of Texas* 55 (1992): 85–92.

31. Charles C. Lund, "The Doctor, the Patient, and the Truth," *Annals of Internal Medicine* 24 (June 1946): 955–959, quote from 958.

32. Nathan S. Kline and Julius Sobin, "The Psychological Management of Cancer Cases," *JAMA* 146 (August 25, 1951): 1547–1551. Kline and Sobin asserted, "Severe and prolonged depression with or without suicidal tendencies may result when the facts of the condition are made known," and that if the depression persists, it should be treated with electric shock therapy. For patients who become obsessively preoccupied with their disease, a prefrontal lobotomy, they said, "usually results in the loss of this preoccupation with self and future" (1551).

33. Leak, 83.

34. Elizabeth Ford Love, "Do All Hands Help Ease the Sting of Death by Tact and Kindliness?" *Hospitals* 18 (December 1944): 47–48.

35. Kasley, 173.

36. E. M. Bluestone, "On the Significance of Death in Hospital Practice," *Modern Hospital* 78 (March 1952): 86–88.

37. Bluestone, 88.

38. Walter C. Alvarez, "The Care of the Dying," *JAMA* 150 (September 13, 1952): 86–91.

39. All of these qualities are also displayed in Alvarez's intriguing autobiography: *Incurable Physician: An Autobiography* (Englewood Cliffs, NJ: Prentice-Hall, 1963).

40. See the discussion of Browne in Chapter 1.

41. Alvarez, "The Care of the Dying," 87, 90, and 91, quote from 87.

42. For example, Alvarez, "The Care of the Dying," 88 and 89.

43. Alvarez, "The Care of the Dying," 88–91.

44. Alvarez, "The Care of the Dying," 87–88.

45. Alvarez, "The Care of the Dying," 86.

46. Alvarez, "The Care of the Dying," 86 and 89–90.

47. Alvarez, "The Care of the Dying," 87.

48. Alvarez, "The Care of the Dying," 87.

49. Alvarez, "The Care of the Dying," 86.

50. Alvarez, "The Care of the Dying," 86–87.

51. Alvarez, "The Care of the Dying," 87.

52. Alvarez, "The Care of the Dying," 87 and 88.

53. Alvarez, "The Care of the Dying," 87.

54. Alvarez, "The Care of the Dying," 89.

55. Alvarez, "The Care of the Dying," 91.

56. Alvarez, "The Care of the Dying," 91.

57. Alvarez, "The Care of the Dying," 89.

58. Alvarez, "The Care of the Dying," 88 and 91.

59. Alvarez, "The Care of the Dying," 90.

60. Alvarez, "The Care of the Dying," 90–91.

61. See the discussion of Marx in Chapter 3; and Carl Friedrich Heinrich Marx, "Medical Euthanasia" (1826), trans. Walter Cane, in *Journal of the History of Medicine and Allied Sciences* 7 (1952): 401–416, esp. 414–416.

62. Alvarez, "The Care of the Dying," 88.

63. Alvarez, "The Care of the

Dying," 88. The history of the terminal care of children is a topic in itself, which is not systematically covered in this book.

64. Alvarez, "Care of the Dying," 88–89.

65. Alvarez, "Care of the Dying," 90.

66. Alvarez, "Care of the Dying," 89 and 91, quote from 91.

67. Walter Alvarez, "Help for the Dying Patient," *Geriatrics* 18 (February 1964): 69.

68. Harrison Sainsbury, *Principia Theapeutica* (London: Methuen, 1906), 224–229. See the discussions of Sainsbury in Chapter 5.

69. See the discussion of Glaister in Chapter 5.

70. Chapman, "He Was in the Prime of Life"; and Peter Pineo Chase and Irving A. Beck, "Making a Graceful Exit," *Rhode Island Medical Journal* 39 (September 1956): 497–499 and 516–525.

71. Chapman, 494–495.

72. See the insightful essay by August M. Kasper, "The Doctor and Death," in *The Meaning of Death*, ed. Herman Feifel (New York: McGraw-Hill, 1959), 259–270. William B. Bean called death "the final frustration" of the good physician and a topic that was being avoided in medical teaching and scientific papers. Bean, 202.

73. Mengert, 99. Several authors in the 1950s and 1960s indicate that physicians at the time equated the death of their patients with personal defeat—so much so, that some doctors would avoid seeing patients who were dying. Chapman, 495; and John J. Farrell, "The Right of a Patient to Die," *Journal of the South Carolina Medical Association* 54 (July 1958): 231, where Farrell says, "As surgeons we all too often consider death a personal defeat."

74. Mengert, 100.

75. Mengert, 99–101.

76. Mengert, 101.

77. See the graphic story of the treatment of a patient with Bright's disease by Chapman (496); and the opposition to "extravagant" maneuvers to keep extant traces of life by Bean (202).

78. Chapman, 496–497.

79. Donald C. Beatty, "Shall We Talk About Death?" *Pastoral Psychology* 6 (1955): 12.

80. Beatty, 11–14, quotes from 13–14.

81. T. N. Rudd, "Family Doctor at the Death-Bed," *Medical World* 85 (July 1956): 51. Rudd says that clergy are frequently excluded from the deathbed in order to maintain "the conspiracy to keep Death out of the picture" (2).

82. William T. Fitts Jr. and I. S. Ravdin, "What Philadelphia Physicians Tell Patients with Cancer," *JAMA* 153 (November 7, 1953): 901–904.

83. Chapman, 495.

84. Kline and Sobin (1951); Bradford J. Murphy, "Psychological Management of the Patient with Incurable Cancer," *Geriatrics* 9 (1953): 130–134; Gerald J. Aronson, "Treatment of the Dying Person," in *The Meaning of Death*, ed. Herman Feifel, 251–258.

85. Geoffrey Gorer, "The Pornography of Death," *Modern Writing* (1965): 56–62. Gorer's essay was a frequent reading in textbooks on death and dying in the 1960s.

86. Sainsbury, 224–229.

87. See Alvarez, "Care of the Dying," 86. Beatty, Rudd, and Chapman describe family members' participation in the "drama of deceit" over keeping loved ones from knowing about their prognosis. Rudd, 51; see also Beatty, 12; and Chapman, 50.

88. Physician-family-patient relationships were multifaceted. It appears that often families were "managed" like patients—encouraged by the hope that "everything possible is being done," told when they could visit their loved ones, and sometimes invited to express their preferences. At times, family members were as optimistic as physicians about the therapeutic promise of aggressive treatments. At other times, their requests for "no more treatment" were overruled by doctors. These quotes are from Gavey, 18–19.

89. "A Way of Dying," *Atlantic Monthly* (January 1957): 53–55.

90. Safar; and Petty, esp. 1–4.

91. For a brief background to the Roman Catholic attention to these questions, as well as Pope Pius's attention to them, see Albert R. Jonsen, *The Birth of Bioethics* (New York: Oxford University Press, 1998), 36–38 and 236–237.

92. The pope gave his response to the anesthesiologists on November 24, 1957. The references here are taken from *The Pope Speaks* 4 (1958): 393–398, which is printed in full as "Pope Pius XII: The Prolongation of Life," in *Ethics in Medicine: Historical Perspectives and Contemporary Concerns*, eds. Stanley Joel Reiser, Arthur J. Dyck, and William J. Curran (Cambridge, MA: MIT Press, 1977), 501–504. The references that follow are from "Pope Pius XII" in Reiser, Dyck, and Curran. The questions are posed on 502 and 503.

93. Pope Pius XII, 501.

94. Pope Pius XII, 502.

95. Pope Pius XII, 503.

96. Pope Pius XII, 503.

97. Pope Pius XII, 504 and 503.

98. Jonsen asserts that "no movement on behalf of patients' rights" emerged until the late 1960s, and Starr states that "rights in health care, such as the right to informed consent" became evident in the 1970s. See Jonsen, 368–369; and Paul Starr, *The Social Transformation of American Medicine* (New York: Basic Books, 1982), 388–391. The American Hospital Association adopted a Patients' Bill of Rights in 1972.

99. See the impressive analysis of Ruth R. Faden and Tom L. Beauchamp, *A History and Theory of Informed Consent* (New York: Oxford University Press, 1986), 53–113, especially 86ff., for the legal import of informed consent in medicine during and after 1957. The factors Faden and Beauchamp list as possible explanations for the medical-legal focus on informed consent during and after 1957 do not include the tradition of palliative care advocacy.

100. Editorial, "Life in Death," *New England Journal of Medicine* 256 (1957): 760.

101. Mengert, 99–103.

102. John J. Farrell, 231–233. Farrell based his article on the address he delivered to the South Carolina chapter of the American College of Surgeons in 1957. For references to the lay press, see Mengert, 102–103.

103. R. Ruff, "Have We the Right to Prolong Dying?" *Medical Economics* 37 (1960): 39–44.

104. These figures are based on a search of the literature beginning with the bibliography by Albert Jay Miller and Michael James Acri, *Death: A Bibliographical Guide* (Metuchen, NJ: Scarecrow Press, 1977).

105. "The Patient's Philosophy, His Heart, and His Bill," *JAMA* 185 (July 13, 1963): 29–30.

106. "E. H. Rynearson of Mayo Clinic," *New York Times*, February 20, 1987, http://nytimes/1987/02/20/obituaries/eh-rynearson-of-mayo-clinic.html (accessed February 7, 2013). Rynearson retired from the Mayo Clinic in 1966.

107. Edward H. Rynearson, "You Are Standing at the Bedside of a Patient Dying of Untreatable Cancer," *CA: A Cancer Journal for Clinicians* 9 (1958): 85–87.

108. That is, euthanasia in S. D. William's sense of actively ending a patient's life. The same meaning was ascribed to euthanasia by Walter Al-varez in 1952. During these years a number of physicians were concerned that if they stopped active treatments to prolong life, they could be charged with "committing passive euthanasia." The dean of a medical school commented to a reporter, "No matter how cautiously we speak [about ceasing curative treatments], we're bound to be accused of advocating euthanasia." The quote is from Lois Mattox Miller, "Neither Life nor Death," *Reader's Digest* (December 1960): 56. The Episcopalian theological ethicist, Joseph Fletcher, for example, equated the terms "direct euthanasia" with mercy killing and ceasing treatments to prolong life with "indirect euthanasia." Fletcher likely believed that that terminology would make his ardent defenses of mercy killing more acceptable. See Joseph Fletcher, "The Patient's Right to Die," *Harper's* 221 (October 1960): 139–143. Catholic authorities placed Fletcher's book *Morals and Medicine* (first published in 1954) on its index of books that should not be read without official permission. David F. Kelly, *The Emergence of Roman Catholic Medical Ethics in North America* (New York: Edwin Mellen Press, 1979), 378; and Fletcher, *Morals and Medicine* (Boston: Beacon Press, 1960 [1954]), 172–210. William B. Bean likely voiced the views of most physicians in the 1940s through the 1960s by commenting that "the possibility that euthanasia will be established as a sensible method of determining who should die, and when, has probably received a mortal stroke from the concentration camps of Europe ... with their orgies of human sacrifice, casual torture, and crude experiment[s]" (Bean, 202).

109. Rynearson, 85.

110. Rynearson, 85.

111. Rynearson cites a text from Father Gerald Kelley, whose first edition of *Medico-Moral Problems* was published in 1958. See Kelly, 352–353, 359–371.

112. Rynearson, 86.

113. Rynearson, 86–87, quotes from 86.

114. Rynearson, 86.

115. Rynearson, 87.

116. Rynearson, 87.

117. Paul Chodoff, "The Dying Patient," *Medical Annals of the District of Columbia* 29 (August 1960): 447–450.

118. "Symposium on Terminal Care," *CA: A Cancer Journal for Clinicians* 10 (1960): 12–24.

119. "Symposium on Terminal Care," 22.

120. "What Others Say in Opposition to Dr. Ruff," *Medical Economics* 37 (1960): 40.

121. "Symposium on Terminal Care," 22–23; and Karnofsky, 9–11.

122. "Cancer and Conscience," *TIME*, November 3, 1961, 60.

123. Lois Mattox Miller, 55 and 59.

Chapter 7

1. Arlo S. Hermreck, "The History of Cardiopulmonary Resuscitation," *American Journal of Surgery* 156 (December 1988): 433–435; and Peter Safar, "History of Cardiopulmonary-Cerebral Resuscitation," in *Cardiopulmonary Resuscitation*, eds. William Kaye and Nicholas G Bircher (New York: Churchill Livingstone, 1989), 1–53, esp. 21ff.

2. Thomas L. Petty, "The Modern Evolution of Mechanical Ventilation," *Clinics in Chest Medicine* 9 (March 1988): 1–10.

3. Claude S. Beck, "Reminiscences of Cardiac Resuscitation," *Review of Surgery* (March–April 1970): 77–86, esp. 85–86.

4. Kevin Mohee, "Cardiac Pacing: A Brief History in the Development of Pacemakers," http://sscts.org/HistoryPacemakers.aspx (accessed November 28, 2011).

5. John Anthony Tercier, *The Contemporary Deathbed: The Ultimate Rush* (New York: Palgrave Macmillan, 2005), 102–106; American Heart Association, "Guidelines for Cardiopulmonary Resuscitation and Emergency Cardiac Care," *JAMA* 268 (October 28, 1992): 2172–2181; and Beck, 86.

6. M. W. L. Gauderer, J. L. Ponsky, and R. J. Izant Jr., "Gastrostomy Without Laparotomy: A Percutaneous Endoscopic Technique," *Journal of Pediatric Surgery* 15 (1980): 872–875.

7. W. B. Kouwenhoven, J. R. Jude, and G. G. Knickerbocker, "Closed Chest Cardiac Massage," *JAMA* 173 (1960): 1064–1067.

8. Safar, "History," 1–53; Peter Safar, ed., *Advances in Cardiopulmonary Resuscitation* (New York: Springer-Verlag, 1975); and Tercier, 31–186.

9. These steps are depicted and described (in light of their histories) in Safar, "History," 3 and 23–36. See also J. H. Hollingsworth, "The Results of Cardiopulmonary Resuscitation: A 3-Year University Hospital Experience," *Annals of Internal Medicine* 71 (September 1969): 459–460.

10. See Tercier's discussion of historical and contemporary CPR (24–48).

11. Tercier, 169. Tercier comments, "Within the hospital, resuscitative protocols, though aiming to revive life, much more commonly ends up diagnosing death. How does the intern know when the patient is dead? When the patient has failed to respond to CPR" (169). Tercier views this definitive determination of as by and large positive. It transforms mourners into survivors, enables them to build new identities, assures them that everything that could have been done medically was done, bestows peace upon the dying, ushers the dead into the realm of transcendent memories, and substantiates the goodness of life in a secular world. Tercier, 170–178. Except for the medical assurance, the same listing applies to deaths by warfare and accidents.

12. Tercier, 167, 174–5, 220–222, and 241, quotes from 175, 222 and 241.

13. Tercier, 159.

14. Safar, "History," 19 and 23.

15. Jatinder Bains, "From Reviving the Living to Raising the Dead: The Making of Cardiac Resuscitation," *Social Science of Medicine* 47, no. 9 (1998): 1341–1349, quote from 1341.

16. Safar, "History," 37; Tercier, 38 and 41–42; and Hollingsworth, 460.

17. Bains, 1343.

18. American Heart Association, 2172–2173.

19. *Emergency!*, broadcast between 1972 and 1978, featured paramedics with an EKG machine and, after four seasons, a defibrillator. *ER*, aired in the United States between 1994 and 2009, depicted full-fledged CPR in ERs, as did *Casualty* in the United Kingdom between 1986 and 1999. See Bains, 1344, and Tercier, 189–218.

20. Tercier, 179.

21. See Barney G. Glaser and Anselm L. Strauss, *Awareness of Dying* (Chicago: Aldine, 1965).

22. Glaser and Strauss, *Awareness*, 194–200, quotes from 194 and 200; another description of CPR is found in their second major book, *Time for Dying* (Chicago: Aldine, 1968), 107–108.

23. Glaser and Strauss, *Time for Dying*, 114–115.

24. Glaser and Strauss, *Awareness*, 201.

25. Glaser and Strauss, *Awareness*, 202–203.

26. Glaser and Strauss, *Awareness*, 219–221. These conditions include internalizing the hospital's life-saving ideal, admiration for a doctor who saved the life of a patient "against low odds for ... survival," and the "*visibility* of her failure to join the life-rescuing effort."

27. Glaser and Strauss, *Awareness*, 99.

28. W. S. Symmers, "Not Allowed to Die," *British Medical Journal* 1 (February 1968): 442.

29. Symmers, 1961, 60.

30. T. T. Jones, "The Right to Live and the Right to Die," *Medical Times* 95 (November 1967): 1176–1177.

31. E. E. Menefee, "The Right to Live and the Right to Die," *Medical Times* 95 (November 1967): 1178–1179.

32. Eugene G. Laforet, "The 'Hopeless' Case," *Archives of Internal Medicine* 112 (September 1963): 318–319 and 325.

33. Jack W. Provonsha, "The Prolongation of Life," *Bulletin of the American Protestant Hospital Association* 35 (Spring 1971): 14–16, quotes from 16.

34. David A. Karnofsky quoted in "Cancer and Conscience," *TIME*, November 3, 1961, 60.

35. Mark M. Ravitch, "Let Your Patient Die with Dignity," *Medical Times* 93 (June 1965): 594–595.

36. Editorial, "When Do We Let the Patient Die?" *Annals of Internal Medicine* 68 (March 1968): 695–700.

37. John B. McClanahan, "The Patient's Right to Die," *Memphis and Mid-South Medical Journal* 38 (August 1963): 303–316, quotes from 313.

38. Charles D. Aring, "Intimations of Mortality: An Appreciation of Death and Dying," *Annals of Internal Medicine* 69 (July 1968): 137–152, quote from 149.

39. Norman K. Brown et al., "The Preservation of Life," *JAMA* 211 (January 5, 1970): 76–82.

40. Thomas P. Hackett and Avery D. Weisman, "The Treatment of the Dying," *Current Psychiatric Therapies* 2 (1962): 121; for dying patients' isolation and assigned inferiority, see Aring, 144–145.

41. Glaser and Strauss's books and articles, including *Awareness of Dying*, were based on grants from the National Institutes of Health that involved three years of fieldwork in six hospitals in the San Francisco Bay area (vii–x and 286). Within a year after its initial publication, *Awareness* was in its third printing.

42. For the U.S. statistics, see Glaser and Strauss, 6; for England, see J. M. Holford, "Terminal Care," *Nursing Times* 69 (January 25, 1973): 113. And for Western Europe, see Josef Mayer-Scheu, "Compas-

sion and Death," in *The Experience of Dying*, eds. Norbert Grienackez and Alois Muller (New York: Herder and Herder, 1974), 111–113. The demographic details of these statistics are complex and reflect the methodologies of respective researchers. The percentages of Americans dying "as hospital inpatients" was judged to be "approximately 54 percent" in 1980 according to the study of James Flory et al., "Place of Death: U.S. Trends Since 1980," *Health Affairs* 23 (2004): 194–200.

43. Glaser and Strauss, *Awareness*, 5 and 29.

44. Glaser and Strauss, *Awareness*, 46–63, quotes from 47.

45. Glaser and Strauss, *Awareness*, 64–78, quotes from 71, 77, and 78.

46. Glaser and Strauss, *Awareness*, 74–77 and 79–99.

47. Glaser and Strauss, *Awareness*, 119–120.

48. Glaser and Strauss, *Awareness*, 98–104.

49. Glaser and Strauss, *Awareness*, 186–197.

50. Glaser and Strauss, *Awareness*, 4–5 and 204–237, quotations from 204 and 237.

51. Glaser and Strauss, *Time for Dying*, 47.

52. Glaser and Strauss, *Awareness*, 223–225.

53. Glaser and Strauss, *Awareness*, 245.

54. See the discussion under the sub-topic "Between Worcester and Alvarez" in Chapter 6.

55. Glaser and Strauss, *Awareness*, 119: 88 percent of the physicians in the study by Oken said that their policy was not to tell patients of they had a malignant disease, even though 60 percent of the physicians questioned said they would want to be told. Donald Oken, "What to Tell Cancer Patients," *JAMA* 175 (April 1, 1961): 1120–1128. J.M. Hinton's impressive discussion of truth telling in England and the United States in 1966 concluded with the words, "It is apparent that most people claim that they would like to be told if they have a potentially fatal illness, but most doctors are reluctant to tell them." J. M. Hinton, "Facing Death," *Journal of Psychosomatic Research* 10 (1966): 22–28, quote from 28.

56. Glaser and Strauss, *Awareness*, 29–39, quotes from 29, 34, and 36.

57. Glaser and Strauss, *Time for Dying*, 168; for limitations of family visiting hours, see *Time for Dying*, 191–193.

58. Hackett and Weisman, 121.

59. Hackett and Weisman, 121–125, quote from 125.

60. Hackett and Weisman, 125.

61. Joan M. Baker and Karen C. Sorensen, "A Patient's Concern with Death," *American Journal of Nursing* 63 (1963): 91.

62. Baker and Sorensen, 90–93.

63. Ramona Powell Davidson, "Let's Talk about Death: To Give Care in Terminal Illness," *American Journal of Nursing* 64 (January 1966): 74–75, quotes from 74.

64. Aring, 137–152, quotes from 40 and 144–145.

65. Leslie J. Blackhall, "Must We Always Use CPR?" *New England Journal of Medicine* 317 (November 12, 1987): 1282.

66. Blackhall, 1283; and A. L. Johnson et al., "Results of Cardiac Resuscitation in 552 Patients," *American Journal of Cardiology* 20 (1967): 831–835.

67. Hollingsworth, 459–466, esp. 464.

68. Blackwell, 1282.

69. These statistics are taken from the following studies published between 1965 and 1977, all of which, of course, do not record the same sets of statistics: A. L. Johnson et al.; Hollingsworth; Jean G. Lemier and Arnold L. Johnson, "Is Cardiac Resuscitation Worthwhile? A Decade of Experience," *New England Journal of Medicine* 286 (May 4, 1972): 970–972; Bernard Messert and Charles E. Quaglieri, "Cardiopulmonary Resuscitation: Perspectives and Problems," *The Lancet* (August 21, 1976): 410–411; and R. C. Peatfield et al., "Survival After Cardiac Arrest in Hospital," *The Lancet* (June 11, 1977): 1223–1225.

70. Blackhall, 1283, and Peatfield, 1224.

71. Messert and Quaglieri, 411.

72. I. Fusgen and J. D. Summa, "How Much Sense Is There in an Attempt to Resuscitate an Aged Person?" *Gerontology* 24 (1978): 37.

73. Nathan Schnaper, "Death and Dying: Has the Topic Been Beaten to Death?" *Journal of Nervous and Mental Disease* 160 (March 1975): 157; and Albert Jay Miller and Michael James Acri, *Death: A Bibliographical Guide* (Metuchen, NJ: Scarecrow Press, 1977).

74. Daniel Leviton, "Death Education," in *New Meanings of Death*, ed. Herman Feifel (New York: McGraw-Hill, 1977), 254–272.

75. Leviton, 235.

76. Peter Steinfels, "Introduction," in *Death Inside Out*, eds. Peter Steinfels and Robert M. Veatch (New York: Harper and Row, 1974), 1.

77. Goeffrey Gorer, *Death, Grief and Mourning* (New York: Doubleday, 1965), 192–199.

78. Leviton, 258. Leviton began promoting death education through articles and films beginning in 1969.

79. Herman Feifel, ed., *The Meaning of Death* (New York: McGraw-Hill, 1959), xiv.

80. Elisabeth Kübler-Ross, *On Death and Dying* (New York: Macmillan, 1969), 1–13, quote from 6–7.

81. See, for example, the groundbreaking studies of Jacques Choron, *Death and Western Thought* (New York: Collier Books, 1963), and Jacques Choron, *Death and Modern Man* (New York: Collier Books, 1964), focused on the "old-fashioned" problems of questions regarding immortality, varieties of death fear, and the meaning of life (or lack of it) in a scientific understanding of the universe (quote from vii). Ernest Becker's Pulitzer Prize–winning *The Denial of Death* (New York: Free Press, 1973) drew upon an impressive range of thinkers in psychology, philosophy, literature, and theology to argue against the "healthy-minded" view that fear of death is "something that society creates" and that can, therefore, be rejected. Becker believed that, in spite of appearances to the contrary, death is universally feared. Its terror, Becker argues in agreement with the theologian Søren Kierkegaard, is all-consuming for all who look full-faced at death. See esp. 13–96. See also the discussion and bibliography on the "theology of death" between the late 1950s and the 1970s in Gisbert Greshake, "Towards a Theology of Dying," in *The Experience of Dying*, eds. Nobert Greenacher and Alios Muller (New York: Herder and Herder, 1974), 80–98.

82. The quote is from the philosopher Bertrand Russell in Choron's *Death and Modern Man*, 196. Within this book, see also Choron's chapters on "Death and Life's Futility," 160–168 and "The Implication of the Scientific View of the World," 194–200.

83. Glaser and Strauss, *Time for Dying*, 251–253.

84. Glaser and Strauss, *Time for Dying*, 251–252, quote from 252.

85. Glaser and Strauss, *Time for Dying*, 253–259.

86. Anselm L. Strauss, Barney Glaser, and Jeanne Quint, "The Nonaccountability of Terminal Care," *Hospitals, J.A.H.A.* 38 (January 16, 1964): 73–87, quotes from 84 and 87.

87. Jeanne C. Quint, Anselm L.

Strauss, and Barney G. Glaser, "Improving Nursing Care of the Dying," *Nursing Forum* 6 (1967): 369–378, quote from 378; and Anselm L. Strauss, "Reforms Needed in Providing Terminal Care in Hospitals," *Archives of the Foundation of Thanatology* 1 (1969): 21–22.

88. Frances Mervyn, "The Plight of Dying Patients in Hospitals," *American Journal of Nursing* 71 (October 1971): 1988–1990, quote from 1990.

89. Kübler-Ross, 21–27 and 249–269.

90. Kübler-Ross, 37–156; also Kübler-Ross, "The Right to Die with Dignity," *Bulletin of the Menninger Clinic* 36 (May 1972): 302–312.

91. See, for example, Jane H. Barsteiner, "Death and Dying," *The Journal of Practical Nursing* 24 (1974): 28–30. For the relationship between Kübler-Ross's five stages and truth telling, see Robert E. Kavanaugh, "Helping Patients Who Are Facing Death," *Nursing* 4 (May 1974): 36.

92. For views of the psychiatrist, see Schnaper, 157–158; and for critiques of the five stages, see, for example, Melvin J. Krant and Alan Sheldon, "The Dying Patient—Medicine's Responsibility," *Journal of Thanatology* 1 (February 1971): 7; and Richard Schulz and David Aderman, "Clinical Research and the Stages of Dying," *Omega* 5 (Summer 1974): 137–143.

93. Loudon Wainwright, "A Profound Lesson for the Living," *LIFE* 67 (November 21, 1969): 34–43.

94. Bernice M. Wagner, "Teaching Students to Work with the Dying," *American Journal of Nursing* 64 (November 1964): 128–131.

95. David Barton et al., "Death and Dying: A Course for Medical Students," *Journal of Medical Education* 47 (December 1972): 945–951.

96. Edward H. Liston, "Education on Death and Dying: A Survey of American Medical Schools," *Journal of Medical Education* 48 (June 1973): 577–578; and George E. Dickinson, "Death Education in U.S. Medical Schools: 1975–1980," *Journal of Medical Education* 56 (February 1981): 111–114, quote from 113.

97. See Cicely Saunders, *Cicely Saunders: Selected Writings*, edited with introduction by David Clark (Oxford: Oxford University Press, 2006), xiv; and Saunder's description of her relationship with Tasma in Sandol Stoddard, *The Hospice Movement* (New York: Stein and Day, 1978), 73–74.

98. Milton J. Lewis, *Medicine and Care of the Dying: A Modern History*

(Oxford and New York: Oxford University Press, 2007), 14–29; and Stoddard, 7–11, 64–66.

99. "St. Joseph's Hospice," *American Journal of Nursing* 65 (March 1965): 7.

100. Cicely Saunders, "Dying of Cancer," *St. Thomas's Hospital Gazette* 56, no. 2 (1958): 37–47, as reprinted in Saunders, *Cicely Saunders: Selected Writings*, 1–11. See especially 3–11.

101. Saunders, xv.

102. In "Dying of Cancer," Saunders refers to the writings of Worcester, Gavey, Hebb, Hoyle, and Leak, all of whom were referenced in Chapter 6. Worcester is discussed in detail in Chapter 5.

103. Saunders, *Cicely Saunders: Selected Writings*, esp. 1–35. In addition to Saunders, see the article by the British physician, Ian Grant, based on over 30 years of general medical practice: "Care for the Dying," *British Medical Journal* 2 (December 28, 1957): 1539–1540.

104. For example, Cicely Saunders, "The Management of Patients in the Terminal Stage," *Cancer* 6, ed. R. Raven (London: Butterworth, 1960), 403–417; and Cicely Saunders, *The Management of Terminal Illness* (London: Hospital Medicine Publications, 1967), 1–29. Both publications are abbreviated and reprinted in *Cicely Saunders: Selected Writings*, 21–35 and 91–114.

105. Saunders, "Dying of Cancer," 11.

106. Saunders, "Distress in Dying," *British Medical Journal* 2 (July–December 1963): 746, reprinted in *Cicely Saunders: Selected Writings*, 65.

107. Cicely Saunders, "The Last Stages of Life," *American Journal of Nursing* 65 (March 1965): 70.

108. Saunders, "The Last Stages of Life," 70–73, quotes from 70 and 71.

109. Saunders, "The Last Stages of Life," 74.

110. Saunders, "The Management of Terminal Illness," 1967, found in *Cicely Saunders: Selected Writings*, 91–114, quotes from 106. In this lengthy article Saunders cites over 150 authors prominent in the medical literature as well as in the death and dying movement. Her references include many authors referenced in this chapter.

111. See, for example, Cicely Saunders, "St. Christopher's Hospice," *British Hospital Journal and Social Service Review* 77 (November 10, 1967): 2127–2130; and Cicely Saunders, "A Place to Die," *Crux* 11 (1973–1974): 24–27.

112. Saunders, "Dimensions of

Death," in *Religion and Medicine*, ed. M. A. H. Melinsky (London: SCM Press, 1975), 113–116, found in *Cicely Saunders: Selected Writings*, 130–131.

113. Saunders's emphasis on hospice as a community was inspired by her years of work with St. Joseph's, which is revealed in Cicely Saunders, "Working at St. Joseph's Hospice in Hackney," *Annual Report of St. Vincent's Dublin* (1962): 37; reprinted in Saunders, *Cicely Saunders: Selected Writings*, 57–60.

114. *St. Christopher's Hospice: Annual Report, 1976–1977* (December 1977), 2–73, esp. 17.

115. These figures are approximations. For the number of hospices in England, see John Agate, "Care of the Dying in Geriatric Departments," *The Lancet* (February 17, 1973): 365; and for the United States, see *St. Christopher's Hospice: Annual Report, 1976–1977*, 11.

116. *St. Christopher's Hospice: Annual Report, 1976–1977*, 23.

117. I have found no definitive biography of Dame Sanders, but am indebted to the brief and impressive review of her life by David Clark in *Cicely Saunders: Selected Writings*, iii–xvi.

118. For the number and visitors and quote, see *St. Christopher's Hospice: Annual Report, 1976–1977*, 17 and 23.

119. Belfour M. Mount, "The Problem of Caring for the Dying in a General Hospital: The Palliative Care Unit as a Possible Solution," *CMA Journal* 115 (June 17, 1976): 119–121; and Dottie C. Wilson, Ina Ajemian, and Balfour M. Mount, "Montreal (1975)—The Royal Victoria Hospital Palliative Care Service," in *The Hospice: Development and Administration*, ed. Glen W. Davidson (Washington: Hemisphere Publishing Corporation, 1978), 3–19.

120. Wilson, Ajemian, and Mount, 8.

121. David Clark, "From Margins to Centre: A Review of the History of Palliative Care in Cancer," *Lancet Oncology* 8 (May 2007): 434.

122. See, for example, the essays on these and other programs in *The Hospice: Development and Administration*, 21–95; Judy Alsofrom, "The 'Hospice' Way of Dying—At Home with Friends and Family," *American Medical News* 20 (February 21, 1977): 7–9; and Claire F. Ryder and Diane M. Ross, "Terminal Care—Issues and Alternatives," *Public Health Reports* 92 (January–February 1977): 20–29.

123. Constance Holden, "The Hospice Movement and Its Implica-

tion," *Annals of the American Academy of Political and Social Sciences* 447 (January 1980): 59–63.

124. Krant and Sheldon, 1–24, quote from 21. Their extensively referenced article recognized the "outstanding" work at St. Christopher's on 16.

125. Melvin J. Krant, "The Organized Care of the Dying Patient," *Hospital Practice* (January 1972): 101–108, quote from 101.

126. The quotes are excerpts from Carol Goffnett, "Your Patient's Dying—Now What?" *Nursing* 9 (November 1979): 31–33. For home care, state and charity sponsored activities of district nurses in England, see Olive Keywood, "Care of the Dying in Their Own Home," *Nursing Times* 70 (September 26, 1974): 1516–1517.

127. Ida M. Martinson, "Why Don't We Let Them Die at Home?" *RN* (January 1976): 58–65; and Mark Jury and Dan Jury, *Gramp* (New York: Grossman, 1976).

128. For example, Kennedy F. Hegland, "Unauthorized Rendition of Lifesaving Medical Treatment," *California Law Review* 53 (August 1965), 863; Ravitch, 594; Norman L. Cantor, "A Patient's Decision to Decline Lifesaving Medical Treatment: Bodily Integrity versus the Preservation of Life," *Rutgers Law Review* 26 (Winter 1973): 228–264, reprinted in *Ethical Issues in Death and Dying,* ed. Robert F. Weir (New York: Columbia University Press, 1977), 265; and Thomas W. Furlow Jr. "Tyranny of Technology," *The Humanist* (July–August 1974): 8.

129. Russell Noyes Jr. and Terry A. Travis, "The Care of Terminally Ill Patients," *Archives of Internal Medicine* 132 (October 1973): 607–611, quote from 610.

130. Furlow, 8.

131. Frank J. Ayd Jr., "The Hopeless Case," *JAMA* 181 (September 29, 1962): 1099–1103, quote from 1102.

132. Ravitch, 94–596, quotes from 595.

133. Vincent J. Collins, "Limits of Medical Responsibility in Prolonging Life," *JAMA* 206 (October 7, 1968): 389–392, quotes from 390 and 391.

134. Sigmund Benham Kahn and Vincent Zarro, "The Management of the Dying Patient," *Seminars in Drug Treatment* 3 (Summer 1973): 37–44, esp. 39.

135. Authors differ in their assessments respecting when the bioethics movement got underway. Albert Jonsen dates it from the early 1960s, David Rothman to the mid–1960s, and Robert Veatch to the years between 1968 and 1972. I basically agree with Veatch. Albert R. Jonsen, *The Birth of Bioethics* (New York: Oxford University Press, 1998); David J. Rothman, *Strangers at the Bedside: A History of How Law and Bioethics Transformed Medical Decision Making* (New York: Basic Books, 1991); and Robert M. Veatch, "The Birth of Bioethics: Autobiographical reflections of a Patient Person," *Cambridge Quarterly of Healthcare Ethics* 11, no. 4 (2002): 344–352.

136. The first major book on the nature of and topics covered by bioethics was by Tom L. Beauchamp and James F. Childress, *Principles of Biomedical Ethics* (New York: Oxford University Press, 1976), which is now in its 7th (2012) major revision. Chapter 1 of the 1976 edition focuses on "Morality and Ethical Theory." For a brief overview of ethical reasoning, see Harold Y. Vanderpool, "Introduction and Overview: Ethics, Historical Case Studies, and the Research Enterprise," in *The Ethics of Research Involving Human Subjects,* ed. Harold Y. Vanderpool (Frederick, MD: University Publishing Group, 1996), 1–30, esp. 2–4. For a much more extensive analysis/overview of ethical theories applied to the topic of a dying patient's right to know the truth, see Robert M. Veatch, *Death, Dying, and the Biological Revolution* (New Haven, CT: Yale University Press, 1976), 206–248.

137. See, for example, Jonsen, *The Birth of Bioethics,* 20–89; for overviews, see Arthur Caplan, "Bioethics," at http://www.encyclopedia.com/topic/bioethics.aspx (accessed July 18, 2013), and Allan M. Brandt, "Bioethics: Then and Now," *Lahey Clinic Medical Ethics* (Spring 2000), http://www.bucklin.org/bioethics-history.htm (accessed July 18, 2013).

138. See Daniel Callahan, "Bioethics as a Discipline," *Hastings Center Studies* 1, no. 1 (1973): 66–73; also Jonsen, *The Birth of Bioethics,* 325–376.

139. Notably, the Hastings Center (first established as the Institute of Society, Ethics and the Life Sciences in 1969) and the Kennedy Institute of Ethics, established at Georgetown University in 1971. From these and other beginnings, (1) courses in biomedical ethics were soon taught in medical and nursing schools, and universities, followed by, (2) departments of medical ethics and the medical humanities, the first of which was the Institute for the Medical Humanities established at the University of Texas Medical Branch in Galveston in 1973, and (3) a host of scholarly journals.

140. For example, Stanley Joel Reiser, Arthur J. Dyck, and William J. Curran, *Ethics in Medicine* (Cambridge, MA: MIT Press, 1977), sections I (ethical dimensions of physicians-patient relationship through history), IV (on truth telling), and VII (suffering and dying), 5–76, 201–254 and 487–550.

141. Veatch, "The Birth of Bioethics," 344–346; and especially Veatch, *Death, Dying, and the Biological Revolution,* 77–248.

142. Noyes and Travis's 1973 survey of Iowa physicians indicated that following discussions with family members and others, the physicians they polled "ultimately regarded themselves as the final authority" (609). See also Menefee, 1178–1178; Collins, 389–391; and Kahn and Zarro, 39.

143. Paul Ramsey, *The Patient as Person: Explorations in Medical Ethics* (New Haven, CT: Yale University Press, 1970). *Patient as Person* was in its 5th printing in 1975. A second edition of this groundbreaking work was published in 2002, 24 years after Ramsey's death. In one of the introductory essays to this new edition, Albert R. Jonsen discusses Ramsey's bioethics training, the dynamics surrounding the Yale lectures, and Ramsey's contributions to bioethics: Albert R. Jonsen, "The Structure of an Ethical Revolution: Paul Ramsey, the Beecher Lectures, and the Birth of Bioethics," in Paul Ramsey, *The Patient as Person: Explorations in Medical Ethics,* 2nd ed. (New Haven, CT: Yale University Press, 2002), xvi–xxviii.

144. Chapter 3 of *Patient as Person* is titled "On (Only) Caring for the Dying," 113–164, quote from 116.

145. Ramsey, 1970, xi–xiii.

146. Ramsey, quotes from 133, 153, and 156.

147. Ramsey, 147. Karnofsky's views and those of physicians who agreed with him are discussed at the end of Chapter 6.

148. Oken, 1120–1128; and Dennis H. Novack et al., "Changes in Physicians' Attitudes toward Telling the Cancer Patient," *JAMA* 241 (March 2, 1979): 897–900. To ensure accuracy in their comparisons, Novack et al. used Oken's questionnaire.

149. Novack et al. discuss how and why physicians in 1979 "are telling their patients about terminal diagnosis" (899).

150. The quotes are from Novack et al., 87 and 89, who also discuss a number of these factors. Reasons for the dramatic change are discussed at length in my unpublished and

archived paper: Harold Y. Vanderpool, "Should Cancer Diagnosis Be Concealed or Revealed? The History and Meaning of a Dramatic Change in American Medicine," January 1992, unpublished manuscript, 28 pages. See also Vanderpool, "The Responsibilities of Physicians toward Dying Patients," in *Medical Complications in Cancer Patients*, eds. J. Klastersky and M. J. Staquet (New York: Raven Press, 1981), 124–133.

151. George L. Spaeth, "Letters: Telling the Cancer Patient," *JAMA* 242 (October 26, 1979): 1847–1848, quote from 1848.

152. Veatch, *Death, Dying, and the Biological Revolution*, quotes from 162 and 163.

153. Veatch, *Death, Dying, and the Biological Revolution*, 104–105.

154. Veatch, *Death, Dying, and the Biological Revolution*, 204–248, quote from 248.

155. See, for example, Leon R. Kass, "Averting One's Eyes or Facing the Music?—On Dignity and Death," in *Death Inside Out*, eds. Peter Steinfels and Robert M. Veatch (New York: Harper and Row, 1974), 101–114; and Schnaper on the indignities of incontinence and other needs of dependent patients (158).

156. See the discussion of Rynearson toward the end of Chapter 6.

157. Harold Y. Vanderpool, "The Ethics of Terminal Care," *JAMA* 239 (February 27, 1978): 850–852. Within months I received over 700 personal requests for copies of this article.

158. Vanderpool, "Ethics of Terminal Care," 851.

159. Vanderpool, "Ethics of Terminal Care," 850–851.

160. Vanderpool, "Ethics of Terminal Care," 851–852.

161. Vanderpool, "Ethics of Terminal Care," 851–852.

162. See the engaging study by David Rothman, *Strangers at the Bedside*. Rothman sets forth numerous reasons for this alienation, including, for example, the virtual disappearance of physician house calls by the 1960s (less than 1 percent of physician-patient contacts), the closures of neighborhood hospitals, how modern hospitals separated physicians into "their own universe" and faced overwhelming pressures to move quickly from one case to the next, the isolating complexities of medicine, feminist critiques of male doctors, and the resulting promulgation of bills of patients rights beginning in 1970 (127–147, endnote quote from 133).

163. Ruth R. Faden and Tom L. Beauchamp, *A History and Theory of Informed Consent* (New York: Oxford University Press, 1986), 34–35 and 125–143; see also David S. Rubsamen, "Doctor and the Law: What Every Doctor Needs to Know about Changes in 'Informed Consent,'" *Medical World News* 14 (February 9, 1973): 66–67.

164. Cantor, 241–269; and Thomas A. Rutledge, "Informed Consent for the Terminal Patient," *Baylor Law Review* 27 (1975); 111–121; and Veatch, *Death, Dying, and the Biological Revolution*, 116–122 and 161–163. Paul Ramsey spoke eloquently about informed consent for subjects of human research, but in *The Patient as Person*, Ramsey based duties to dying persons on charity and the moral and religious value of human beings. See Ramsey, 2–10.

165. The quotes are from Joseph E. Simonaitis, "Law and Medicine: More About Informed Consent," *JAMA* 224 (June 25, 1973): 1831–1832. See also the series of articles by Angela Roddey Holder, "Informed Consent: Its Evolution," *JAMA* 214 (November 9, 1970): 1181–1182; "Informed Consent: The Obligation," *JAMA* 214 (November 16, 1970): 1383–1384; and "Informed Consent: Limitations," *JAMA* 214 (November 23, 1970): 1611–1612.

166. "AMA Passes 'Death with Dignity' Resolution," *Science News* 24 (December 15, 1973): 375.

167. "AMA Grams: The Physician and the Dying Patient," *JAMA* 227 (February 18, 1974): 728.

168. Robert M. Veatch, "Death and Dying: The Legislative Options," *Medical Communications* 6 (Winter 1977/Spring 1978): 23–29, quote from 25. See also Robert M. Veatch, "Choosing Not to Prolong Dying," *Medical Dimensions Magazine* (December 1972): 8–10 and 40. In "Death and Dying: The Legislative Options," 26, Veatch spoke of the "obvious variation in views about what treatment is appropriate for a terminally ill patient."

169. Veatch, "Death and Dying: The Legislative Options," 25.

170. Veatch, "Death and Dying: The Legislative Options," 26. For his analysis of other state bills based on the right to refuse treatment, see Veatch, *Death, Dying, and the Biological Revolution*, 197–203.

171. The quote is from Veatch, "Death and Dying: The Legislative Options," 29.

Chapter 8

1. Richard Henry Dana, Jr., *Two Years Before the Mast* (New York: New American Library, 1964 [1869]), 29–30, abbreviated. An attempt to round the Horn has been immortalized in the adaptations of *Mutiny on the Bounty*.

2. See the first pages of Chapter 7 for the invention of the PEG in 1980, and Michael W. L. Gauderer, "Percutaneous Endoscopic Gastrostomy—20 Years Later: A Historical Perspective," *Journal of Pediatric Surgery* 36 (January 2001): 217–219.

3. The literature on these topics is vast. See, for example, J. D. Young and M. K. Sykes, "Artificial Ventilation: History, Equipment, and Techniques," *Thorax* 14 (1990): 753–758; Nitin Puri, Vinod Puri, and R. P. Dellinger, "History of Technology in the Intensive Care Unit," *Critical Care Clinics* 25 (2009): 185–200; and Eduardo Mireles-Cabodevila et al., "Alternative Modes of Mechanical Ventilation: A Review for the Hospitalist," *Cleveland Clinic Journal of Medicine* 76 (July 2009): 417–430.

4. Commonly caused by sepsis, ARDS was uniformly defined in 1992 and in 1997 carried the mortality risk of 40 percent. Ramesh C. Sachdeva and Kalpalatha K. Guntupalli, "Acute Respiratory Distress Syndrome," *Critical Care Clinics* 13 (July 1997): 502–521.

5. COPD includes emphysema (destruction and rigidity of the lungs alveoli [air sacs]), chronic bronchitis, and asthmatic bronchitis. Its prevalence alone illustrates why ICU care expanded and highlighted life-sustaining treatment. In 1995 500,000 persons in the United States were hospitalized for COPD, and in 1997 approximately 4.3 percent of the population died from COPD, the most common cause of which was cigarette smoking. See esp. Thomas L. Petty, "The History of COPD," *International Journal of Chronic Obstructive Pulmonary Disease* 1 (March 2006): 3–14; and COPD International, "COPD Statistical Information," at http://www.copd-international.com/library/statistics.htm (accessed March 25, 2012).

6. The primary immediate causes of acute renal disease or chronic kidney failure for patients on dialysis are cardiac disease and infection/sepsis, which, of course, require critical care. Laura M. Dember, "Critical Care Issues in the Patient with Chronic Renal Failure," *Critical Care Clinics* 18 (2000): 421–440.

7. Over 192,000 pacemakers were implanted in patients in the United States by 1997, and their costs exceeded $2 billion by 2000. Kevin

Mohee, "Cardiac Pacing: A Brief History in the Development of Pacemakers," http://ssct.org/HistoryPacemakers.aspx (accessed November 28, 2011).

8. Worldwide attention to critical care medicine occurred throughout the 1980s and 1990s. Intensive care units (ICUs) continued to vary greatly across the United States and in other nations, many based on teams of doctors and nurses with and without specialized training in intensive medicine. Comparative studies in the late 1980s indicated that full-time intensivists reduced ICU mortality, patient's medical complications, and time spent in ICUs, but turf wars continued between physicians throughout the 1990s. Ed Marchan et al., "The Intensivist," *JHN Journal* 5 (2010): 20–22; and R. W. Carlson, E. E. Weiland, and K. Srivathsan, "Does a Full-time, 24 Hour Intensivist Improve Care and Efficiency?" *Critical Care Clinics* 12 (July 1996): 525–551. See also comparisons of critical care between the United States, Canada, Australia and New Zealand, Europe and Japan: W. J. Sibbald and T. Singh, "Critical Care in Canada: The North American Difference," *Critical Care Clinics* 13 (April 1997): 347–362; G. J. Dobb, "Intensive Care in Australia and New Zealand: No Nonsense 'Down Under,'" *Critical Care Clinics* 13 (April 1997): 299–316; and D. C. Angus, C. A. Sirio, and J. Bion, "International Comparisons of Critical Care Outcome and Resource Consumption," *Critical Care Clinics* 13 (April 1997): 389–408.

9. Ulrich Sigwart et al., "Intravascular Stents to Prevent Occlusion and Restenosis after Transluminal Angioplasty," *New England Journal of Medicine* 316 (March 19, 1987): 701–706. By 1999 nearly 85 percent of intra-artery procedures via skin punctures into the arteries included intracoronary stents.

10. Comparisons between the more effective positive-and-negative (biphasic), lower electric shock AEDs and the older monophasic AEDs began in 1989. G. Ristagno, Wanchun Tang, and Max Harry Weil, "Cardiopulmonary Resuscitation: From the Beginning to the Present Day," *Critical Care Clinics* 25 (2009): 133–151, esp. 142–148; and American Heart Association Scientific Statement, "Low-Energy Biphasic Waveform Defibrillation: Evidence-Based Review Applied to Emergency Cardiovascular Care Guidelines," *Circulation* 97 (1998): 1654–1667.

11. *Index Medicus* replaced previous cumulative indexes and was published by the National Library of Medicine between 1960 and 2004, at which time PubMed and MEDLINE assumed the responsibility of identifying the ever-increasing volume of medical and medical-related literature.

12. Kenneth C. Calman, "Palliative Medicine: On the Way to Becoming a Recognized Discipline," *Journal of Palliative Care* 4 (1988): 12–14.

13. Ira R. Byock, "Hospice and the Family Physician," *Journal of Family Practice* 18 (1984): 781–784.

14. Josefina B. Magno, "USA Hospice Care in the 1990s," *Palliative Medicine* 6 (1992): 162.

15. Magno, 162.

16. Nathan Schnaper and Peter H. Wiernick, "The Hospice: New Wine in Old Bottles?" *Maryland State Medical Journal* 32 (1983): 102–104. Schnaper and Wiernick's tirade charged the hospice movement with reinstituting "a church rather than medicine," with being "comforters" instead of modern medical practitioners (quotes from 102).

17. Magno, 162–163. Similar concerns about the low status of physicians involved with hospice care were voiced by the Scottish palliative care physician Derek Doyle, who in 1987 spoke of those entering palliative care as lacking "professional credibility with [their] 'academic' colleagues." Derek Doyle, "Education and Training in Palliative Care," *Journal of Palliative Care* 2 (1987): 5–7.

18. Magno, 163.

19. David Clark, "From Margins to Centre: A Review of the History of Palliative Care in Cancer," *Lancet Oncology* 8 (2007): 430–438, esp. 433.

20. Marjorie C. Dobratz, "Hospice Nursing: Present Perspectives and Future Directives," *Cancer Nursing* 13 (1990): 116–122.

21. "Palliative Medicine: Meeting a Critical Need," http://www.cfps.ca/archive/communic/newsreleases/nr05october1999.asp (accessed February 20, 2003).

22. Cicely Saunders, "Origins: International Perspectives, Then and Now," *Hospice Journal* 14 (1999), reprinted in Cicely Saunders, *Cicely Saunders: Selected Writings 1958–2004*, edited with introduction by David Clark (Oxford: Oxford University Press, 2006), 247.

23. Clark, 434–436.

24. See, for example, the fascinating study of a program of palliative care teaching and training in Zimbabwe: T. Buchan and T. Page, "Teaching the Management of Terminal Illness in Zimbabwe," *Central African Journal of Medicine* 31 (April 1985): 82–85.

25. See the discussion of the development of hospice programs in Chapter 7. See also Carolyn Cook Gotay, "Models of Terminal Care: A Review of the Research Literature," *Clinical and Investigative Medicine* 6 (1983): 131–141; and Inge B. Corless, "Implications of the New Hospice Legislation and the Accompanying Regulations," *Nursing Clinics of North America* 20 (June 1985): 283 and 284.

26. Paul R. Torrens, "Hospice Care: What Have We Learned?" *American Review of Public Health* 5 (1985): 65 and 80.

27. Peter C. Raich, Richard John C. Pearson, and Richard M. Iammarino, "Hospices Are Developing in West Virginia: What Physicians Need to Know," *West Virginia Medical Journal* 79 (June 1983): 116–119; Lenora Finn Paradis, ed., *Hospice Handbook: A Guide for Managers and Planners* (Rockville, MD: Aspen Systems Corporation, 1985), 3–4; Corless, 282.

28. Paul T. Werner, "Hospice Care—An Alternative," *Journal of the Medical Association of Georgia* 71 (1982): 693–694; and Richard M. Dupree, "Hospice—Compassionate, Comprehensive Approach to Terminal Care," *Postgraduate Medicine* 72 (1982): 239–246.

29. Paradis, 5.

30. Anthony M. Smith, "Palliative Care Services in Britain and Ireland 1990—An Overview," *Palliative Medicine* 6 (1992): 277–291.

31. Llora Finlay, "UK Strategies for Palliative Care," *Journal of the Royal Society of Medicine* 94 (September 2001): 437–441; and "Help the Hospices: Facts and Figures," at http://www.helpthehospices.org.uk/about-hospice-care/facts-figures/ (accessed August 25, 2013).

32. Torrens, 68; and Lynn B. Podell, "Medicare Coverage of Hospice Care," *American Journal of Hospital Pharmacy* 41 (May 1984): 942–944.

33. Paradis, 363.

34. [Congressman] Matthew J. Rinaldo, "Medicare to Cover Hospice Services," *Journal of the Medical Society of New Jersey* 79 (December 1982): 1015–1016; Torrens, 68–69; and Jill Rhymes, "Hospice Care in America" *JAMA* 264 (July 18, 1990): 369–372.

35. Torrens, 68; and Magno, 159. Questions over the degrees to which Medicare coverage of hospice home care was or was not more cost effective than conventional hospital care

and hospice-based hospital care is a topic in itself. A number of studies found that hospice home care was indeed less expensive than hospital-based hospice care, not to speak of conventional care. Other studies noted that such conclusions were not definitive because their methodological flaws—such as inadequate controls with respect to the types and severities of the terminal illnesses of the patients who were being investigated in different setting and the lengths of time over which patients were studied in institutional settings that were being compared with one another. See, for example, Torrens, 72–76; and Rhymes, 370. Other studies that carefully controlled for the types of care settings under investigation and the lengths of stays of the patients in these settings found that the costs of caring for patients in both home care hospices and hospital-based hospices were lower than conventional hospital costs for similar sets of patients. See, for example, Vincent Mor and David Kidder, "Cost Savings in Hospice: Final Results of the National Hospice Study," *HSR: Health Services Research* 20 (October 1985): 407–422.

36. Torrens, 68–69; Magno, 159–162; and Corless, 285–295.

37. Podell, 942–943.

38. The four points that follow accord with the official legislation: Department of Health and Human Services: Medicare Program; Hospice Care, Final Rule; *Federal Register* 48 (December 16, 1983): 56008–56036.

39. Corless, 284–286; Podell, 942–943; and Torrens, 67–69.

40. The quote is from Magno, 161.

41. Anne Gilmore, "Treating the Terminal Patient: 'Ignorance Is Rife,'" *Canadian Medical Association Journal* 135 (August 1, 1986): 235–236; Andrew B. Adams, "Dilemmas of Hospice: A Critical Look at Its Problems," *CA: A Cancer Journal for Clinicians* 34 (July/August 1984): 188; and Wayne H. Thalhuber, "Overcoming Physician Barriers to Hospice Care," *Minnesota Medicine* 78 (February 1995): 18–22, esp. 19–20.

42. Cicely Saunders, "Evaluation of Hospice Activities," *Journal of Chronic Diseases* 37 (1984): 871.

43. *Federal Register*, Section III, E.

44. Adams, 188; and Rhymes, 371.

45. Howard Brody and Joanne Lynn, "The Physician's Responsibility Under the New Medicare Reimbursement for Hospice Care," *New England Journal of Medicine* 310 (April 5, 1984): 920–922.

46. Dobratz, 118; and Nicholas A.

Christakis, "Timing of Referral of Terminally Ill Patients to an Outpatient Hospice," *Journal of General Internal Medicine* 9 (June 1994): 314–320.

47. Byrock, 781–784.

48. Coreless, 284 and 296.

49. Magno, 161; see also the comments by Raich et al. about West Virginia (116), and the discussion of Magno about the 5 years of struggle the Hospice of Southeastern Michigan endured before its program was stabilized (161–162).

50. Rhymes, 369–371.

51. Torrens, 76–77.

52. Torrens, 68 and 79.

53. These figures are taken from the authoritative articles by Magno, 159–169, and Rhymes, 369 and 371. Other authors offered somewhat differing statistics, and Ann MacGregor spoke of 1,683 "hospice programs" in 1987. See Ann MacGregor, "Hospice, A Special Kind of Caring," *Iowa Medicine* 78 (August 1988): 362.

54. Marilyn J. Field and Christine K. Cassel, eds., *Approaching Death: Improving Care at the End of Life* (Washington, D.C.: National Academy Press, 1997), 39–40. Because the data on hospice deaths was published by the National Hospice Organization, it apparently dealt with out-of-hospital hospice deaths.

55. Rhymes, 369 and 370.

56. Sandol Stoddard, "Hospice in the United States: An Overview," *Journal of Palliative Care* 5 (1989): 10–19, quotes from 13 and 17.

57. See "Porter Storey, MD," in http:///www.reachmd.com/xmradioguest.aspx?pid-70632 (accessed September 29, 2011); "A Word with the Authors: Primer Tracks Growth in the Field" http://aahpm.org/apps/blog/?tag=primer (accessed September 29, 2011); and Timothy E. Quill et al., *Primer of Palliative Care*, 5th ed. (Glenview, IL: American Academy of Hospice and Palliative Medicine, 2010).

58. Porter Storey, "Goals of Hospice Care," *Texas Medicine* 86 (February 1990): 50–54. Storey listed 40 Texas hospices, 33 of which were Medicare-certified.

59. Magno, 164.

60. For example, Marcy A. Fraser and Jerilyn Hesse, "AIDS Homecare and Hospice in San Francisco: A Model for Compassionate Care," *Journal of Palliative Care* 4 (1988): 116–118; Karen Gardner, "The Hospice Response to AIDS," *Quality Review Bulletin* 14 (June 1988): 198–200; Carol S. Dukes, B. A. Turpin, and J. R. Atwood, "Hospice Education about People with AIDS as Ter-

minally Ill Patients: Coping with a New Epidemic of Death," *American Journal of Hospice and Palliative Care* 12 (January/February 1995): 25–31; and for challenges in Canada, Frank J. Foley et al., "AIDS Palliative Care—Challenging the Palliative Paradigm," *Journal of Palliative Care* 11 (1995): 19–22.

61. Stoddard then outlined why and how hospices should care for persons with AIDS. Stoddard, 18–19.

62. Rhymes, 367.

63. Doyle, 5–7; Dorothy Brockopp, "Palliative Care: Essential Concepts in the Education of Health Professionals," *Journal of Palliative Care* 2 (1987): 18–23; and Dobratz, 116–122.

64. Rodger Carlton and Elaine Ford, "Medical Education in Palliative Care," *Academic Medicine* 70 (April 1995): 258–259, quote from 258.

65. Thalhuber, 18–22.

66. This survey is discussed by Alan C. Mermann et al., "Learning to Care for the Dying: A Survey of Medical Schools and a Model Course," *Academic Medicine* 66 (January 1991): 35–38.

67. The quote is from Barrie R. Cassileth et al., "Medical Students' Reactions to a Hospice Preceptorship," *Journal of Cancer Education* 4 (1989): 261.

68. Margaret B. Coolican et al., "Education about Death, Dying, and Bereavement in Nursing Programs," *Nurse Educator* 19 (November/December 1994): 35–40.

69. Cassileth et al., 261–263. This course was initiated in 1986.

70. Mermann et al., 35–38. This course was also begun in 1986.

71. T. Patrick Hill, "Treating the Dying Patient: The Challenge for Medical Education," *Archives of Internal Medicine* 155 (June 26, 1995): 1265–1269.

72. Field and Cassel, 329–330, 343, and 351. The goals of the ABIM were to identify and promote physician competency in the care of dying patients during internal medicine residency and subspecialty fellowship training.

73. Eloise M. Harman, "Acute Respiratory Distress Syndrome: Prognosis," *Medscape*, http://emedicine.medscape.com/article/165139-overview (accessed February 18, 2014).

74. See, for example, this book's previous discussions of Theophile Bonet in late 17th century, John Ferriar in 1789, Carl F. H. Marx in 1826, Hugh Noble in 1854, and William Munk in the late 19th century.

75. Sherwin B. Nuland, *How We*

Die (New York: Vintage Books, 1993), 27–28, 225–227, and quote from 254.

76. Nuland, 257–258 (on the riddle), 142–143 (excessive treatments), and 265–266 (last-ditch fights and family doctors).

77. Nuland, 142, 195, 255, 267–268.

78. Nuland, 268.

79. Nuland, xvi–xvii.

80. Nuland, 265.

81. Nuland, 251–259, quotes from 251, 253, and 259.

82. John A. Beall, "Mercy—for the Terminally Ill Cancer Patient!" *JAMA* 249 (June 3, 1983): 2883. The text is abbreviated and slightly amended.

83. Sidney H. Wanzer et al., "The Physician's Responsibility toward Hopelessly Ill Patients: A Second Look," *New England Journal of Medicine* 320 (March 30, 1989): 846.

84. Andrew L. Evans and Baruch A. Brody, "The Do-Not-Resuscitate Order in Teaching Hospitals," *JAMA* 253 (April 19, 1985): 2236–2239; L. J. Blackhall, "Must We Always Use CPR?" *New England Journal of Medicine* 317 (November 12, 1987): 1281–1285; George E. Taffet, Thomas A. Teasdale, and Robert Luchi, "In-Hospital Cardiopulmonary Resuscitation," *JAMA* 260 (October 14, 1988): 2069–2072, esp. 2071; and T. Patrick Hill, 1265–1269, who discusses studies about providers' violating their conscience with respect to "overly burdensome treatment."

85. Evans and Brody, 2238.

86. Blackhall, 1282.

87. See Blackhall, 1282–1283, and Taffet et al., who conclude at the end of their study that an average of 10 percent of patients receiving CPR in general hospital settings survive to discharge (2069–2072, esp. 2011).

88. See the concluding sections of Chapter 7.

89. President's Commission for the Study of Ethical Problems in Medicine and Biomedical and Behavioral Research, *Deciding to Forego Life-Sustaining Treatment* (Honolulu, HI: University Press of the Pacific, 2006 [1983]). The President's Commission published a number of reports in addition to *Deciding to Forego*, all of which were filled with extensive medical, ethical, legal, and health policy analysis. The commission comprised 12 members whose careers embraced medicine, bioethics, theology, sociology, economics and the law. See the discussion of Albert R. Jonsen, a member of the commission, in *The Birth of Bioethics* (New York: Oxford University Press, 1998), 99–118.

90. *Deciding to Forego*, 231–246.

91. *Deciding to Forego*. For the emphasis on self-determination in informed consent, see 43–46, 50–51, and the chart on 244—regarding the powerful roles of physicians in the consenting process, see 45, 240–245, where the use of the chart is questioned. See 236–238 and 248–252 on DNR orders; and 136–148 on advanced directives.

92. *Deciding to Forego*, 49.

93. The quotes are from Michael Gordon, "Resuscitation of the Terminally Ill," *Canadian Medical Association Journal* 142 (1990): 531, and from Wanzer et al., 844.

94. For the establishment of DNR policies, see Nancy S. Jecker, "Calling It Quits: Stopping Futile Treatment and Caring for Patients," *Journal of Clinical Ethics* 5 (Summer 1994): 138–142.

95. Donald J. Murphy and Thomas E. Finucane, "New Do-Not-Resuscitate Policies: A First Step in Cost Control," *Archives of Internal Medicine* 153 (July 26, 1993): 1641–1648, esp. 1645.

96. Murphy and Finucane, 1645–1646; Steven H. Miles, "Medical Futility," *Law, Medicine & Health Care* 20 (1992): 312–313; and Jecker, 139 with quote.

97. Murphy and Finucane emphasize cost-effectiveness throughout their article (1641–1648). Other authors strongly opposed entangling futility judgments with cost containment considerations. See especially Lawrence J. Schneiderman, Nancy S. Jecker, and Albert R. Jonsen, "Medical Futility: Its Meaning and Ethical Implications," *Annals of Internal Medicine* 112 (June 15, 1990): 953, and Tomlinson and Brody, 1280.

98. *Deciding to Forego*, 249.

99. Yale New Haven Hospital: Committee on Policy for DNR Decisions, "Report on Do Not Resuscitate Decisions," *Connecticut Medicine* 47 (August 1983): 477–483.

100. Like other Hastings Center reports, this set of guidelines reflected a consensus of some thirty project members and the participation of 80 or more meeting participants. Hastings Center, *Guidelines on the Termination of Life-Sustaining Treatment and the Care of the Dying* (Bloomington: Indiana University Press, 1987).

101. Hastings Center, 40 and 47–50, quote from 50.

102. Hastings Center, 38–40 (ventilators), 49–50 (CPR), and 65–66 (use of antibiotics); and *Deciding to Forego*, 240–241.

103. Hastings Center, 19, 32, 38, and 65.

104. Blackhall, 1283–1284. During his discussion Blackhall uses the term "futile" (1283).

105. The first of the three phrases is from Tom Tomlinson and Howard Brody, "Futility and the Ethics of Resuscitation," *JAMA* 264 (September 12, 1990); 1278; and the second and third are from Schneiderman, et al., 950.

106. John D. Lantos et al., "The Illusion of Futility in Clinical Practice," *American Journal of Medicine* 87 (July 1989): 81–84; and Robert D. Truog et al., "The Problem with Futility," *New England Journal of Medicine* 326 (June 4, 1992): 1560–1563.

107. Schneiderman et al., 949–953, quotes from 951 and 952.

108. See, for example, the references in Miles, 311. Note the critique of that view on 312.

109. Tomlinson and Brody, 1279. They soften the finality of a decision not to resuscitate by saying that out of empathy for a patient's desperation, a doctor can agree to CPR. In their discussion of the ethics of futility in 1994, Tom L. Beauchamp and James F. Childress agree with Tomlinson and Brody's basic points: *Principles of Biomedical Ethics*, 4th ed. (New York: Oxford University Press, 1994), 288–291.

110. Miles, 310–313, quote from 313.

111. George D. Lundberg, "American Health Care System Management Objectives," *JAMA* 269 (May 19, 1993): 2555.

112. See Jecker, 139, who, in contrast to almost all the other authors referenced in these last four subsections, emphasizes that the topic of palliative care moves far beyond discussions of "futility." For the Denver project and Donald Murphy's role (the co-author of the Murphy and Finucane article) in that project, see also Rosemarie Tong, "Towards a Just, Courageous, and Honest Resolution of the Futility Debate," *Journal of Medicine and Philosophy* 20 (1995): 178–179, and 183.

113. See the excellent overview of these issues and an analysis of existing state legislation in the President's Commission, *Deciding to Forego*, 136–153, and 389–422.

114. *Deciding to Forego*, 153; Yale New Haven Hospital, 431; New York Academy of Medicine, "Joint Subcommittee on the Care of Patients with Terminal Illness," *Bulletin of the New York Academy of Medicine* 63 (May 1987): 417; Hastings Center, 78; and, regarding the House of Lords, I. G. Finlay, "Palliative Medicine Overtakes Euthanasia," *Palliative Medicine* 8 (1994): 271–272.

115. Wanzer et al., 844–845.

116. Panagiota V. Caralis and Jeffrey S. Hammond, "Attitudes of Medical Students, House Staff, and Faculty Physicians toward Euthanasia and Termination of Life-Sustaining Treatment," *Critical Care Medicine* 20 (May 1992): 683–690, esp. 686.

117. Tamar Lewin, "Nancy Cruzan Dies, Outlived by a Debate Over the Right to Die," *New York Times*, December 27, 1990, http://www.nytimes.com/1990/12/27/US/nancy-cruzon-dies-outlived-by-a-debate-over-the-right-to-die (accessed April 17, 2012).

118. Beauchamp and Childress, 9, emphasis mine.

119. George J. Annas, "The Health Care Proxy and the Living Will," *New England Journal of Medicine* 324 (April 25, 1991): 1211. Similar to the President's Commission in 1983, Annas effectively argued that DPAs were far preferable compared to living wills (1210–1213).

120. Ezekiel J. Emanuel et al., "How Well Is the Patient Self-Determination Act Working? An Early Assessment," *American Journal of Medicine* 95 (December 1993): 619–628.

121. R. Sean Morrison, Elizabeth Morrison, and Denise Glickman, "Physician Reluctance to Discuss Advance Directives," *Archives of Internal Medicine* 154 (October 24, 1994): 2311–2318.

122. Ann Fade and Karen Kaplan, "Managed Care and End of Life Decisions," *Trends in Health Care, Law & Ethics* 10 (Winter/Spring 1995): 99.

123. The SUPPORT Principle Investigators, "A Controlled Trial to Improve Care for Seriously Ill Hospitalized Patients: The Study to Understand Prognoses and Preferences for Outcomes and Risks of Treatments (SUPPORT)," *Journal of the American Medical Association* 274 (November 22/29, 1995): 1591–1598.

124. SUPPORT Investigators, 1591 and 1594.

125. SUPPORT Investigators, 1592 and 1594.

126. SUPPORT Investigators, 1596.

127. SUPPORT Investigators, 1594–1598, quotes from 1596 and 1597.

128. Bernard Lo, "End-of-Life Care after Termination of SUPPORT," SPECIAL SUPPLEMENT, *Hastings Center Report* 25 (November–December 1995): S6-S8.

129. Patricia A. Marshall, "The SUPPORT Study: Who's Talking?" SPECIAL SUPPLEMENT, *Hasting Center Report* 25 (November–December 1995): S9-S11.

130. George J. Annas, "How We Lie," SPECIAL SUPPLEMENT, *Hastings Center Report* 25 (November–December 1995): S12–S14, quotes from S12.

131. James A. Tulsky, Margaret A. Chesney, and Bernard Lo, "How Do Medical Residents Discuss Resuscitation with Patients?" *Journal of General Internal Medicine* 10 (1995): 436–442.

132. Calls for systematic reform are found in the articles by Marshall, "The SUPPORT Study," and Lo, "End-of-Life Care." The italics are mine. Notably, the first recognition of the need of systematic reform was voiced by Barney G. Glaser, Anselm L. Strauss, and Jeanne C. Quint in 1968. See my discussion of their proposals in Chapter 7.

133. Annas, "How We Lie," S11.

134. Marshall, S11; Kathryn A. Koch, "The Language of Death: Euthanatos Et Mors," *Critical Care Clinics* 12 (January 1996): 1–14; Joanne Lynn, "An 88-Year-Old Woman Facing the End of Life," *JAMA* 277 (May 28, 1997): 1633–1640, quote from 1639; Ezekiel J. and Linda L. Emanuel, "The Promise of a Good Death," *The Lancet* 351 (May 1998): su21–su29.

135. See "About the IOM," at http://www.iom.edu/about-IOM.aspx (accessed August 5, 2013). The present author served on the IOM's Committee on Xenograft Transplantation (living cells and tissues from animals into humans): Institute of Medicine, *Xenotransplantation: Science, Ethics, and Public Policy* (Washington, D.C.: National Academy Press, 1996). Reports are generated after a series of committee meetings, forums, invited studies by noted scholars, and roundtable, cross-disciplinary discussion.

136. Field and Cassel, ix–xi (for expert contributors, staff, and organizations), 17–18, 70–72 (for quotes), and 87–121 (on the health care system).

137. Field and Cassel, 4–7, quotes from 3 and 4.

138. Field and Cassel, 73–83 (for excellent discussion on the four dimensions of care).

139. Field and Cassel, 7–13.

140. Field and Cassel, vii, 1, 7–13, and 259.

141. Field and Cassel, 327–357; Andrew A. Skolnick, "End-of-Life Care Movement Growing," *JAMA* 278 (September 24, 1997): 967–969; and Last Acts, *Means to a Better End: A Report on Dying in America Today* (Princeton, NJ: Last Acts, 2002), 1–3.

142. Rosemary Gibson, "The Robert Wood Foundation Grant-making Strategies to Improve Care at the End of Life," *Journal of Palliative Care* 1 (1998): 415–417.

143. Christine K. Cassel and Kathleen M. Foley, *Principles for Care of Patients at the End of Life: An Emerging Consensus among the Specialties of Medicine* (New York: Milbank Memorial Fund, 1999), 1–15.

144. J. Andrew Billings, "What Is Palliative Care?" *Journal of Palliative Medicine* 1, no. 1 (1998): 73–81, esp. 75.

145. Billings, 73, 78–79.

146. Cynthia X. Pan et al., "How Prevalent Are Hospital-Based Palliative Care Programs? Status Report and Future Directions," *Journal of Palliative Medicine* 4, no. 3 (2001): 320.

147. Ira Byock, "Hospice and Palliative Care: A Parting of the Ways or a Path to the Future?" *Journal of Palliative Medicine* 2, no. 2 (1998): 170–172.

148. Timothy E. Quill and J. Andrew Billings, "Palliative Care Textbooks Come of Age," *Annals of Internal Medicine* 129 (October 1998): 590–594.

149. Barbara Sadick, "What Is Palliative Care? And Why Is It So Rare?" *Wall Street Journal*, September 15, 2014, R2.

150. Hermann Boerhaave, *Dr. Boerhaave's Academical Lectures on the Theory of Physic*, Vol. VI (London: J. Rivington, 1757), 432–440. These volumes were based on Boerhaave's *Institutiones Medicae*, published initially in Latin in 1708 and translated into many languages.

151. David E. Weissman, "The Growth of Hospital-Based Palliative Care," *Journal of Palliative Medicine* 4, no. 3 (2001): 307.

152. Pan et al., 315–324.

153. Byock, 168; Pan et al., 320.

154. Margaret L. Campbell and Robert R. Frank, "Experience with an End-of-Life Practice at a University Hospital," *Critical Care Medicine* 25 (1997): 197–202.

155. Stephen R. Connor, "New Initiatives Transforming Hospice Care," *Hospice Journal* 14 (1999): 199–200.

156. Tom M. George, "The Next Frontier in End-of-Life Care," *Michigan Medicine* 98 (November 1999): 24–26, quote from 24.

157. Field and Cassel, 224–227, quote from 227. See also the discussion of specialized training for nurses (227–229).

158. Robert A. Burt, "The Supreme Court Speaks: Not Assisted Suicide But a Constitutional Right to Palliative Care," *New England*

Journal of Medicine 337 (October 23, 1997): 1234–1236.

159. Linda L. Blank, "Defining and Evaluating Physician Competence in End-of-Life Patient Care," *Western Journal of Medicine* 163 (September 1995): 297–301, quote from 301.

160. See the discussion of the rapidly expanding number of articles and subjects in the *Index* in the first pages of this chapter.

161. See the discussion above about approval of the national hospice Medicare coverage program.

162. The statistics are from Connor, 193; Emanuel and Emanuel, su26; and the outstanding study by Carol Raphael, Joann Ahrens, and Nicole Fowler, "Financing End-of-Life Care in the USA," *Journal of the Royal Society of Medicine* 94 (September 2001): 458–461. See also John J. Mahoney, "The Medicare Hospice Benefit—15 Years of Success," *Journal of Palliative Medicine* 1, no. 2 (1998): 139–146.

163. See Raphael et al., 458; and Nicholas A. Christakis, *Death Foretold: Prophecy and Prognosis in Medical Care* (Chicago: University of Chicago Press, 1999), 177–178.

164. Harold Y. Vanderpool, "Life Sustaining Treatment and Euthanasia: II. Historical Aspects of," *Bioethics*, 4th ed., ed. Bruce Jennings (Farmington Hills, MI: Macmillan Reference USA, 2014), Vol. 4, 1849–1863. The term *euthanasia* also indicated other practices over time, including extinguishing the lives of unwanted persons (the Nazi eugenics euthanasia program) and withdrawing medical treatment (indirect or passive euthanasia).

165. Cicely Saunders, "On Dying Well," *Cambridge Review* (February 27, 1984): 49–52, reprinted in Cicely Saunders, *Cicely Saunders: Selected Writings 1958–2004*, edited with introduction by David Clark (Oxford: Oxford University Press, 2006), 197–202.

166. Koch, 1–12.

167. Storey, 50–54, quotes from 51 and 52.

168. This point expands on Storey's article.

169. Storey, 51 and 52.

170. Skolnick, 969.

171. Daniel Callahan, *The Troubled Dream of Life: Living with Mortality* (New York: Simon & Schuster, 1993), which was published in 1994 and thereafter with the new subtitle "In Search of a Peaceful Death." The page references here and below are from the Georgetown University Press edition of this text, with its designated publishing date as 2000.

See 54–89 and 189–219, especially, for example, 54 and 189–192.

172. Callahan, 195–196.

173. Callahan, 191–194.

174. Diane E. Meier, "Book Review: *The Troubled Dream of Life: Living with Mortality*," *New England Journal of Medicine* 329 (1993): 2042–2043, quote from 2042. For Meier's impressive career, see Diane E. Meier, "Finding My Place," *Journal of Palliative Medicine* 12, no. 4 (2009): 331–335.

175. Field and Cassel, 4–5 and 24–25, quote from 24, which includes opposition to imposition of elements of good death on dying patients.

176. Emanuel and Emanuel, "The Promise of a Good Death," su21–su29.

177. Beyond the opposition to euthanasia in Jewish and Christian and Western law, euthanasia was opposed as antithetical to the bottom-line healing and life-saving roles of physicians and to medicine's reverence for human life, as eroding the public's trust in medicine, as against the welfare of society, and as subject to grave abuses. See, for example, Harold Y. Vanderpool, "Doctors and the Dying of Patients in American History," in *Physician-Assisted Suicide*, ed. Robert F. Weir (Bloomington: Indiana University Press, 1997), 33–66.

178. Timothy E. Quill, "Death with Dignity: A Case of Individualized Decision Making," *New England Journal of Medicine* 324 (March 7, 1991): 691–694.

179. Timothy E. Quill, Christine K. Cassel, and Diane E. Meier, "Care of the Hopelessly Ill: Proposed Clinical Criteria for Physician-Assisted Suicide," *New England Journal of Medicine* 327 (November 5, 1992): 1380–1384.

180. Christine K. Cassel and Diane E. Meier, "Morals and Moralism in the Debate Over Euthanasia and Assisted Suicide," *New England Journal of Medicine* 323 (September 13, 1990): 750–752.

181. For example, Howard Brody, "Assisted Death—A Compassionate Response to a Medical Failure," *New England Journal of Medicine* 327 (November 5, 1992): 1384–1388; and Tom L. Beauchamp and James F. Childress, *Principles of Biomedical Ethics*, 4th ed. (New York: Oxford University Press, 1994), 225–241.

182. See the pro-and-con exchanges between prominent supporters and opponents of PAS in Robert F. Weir's edited collection which includes a chapter by Ira R. Byock, "Physician-Assisted Suicide

is *Not* an Acceptable Practice for Physicians," in *Physician-Assisted Suicide*, ed. Robert F. Weir (Bloomington: Indiana University Press, 1997), 107–135.

183. This is a topic in itself. For an overview, see Harold Y. Vanderpool, "Life-Sustaining Treatment and Euthanasia: II. Historical Aspects of." See also Vanderpool, "Doctors and the Dying of Patients," 55–58.

184. Sidney H. Wanzer et al., "The Physician's Responsibility toward Hopelessly Ill Patients: A Second Look," *New England Journal of Medicine* 320 (March 30, 1989): 844–849.

185. Cassel and Meier, "Morals and Moralism," 750–752, quote from 751.

186. Quill, "Death with Dignity." For the influence of this article, see Quill, Cassel, and Meier, "Care of the Hopeless Ill," 1380; Brody, "Assisted Death—A Compassionate Response," 1386; and Beauchamp and Childress, 239–240.

187. Quill, Cassel, and Meier, "Care of the Hopelessly Ill," 1380–1383.

188. Brody, "Assisted Death," 1385–1386.

189. Timothy E. Quill, *A Midwife Through the Dying Process* (Baltimore: Johns Hopkins University Press, 1996), 213 and 219.

190. Diane E. Meier et al., "A National Survey of Physician-Assisted Suicide and Euthanasia in the United States," *New England Journal of Medicine* 338 (April 23, 1998): 1193–1200.

191. For the statistics, see Emanuel and Emanuel, su25.

192. Kathy Faber-Langendoen, "A Multi-Institution Study of Care Given to Patients Dying in Hospitals," *Archives of Internal Medicine* 156 (October 14, 1996): 2130–2136; and Campbell and Frank, 198.

193. See Howard Brody et al., "Withdrawing Intensive Life-Sustaining Treatment—Recommendations for Compassionate Clinical Management," *New England Journal of Medicine* 336 (February 27, 1997): 652–657.

194. Emanuel and Emanuel, su21–su29; and Lynn, 1633–1640.

195. Susan Deim et al., "Cardiopulmonary Resuscitation on Television: Miracles and Misinformation," *New England Journal of Medicine* 334 (June 13, 1996): 1578–1582; for end-of-life care in the news media, see Quill and Billings, 1998, 590.

196. Deim et al., 1578–1581, quote from 1581.

197. Thomas J. Prendergast and John M. Luce, "Increasing Incidence of Withholding and Withdrawal of Life Support from the Critically Ill," *American Journal of Respiratory and Critical Care Medicine* 155 (1997): 15–20, esp. 19.

198. Timothy E. Quill and Howard Brody, "Physician Recommendations and Patient Autonomy: Finding a Balance between Physician Power and Patient Choices," *Annals of Internal Medicine* 125 (November 1, 1996): 763–769, quotes from 766.

199. Alan Maisel and Mark Kuczewski, "Legal and Ethical Myths about Informed Consent," *Archives of Internal Medicine* 156 (December 9/23, 1996): 2521–2526, quote from 2522.

200. Fiona Randall and R. S. Downie, *Palliative Care Ethics* (Oxford: Oxford University Press, 1999), 6–10, quote from 8. The first edition was published in 1996 and reprinted in 1998, with the second edition in 1999.

201. S. Moratti, "The Development of 'Medical Futility,'" *Journal of Medical Ethics* 35 (2009): 369–372.

202. Chapter 166 of the Texas Health and Safety Code; see also James L. Bernat, "Medical Futility," *Neurocritical Care* 2 (2005): 198–205, esp. 204.

203. American Medical Association Council on Ethical and Judicial Affairs, "Medical Futility in End-of Life Care," *JAMA* 281 (March 10, 1999): 937–941.

204. Moratti, 372.

205. Field and Cassel, quotes from 6, 207, and 227–228; for greater detail on these judgments, see 232–233.

206. J. Andrew Billings and Susan Block, "Palliative Care in Undergraduate Medical Education," *JAMA* 278 (September 3, 1997): 733–738; Hill, 1265.

207. Pam Malloy et al., "Evaluation of End-of-Life Nursing Education for Continuing Education and Clinical Staff Development Educators," *Journal for Nurses in Staff Development* 22 (January/February 2006): 31.

208. Hill, 1265–1267; and Billings and Block, 734–735.

209. For outstanding medical school courses and the description of the "educational program in end-of-life care" at the Medical College of Wisconsin, see Mermann et al.; Field and Cassel, 212–217 and 408–412; David E. Weissman, "End-of-Life Physician Education: Is Change Possible?" *Journal of Palliative Care* 1 (1998): 401–407. See also Sharon

Abele Meekin et al., "Development of a Palliative Education Assessment Tool for Medical Student Education," *Academic Medicine* 75 (October 2000): 986–992; Barbara Barzansky, J. J. Veloski, R. Miller, and H. S. Jonas, "Education in End-of-Life Care during Medical School and Residency Training," *Academic Medicine* 7 (October Supplement 1999): S102-S104; and Kenneth R. White, Patrick J. Coyne, and Urvashi B. Patel, "Are Nurses Adequately Prepared for End-of-Life Care?" *Journal of Nursing Scholarship* 33 (Second Quarter 2001): 147–151. For the examples of positive assessments, see Meekin, 987, and Ellen Fox, "Predominance of the Curative Model of Medical Care," *JAMA* 278 (September 3, 1997): 761–763.

210. Field and Cassel, 216–217.

211. Blank, 297; Felicity Audino and Kathleen Foley, "Professional Education in End-of-Life Care: A U.S. Perspective," *Journal of the Royal Society of Medicine* 94 (September 2001): 472–476. For the End-of-Life Nursing Education Consortium, see Malloy et al., 31–36.

212. Quill and Billings, 590–591.

213. Michael W. Rabow et al., "A Failing Grade for End-of-Life Content in Textbooks: What Is to Be Done?" *Journal of Palliative Medicine* 2, no. 2 (1999): 153–155.

214. Rabow et al., 154–155.

215. Quill and Billings, 590.

216. Quill and Billings, 590–594.

217. David E. Weissman, "A New Journal," *Journal of Palliative Medicine* 1, no. 1 (1998): 1–2.

218. See especially Billings and Block, 735; Weissman, "End of Life Physician Education," 401; and Fox, 781–763.

219. Billings and Block, 735.

220. Byock, 166–167, quote from 166.

221. Jordan J. Cohen, "Dying Patients Need Better Doctoring," *Academic Medicine* 72 (August 1997): 704.

Chapter 9

1. Frederick C. Grant, ed., *Hellenistic Religions: The Age of Syncretism* (New York: Liberal Arts Press, 1953), 55–59.

2. Atul Gawande, "Letting Go," *New Yorker*, August 2, 2010, 7–8; see also F. H. Epstein, "The Role of the Physician in the Preservation of Life," *QJM* 100 (2007): 585–589, esp. 588.588.

3. Ira Byock, *The Best Care Possible* (New York: Avery, 2012), 126–147, quote from 147.

4. These tissue plasminogen activator (tPA) drugs included the FDA approval of Tenecteplase in 2000 and the issuing of official guidelines for their use by the American College of Chest Physicians in 2004. Frederick R. Rickles, "Thrombolytic (Fibrinolytic) Drugs and Progress in Treating Cardiovascular Disease," *FASEB Journal* 19, no. 6 (2005), at http://www.fasebj.org/content/19/6/671.full (accessed November 1, 2012); and Venu Menon et al., "Thrombolysis and Adjunctive Therapy in Acute Myocardial Infarction," *Chest* 126 (September 2004, Supplement): 549S-575S.

5. Imatinib is the first-line treatment for a form of chronic myelogenous leukemia (CMS), gastrointestinal stromal tumors (GISTs) and other diseases. By 2011 Gleevec had been approved by the FDA to treat ten types of cancer. See Lauren Cox, "The Top 10 Medical Advances of the Decade," ABC News Unit, December 17, 2009, at http://www.medpagetoday.com/InfectiousDisease/PublicHealth/17594 (accessed November 1, 2012); see also the stories of curing cancers with other experimental drugs by Ron Winslow, Amy Dockser Marcus, and Christopher Weaver, "The Future of Medicine Is *Now*," *Wall Street Journal*, December 29, 2012, C1 and C2.

6. At the present time, about 5.7 million Americans suffer from chronic heart failure (CHF), over 280,000 die each year, and only 2,100 receive heart transplants per year. Andrew L. Rosenberg and Ravi S. Tripathi, "Perioperative Management for Patients Receiving Ventricular Assist Devices and Mechanical Circulatory Support: A Systems-Oriented Approach," *Contemporary Critical Care* 7, no. 12 (May 2010): 1–12, quote from 11.

7. Daniela Lamas and Lisa Rosenbaum, "Freedom from the Tyranny of Choice: Teaching the End-of-Life Conversation," *New England Journal of Medicine* 366 (May 3, 2012): 1657.

8. Sarah Elizabeth Harrington and Thomas J. Smith, "The Role of Chemotherapy at the End of Life: When Is Enough, Enough?" *JAMA* 299 (June 22, 2008): 2667–2677, quote from 2669.

9. These words are from a poem by Doctor Ronald Lands, "Natural Death," *Journal of Palliative Medicine* 12, no. 10 (2009): 959.

10. John Hardwig, "Families and Futility: Forestalling Demands for Futile Treatment," *Journal of Clinical Ethics* 16 (Winter 2005): 337.

11. Alexi A. Wright and Ingrid T.

Katz, "Letting Go of the Rope—Aggressive Treatment, Hospice Care and Open Access," *New England Journal of Medicine* 357 (July 26, 2007): 324–327, esp. 325–326.

12. Thomas J. Smith and Lowell J. Schnipper, "The American Society of Clinical Oncology Program to Improve End-of-Life Care," *Journal of Palliative Medicine* 1, no. 2 (1998): 221.

13. Kathryn L. Tucker, "Ensuring Informed End-of-Life Decisions," *Journal of Palliative Medicine* 12, no. 2 (2009): 119.

14. S. Yousuf Zafar et al., "Chemotherapy Use and Patient Treatment Preferences in Advanced Colorectal Cancer," *Cancer*, pre-publication online issue (September 12, 2012), 1–28, at http://onlinelibrary.wiley.com.libux.utmb.edu/doi/10.1002/cncr.27815/full (accessed September 27, 2012).

15. Diane E. Meier, "'I Don't Want Jenny to Think I'm Abandoning Her': Views on Overtreatment," *Health Affairs* 33, no. 5 (May 2014): 895–898.

16. Teresa Brown, "When It's the Doctor Who Can't Let Go," *New York Times*, September 7, 2014.

17. Quoted from a cancer researcher in Thomas G. Roberts et al., "Trends in the Risks and Benefits of Patients with Cancer Participating in Phase 1 Cancer Trials," *JAMA* 292 (November 3, 2004): 2130–2140, quote from 2139.

18. Charles F. von Gunten, "Oncologists and End-of-Life Care," *Journal of Palliative Medicine* 11, no. 6 (2008): 813; and Biren Saraiya, "Oncologists and End-of-Life Care: Letter to the Editor," *Journal of Palliative Medicine* 12, no. 2 (2009): 116.

19. For a detailed and first-hand analysis of the real world of chemotherapeutic experimentation, see Harold Y. Vanderpool, "The Ethics of Clinical Experimentation with Anticancer Drugs," in *Cancer Treatment and Research in Humanistic Perspective*, eds. Steven C. Gross and Solomon Garb (New York: Springer, 1985), 16–46.

20. Some 90 percent of the agents tested in Phase I trials fail to become approved by the FDA for additional phases of testing. Roberts et al., 2130–2140; Steven Joffe and Franklin G. Miller, "Rethinking Risk-Benefit Assessment for Phase I Cancer Trials," *Journal of Clinical Oncology* 24 (July 1, 2006): 2987–2990; and "Steve's *Strategic* Guide to Phase I Cancer Clinical Trials," at http://cancerguide.org/trials_phase1.html (accessed September 27, 2012).

21. Sometimes Phase II trials enable patients to become cancer free. See Suleika Jaquoa, "Life, Interrupted: A Test of Faith," *Well* (blog), August 22, 2013, at http://well.blogs.nytimes.com/2013/08/22/life-interrupted-a-test-of-faith/?_r=0 (accessed August 28, 2013).

22. MD Anderson Cancer Center, "What are the Phases of Clinical Trials?" at http://www.mdanderson.org/patient-and-cancer-information/cancer-information/clinical-trials (accessed September 27, 2012); and Vanderpool, 1985, 20–22 and 36–37.

23. Roberts et al., esp. 2134–2140.

24. Harrington and Smith, 2667–2677, quote from 2669.

25. "Steve's *Strategic* Guide," 5.

26. Gawande, 1–2, 7–8 and 12, quotes from 7 and 8.

27. Gawande, 12.

28. Byock, 34–57 and 90, esp. 57.

29. Byock, 91.

30. Robert Arnold, "Ambivalence and Ambiguity in Hospitalized, Critically Ill Patients and Its Relevance to Palliative Care," *Journal of Palliative Medicine* 3, no. 1 (2000): 17–22.

31. Byock, 46–49 and 60.

32. Pew Research, Religion and Public Life Project, "Views on End-of-Life Medical Treatments," November 21, 2013, at http://www.pewforum.org/2013/11/21/views-on-end-of-life-medical-treatments/ (accessed November 25, 2013).

33. These figures are taken from Diane E. Meier, "Increased Access to Palliative Care and Hospice Services: Opportunities to Improve Value in Health Care," *Milbank Quarterly* 89, no. 3 (2011): 343–380, esp. 348; Gawande, 2; Bill First, "How Do You Want to Die?" at http://theweek.com/bullpen/column/33111/how-do-you-want-to-die (accessed September 14, 2012); Diane E. Meier et al., "Palliative Medicine: Politics and Policy," *Journal of Palliative Medicine* 13, no. 2 (2010): 141–46; and Anne M. Walling et al., "The Quality of Care Provided to Hospitalized Patients at the End of Life," *Archives of Internal Medicine* 170 (June 28, 2010): 1057–1063.

34. Byock, 221–238.

35. Byock, 235–236.

36. Francis Weld Peabody, "The Care of the Patient," *JAMA* 88 (1927): 877–882, quote from 882.

37. See the inspiration Dame Cicely Saunders drew from Peabody's 1927 essay in, for example, 1998 and 2000: Cicely Saunders, *Cicely Saunders: Selected Writings 1958–2004*, edited with introduction by David Clark (Oxford: Oxford University Press, 2006), 243 and 254.

38. See, for example, Cecilia Sepulveda et al., "Palliative Care: The World Health Organization's Global Perspective," *Journal of Pain and Symptom Management* 24 (August 2002): 91–95; D. Doyle, "Palliative medicine: the first 18 years of a New Sub-specialty of General Medicine," *Journal of the Royal College of Physicians of Edinburgh* 35 (2005): 199–205; Timothy E. Quill et al., *Primer of Palliative Care*, 5th ed. (Glenview, IL: American Academy of Hospice and Palliative Medicine, 2010), 1–5; and C. Porter Storey, "Hospice and Palliative Medicine (HPM)," *Academic Medicine* 87 (September 2012): 1305.

39. World Health Organization, *National Cancer Control Programmes* (Geneva, Switzerland: World Health Organization, 2002).

40. David Clark, "The International Observatory on End of Life Care: A New Initiative to Support Palliative Care Development Around the World," *Journal of Pain and Palliative Care Pharmacotherapy* 17, no. 3/4 (2003): 231–238.

41. National Consensus Project, *Clinical Practice Guidelines for Quality Palliative Care*, 2nd ed. (Pittsburgh, PA: National Consensus Project for Quality Palliative Care, 2009), iv–71, quote from v.

42. Diane E. Meier, "Finding My Place," *Journal of Palliative Medicine* 12, no. 4 (2009): 331–335, quote from 333.

43. National Consensus Project, 6.

44. See, for example, Doyle, 204; and Meier et al., "Palliative Medicine: Politics and Policy," 5.

45. See James Hallenbeck's outstanding discussion of the most important components of palliative care in James L. Hallenbeck, *Palliative Care Perspectives* (Oxford: Oxford University Press, 2003).

46. National Consensus Project, 13, 18–22, 28–68. The above summary is a succinct outline of the more complex presentation of the NCP's domains of palliative care.

47. For example, National Consensus Project, 28–37; and Betty R. Ferrell and Nessa Coyle, eds., *Oxford Textbook of Palliative Nursing*, 3rd ed. (Oxford: Oxford University Press, 2010), 137–578.

48. J. Andrew Billings and Eric L. Krakauer, "On Patient Autonomy and Physician Responsibility in End-of-Life Care," *Archives of Internal Medicine* 171 (May 9, 2011): 849–853. These issues are discussed at length in the two preceding chapters of this book.

49. Laura C. Hanson, "Commu-

nication Is Our Procedure," *Journal of Palliative Medicine* 14, no. 10 (2011): 1084–1085, quote from 1084; see also Hallenbeck, 159–190; and Byock, 44.

50. Timothy E. Quill, "Initiating End-of-Life Discussions with Seriously Ill Patients: Addressing the 'Elephant in the Room,'" *JAMA* 284 (November 15, 2000): 2502–2507, esp. 2503; see, for example, Byock's discussion of the case of Mrs. Maxwell and her family (40–50 and 60–65).

51. Dale G. Larson and Daniel R. Tobin, "End-of Life Conversations Evolving Practice and Theory," *JAMA* 284 (September 27, 2000): 1573–1574.

52. Ezekiel J. Emanuel et al., "Talking with Terminally Ill Patients and Their Caregivers about Death, Dying, and Bereavement: Is It Stressful? Is It Helpful?" *Archives of Internal Medicine* 164 (October 11, 2004): 1999–2004.

53. Harrington and Smith, 2671–2673.

54. Wendy G. Anderson and Nathan E. Goldstein, "Update in Hospice and Palliative Care," *Journal of Palliative Medicine* 13, no. 2 (2010): 197–202.

55. Quill, "Initiating," 2502–2507; and Quill et al., *Primer*, 110–111.

56. See, for example, R. Sean Morrison and Diane E. Meier, "Palliative Care," *New England Journal of Medicine* 350 (June 17, 2004): 2582–2590; Harrington and Smith, 2667–2678; Billings and Krakauer, 849–853; and Gabrielle R. Goldberg and Diane E. Meier, "A Swinging Pendulum," *Archives of Internal Medicine* 171 (May 9, 2011): 854.

57. David J. Casarett and Timothy E. Quill, "'I'm Not Ready for Hospice': Strategies for Timely and Effective Hospice Discussions," *Annals of Internal Medicine* 146 (March 20, 2007): 443–449.

58. A stunning model of an indepth study of the interplay between Western medicine and a cultural tradition is found in Anne Fadiman, *The Spirit Catches You and You Fall Down: A Hmong Child, Her American Doctors, and the Collision of Two Cultures* (New York: Farrar, Straus and Giroux, 1997). This study is supplemented by Kathleen A. Culhane-Pera et al., eds., *Healing by Heart: Clinical and Ethical Case Stories of Hmong Families and Western Providers* (Nashville: Vanderbilt University Press, 2003). See also the brief bibliographical overview of a variety of cultural heritages in National Consensus Project, 56–59.

59. See, for example, Sharon W. Williams et al., "Communication, Decision Making, and Cancer: What African Americans Want Physicians to Know," *Journal of Palliative Medicine* 11, no. 9 (2008): 1211–1226; Mythili Raghavan, Alexander K. Smith, and Robert M. Arnold, "African Americans and End-of-Life Care," *Journal of Palliative Medicine* 13, no. 11 (2008): 1384–1385; F. Amos Bailey et al., "Do-Not-Resuscitate Orders in the Last Days of Life," *Journal of Palliative Medicine* 15, no. 7 (2012): 751–759; Mohammad Zafir al–Shahri and Abdulla al–Khenaizan, "Palliative Care for Muslim Patients," *Journal of Supportive Oncology* 3 (November/December 2005): 432–436; Rajeev Agarwal, "Palliative Care—Hinduism," *Dolentium Hominum* 20 (2005): 91–93; and David E. Weissman, "Talking about Dying: A Clash of Cultures," *Journal of Palliative Medicine* 3, no. 2 (2000): 134–147.

60. Pew Research, Religion, and Public Life Project, 8–9.

61. Susan Descharnais et al., "Lack of Concordance between Physician and Patient: Reports on End-of-Life Care Discussions," *Journal of Palliative Medicine* 10, no. 3 (2007): 728–740.

62. National Consensus Project, 38–55.

63. National Consensus Project, 9–18; see also Judith Gedney Baggs et al., "The Dying Patient in the ICU: The Role of the Interdisciplinary Team," *Critical Care Clinics* 20 (2004): 525–540.

64. Christopher A. Gibson et al., "Psychologic Issues in Palliative Care," *Anesthesiology Clinics of North America* 24 (2006): 61–80.

65. National Consensus Project, 45–48.

66. See Vanderpool's 1978 article on these dimensions of human well being for palliative care at the end of Chapter 7.

67. Maryjo Prince-Paul, "Understanding the Meaning of Social Well-Being at the End of Life," *Oncology Nursing Forum* 35, no. 3 (2008): 365–371, quote from 365.

68. Nessa Coyle, "Introduction of Palliative Nursing Care," in *Oxford Textbook of Palliative Nursing*, 3rd ed., eds. Betty R. Ferrell and Nessa Coyle (Oxford: Oxford University Press, 2010), 3.

69. Anthony L. Back et al., "Abandonment at the End of Life from Patient, Caregiver, Nurse, and Physician Perspectives," *Archives of Internal Medicine* 169 (March 9, 2009): 474–479, quote from 477.

70. Religion refers to a complex, yet harmonized, understanding or worldview concerning beliefs about sacred reality, moral values, symbols, moods and motivations, and community structures and relationships. Existential concerns focus on meaning, well-being, grounds for hope and other matters common to human existence. Broadly speaking, spirituality is used to embrace all of the above. For an overview of recent scholarly thinking about what religion is, see Harold Y. Vanderpool, "The Religious Features of Scientific Medicine," *Kennedy Institute of Ethics Journal* 18 (September 2008): 203–234, esp. 203–208.

71. This literature and its place in palliative care are extensively discussed. See, for example, Timothy P. Daaleman and Larry VandeCreek, "Placing Religion and Spirituality in End-of-Life Care," *JAMA* 284 (November 15, 2000): 2514–2517; Christina Puchalski, "Spirituality in Health: The Role of Spirituality in Critical Care," *Critical Care Clinics* 20 (2004): 487–504; Tomasz R. Okon, "*Palliative Care Review:* Spiritual, Religious, and Existential Aspects of Palliative Care," *Journal of Palliative Medicine* 8, no. 2 (2005): 392–414, discusses the main easily used models of taking spiritual histories on 401–402.

72. Christina Puchalski et al., "Improving the Quality of Spiritual Care as a Dimension of Palliative Care: The Report of the Consensus Conference," *Journal of Palliative Medicine* 12, no. 19 (2009): 885–904; Karen E. Steinhauser et al., "'Are You At Peace?' One Item to Probe Spiritual Concerns at the End of Life," *Archives of Internal Medicine* 166 (January 9, 2006): 101–105.

73. For example, Storey, "Hospice and Palliative Medicine (HPM)," 1305.

74. National Consensus Project, 18; and Joan M. Teno and Stephen R. Connor, "Referring a Patient and Family to High-Quality Palliative Care at the Close of Life," *JAMA* 301 (February 11, 2009): 651–659; see also Harrington and Smith, 2673–2674.

75. Morrison and Meier, 2585–2590.

76. Sepulveda et al., 94.

77. For the roles of nurses, see Ferrell and Coyle, 567–628.

78. National Consensus Project, 9.

79. Linda J. Kristjanson and Samar Aoun, "Palliative Care for Families: Remembering the Hidden Patients," *Canadian Journal of Psychiatry* 49 (June 2004): 359–365; and "Working With Families," at http://www.caresearch.com.au/caresearch/tabid/

1445/Default.aspx (accessed January 11, 2013).

80. Hardwig, 340–341.

81. Hardwig, 342–343; and Byock, 42–50, 90–93, and 245–247.

82. See, for example, Center for Bioethics, University of Minnesota, *End of Life Care: An Ethical Overview* (Minneapolis: University of Minnesota's Center for Bioethics, 2005), 1–75; the National Consensus Project, 63–71, which includes an extended list of publications; and the thoughtful book by Joseph J. Fins, *A Palliative Ethics of Care* (Sudbury, MA: Jones and Bartlett, 2006).

83. The literature on terminal sedation is rather extensive. See especially Paul Rousseau, "The Ethical Validity and Clinical Experience of Palliative Sedation," *Mayo Clinic Proceedings* 75 (October 2000): 1064–1069; Joakim Engstrom et al., "Palliative Sedation at the End of Life—A Systematic Literature Review," *European Journal of Oncology Nursing* 11 (2007): 26–35; and Jeffrey T. Berger, "Rethinking Guidelines for the Use of Palliative Sedation," *Hasting Center Report* (May–June 2010): 32–38.

84. These topics have been fervently and extensively discussed over time. See, for example, the extensively documented book chapter and encyclopedia article by Harold Y. Vanderpool, "Doctors and the Dying of Patients in American History," in *Physician-Assisted Suicide*, ed. Robert F. Weir (Bloomington: Indiana University Press, 1997), 33–66; Milton J. Lewis, *Medicine and Care of the Dying* (Oxford and New York: Oxford University Press, 2007); and Vanderpool, "Life-Sustaining Treatment and Euthanasia: II. Historical Aspects of," in *Encyclopedia of Bioethics*, 4th ed., ed. Bruce Jennings (Farmington Hills, MI: Macmillan Reference USA, 2014), vol. 4, 1849–1863.

85. Richard A. Parker, "Caring for Patients at the End of Life: Reflections after 12 Years of Practice," *Annals of Internal Medicine* 136 (January 1, 2002): 72–75, quotes from 72 and 75.

86. John Ellershaw and Chris Ward, "Care of the Dying Patient: The Last Hours or Days of Life," *British Medical Journal* 326 (January 4, 2003): 30–34; and Doyle, 199–205.

87. Christine Schiessl et al., "Undergraduate Curricula in Palliative Medicine: A Systematic Analysis Based on the Palliative Education Assessment Tool," *Journal of Palliative Medicine* 16, no. 1 (2013): 20–30.

88. For example, Eduardo Mario Mutto et al., "Teaching Dying Patient Care in Three Universities in Argentina, Spain, and Italy, *Journal of Palliative Medicine* 12, no. 7 (2009): 603–607; and Doreen Oneschuk et al., "The Status of Undergraduate Palliative Medicine Education in Canada: A 2001 Survey," *Journal of Palliative Care* 20, no. 1 (2004): 32–37.

89. Marcos Montagnini, Basil Varkey, and Edmund Duthie, Jr., "Palliative Care Education Integrated into a Geriatrics Rotation for Resident Physicians," *Journal of Palliative Medicine* 7, no. 5 (2004): 652–653.

90. Heather C. Fraser, Jean S. Kutner, and Mark P. Pfeifer, "Senior Medical Students' Perception of the Adequacy of Education on End-of-Life Issues," *Journal of Palliative Medicine* 4, no. 3 (2001): 337–343; and the more thorough analysis by Martha E. Billings et al., "Determinants of Medical Students' Perceived Preparation to Perform End-of-Life Care, Quality of End-of-Life Care Education, and Attitudes toward End-of-Life Care," *Journal of Palliative Medicine* 13, no. 3 (2010): 319–326 (see page 323 on whether patients' deaths denote medical failure).

91. Emily S. Van Aalst-Cohen et al., "Palliative Care in Medical School Curricula: A Survey of United States Medical Schools," *Journal of Palliative Medicine* 11, no. 9 (2008): 1200–1202.

92. Pam Malloy et al., "Evaluation of End-of-Life Nursing Education for Continuing Education and Clinical Staff Development Educators," *Journal for Nurses in Staff Development* 22, no. 1 (2006): 31–36; and Pam Malloy et al., "End-of-Life Nursing Educational Consortium: 5 Years of Educating Graduate Nursing Faculty in Excellent Palliative Care," *Journal of Professional Nursing* 24, no. 6 (October–November 2008): 352–357.

93. Joseph J. Fins and Elizabeth G. Nilson, "An Approach to Educating Residents about Palliative Care and Clinical Ethics," *Academic Medicine* (June 2000): 662–665; Douglas D. Ross, Heather C. Fraser, and Jean S. Kutner, "Institutionalization of a Palliative and End-of-Life Care Educational Program in a Medical School Curriculum," *Journal of Palliative Medicine* 4, no. 4 (2001): 512–518; Montagnini et al.; and Katya Robinson et al., "Assessment of the Education for Physicians on End-of-Life Care (EPEC) Project," *Journal of Palliative Medicine* 7, no. 5 (2004): 637–645.

94. National Consensus Project, 7; and Meier, 2006, 22–24.

95. D. Doyle, 199–203.

96. Kathleen M. Foley, "The Past and Future of Palliative Care," *Hastings Center Special Report* 35, no. 6 (2005): S42–S46; and Ronald Schonwetter, "Hospice and Palliative Medicine Goes Mainstream," *Journal of Palliative Medicine* 9, no. 6 (2006): 1240–1242.

97. Ferrell and Coyle, 61–65, 137–649, and 1121–1130.

98. See, for example, David J. Cassarett, "The Future of the Palliative Medicine Fellowship," *Journal of Palliative Medicine* 3, no. 2 (2000): 151–155; Schonwetter, 1241; Storey, "Hospice and Palliative Medicine (HPM)," 1305; and websites on certification.

99. Lydia Zuraw, "As Palliative Care Need Grows, Specialists Are Scarce," *New America Media*, at http://www.npr.org/blogs/health/2013/or/o3/176121004/as-pallia tive-care-need-grows (accessed July 5, 2013). Zuraw claims that there was a shortage of a whopping 18,000 palliative care physicians in 2013.

100. Bonnie Darves, "Palliative Medicine Career Paths," NEJM Career Center (October 2008), at http://www.nejmjobs.org/career-resou rces/palliative-medicine.aspx (accessed September 2); and Storey, "Hospice and Palliative Medicine (HPM)," 1305.

101. Robert Wood Johnson Foundation Surgeons Palliative Care Workgroup, "Office of Promoting Excellence in End-of-Life Care: Surgeons' Palliative Care Workgroup Report from the Field," *Journal of American College of Surgery* 197 (October 2003): 661–686, quote from 666.

102. Geoffrey Dunn, "Palliative Medicine and the Surgeon," *Journal of Palliative Medicine* 13, no. 5 (2011): 538.

103. Kathy Faber-Langendoen and Paul N. Lanken, "Dying Patients in the Intensive Care Unit: Forgoing Treatment, Maintaining Care," *Annals of Internal Medicine* 133 (December 5, 2000): 886–893, quote from 891.

104. Derek C. Angus et al., "Use of Intensive Care at the End of Life in the United States: An Epidemiologic Study," *Critical Care Medicine* 32, no. 3 (2004): 638–643; Gordon D. Rubenfeld, "Principles and Practice of Withdrawing Life-Sustaining Treatments," *Critical Care Clinics* 20 (2004): 435–451; James E. Szalados, "Discontinuation of Mechanical Ventilation at End-of-Life: The Ethical and Legal Boundaries of

Physician Conduct in Termination of Life Support," *Critical Care Clinics* 23 (2007): 317–337; and Judith E. Nelson, moderator, "Palliative Care in the ICU," *Journal of Palliative Medicine* 15, no. 2 (2012): 168–174.

105. Tom M. George, "The Next Frontier in End-of-Life Care," *Michigan Medicine* 98 (November 1999): 24–26, quote from 24; and Cynthia X. Pan et al., "How Prevalent Are Hospital-Based Palliative Care Programs? Status Report and Future Directions," *Journal of Palliative Medicine* 4, no. 3 (2001): 315–324.

106. Benjamin Goldsmith et al., "Variability in Access to Hospital Palliative Care in the United States," *Journal of Palliative Medicine* 11, no. 8 (2008): 1094–1099; and Howard Gleckman, "Palliative Care Expanding In Hospitals," *Forbes*, at http://www.forbes.com/sites/howardgleckman2011/10/15/palliative-care-expanding (accessed August 29, 2012).

107. Christine S. Ritchie et al., "Palliative Care Programs: The Challenges of Growth," *Journal of Palliative Medicine* 13, no. 9 (2010): 1065–1070, quote from 1965; and David E. Weissman, "Next Gen Palliative Care," *Journal of Palliative Medicine* 15, no. 1 (2012): 2–4.

108. Richard Franki, "More Hospitals House Palliative Care Teams," *Oncology Report*, August 30, 2012, at http://www.oncologypractice.com/single-view/more-hospitals-house-palliative-care-teams/b92d4063830dcdb16e0f56da16c1f21c.html (accessed September 5, 2012).

109. Goldsmith et al.

110. Richard Franki, "More Hospitals Providing Palliative Care," *Oncology Report*, at http://www.oncologypractice.com/index.php?id=6016&type=98&tx_ttnews[tt_news]=2142 (accessed August 6, 2012).

111. David Clark and Carlos Centeno, "Palliative Care in Europe: An Emerging Approach to Comparative Analysis," *Clinical Medicine* 6 (March/April 2006): 197–201; Michael Wright et al., "Mapping Levels of Palliative Care Development: A Global View," *Journal of Pain Symptom Management* 35, no. 5 (May 2008): 469–485; and Geoffrey W. Hanks, "The Mainstreaming of Palliative Care," *Journal of Palliative Medicine* 11, no. 8 (2008): 1063–1064.

112. David Clark, "End-of-Life Care Around the World: Achievements to Date and Challenges Remaining," *OMEGA* 56, no. 1 (2007–2008): 101–110.

113. Kathryn Towns et al., "Availability of Services in Ontario Hospices and Hospitals Providing Inpatient Palliative Care," *Journal of Palliative Medicine* 15, no. 5 (2012): 527–534.

114. Nelson et al., 168–174, especially 168 and 170, quote from 168.

115. Cicely Saunders, "The Evolution of Palliative Care" (2003): 265, in *Cicely Saunders: Selected Writings 1958–2004*, edited with introduction by David Clark (Oxford: Oxford University Press, 2006), 263–268.

116. Clark, 2007–2008, 101–110, quote from 107.

117. These data are taken from National Consensus Project, 1; David J. Casarett, "Rethinking Hospice Eligibility Criteria," *JAMA* 305 (March 9, 2011): 1031–1032; and David G. Stevenson, "Growing Pains for the Medicare Hospital Benefit," *New England Journal of Medicine* 367 (November 1, 2012): 1683–1685.

118. This correction is important because the "lucky few" reference is made by an experienced professional in cardiopulmonary resuscitation who wrote the graphic and impressive book on the history and nature of CPR extensively referenced in Chapter 8. John Anthony Tercier, *The Contemporary Deathbed: The Ultimate Rush* (New York: Palgrave Macmillan, 2005), 241.

119. Stevenson, 1685.

120. Wright and Katz, 325; Meier, 2011, 349; and Stevenson, 1684.

121. See Wright and Katz, 324–327, and the detailed exemplary case discussion in Teno and Connor, 651–659.

122. Byock, 105–107 and 244.

123. Morrison and Meier, 2582; and Casarett and Quill, 443–449.

124. Wright and Katz, 327.

125. Claire M. Spettell et al., "A Comprehensive Case Management Program to Improve Palliative Care," *Journal of Palliative Medicine* 12, no. 9 (2009): 827–832.

126. Wright and Katz, 327.

127. Stevenson, 1683–1685.

128. Darves, 4.

129. National Consensus Project, 18–71.

130. Doyle, 109–203.

131. J. Randall Curtis and R. Sean Morrison, "The Future of Funding for Palliative Care Research: Suggestions for Our Field," *Journal of Palliative Medicine* 12, no. 1 (2009): 26–28; Meier et al., 2010, 1–6; and Meier, "Increasing Access to Palliative Care," 364–365.

132. For example, the full program for attendees to the 18th International Conference on Palliative Care covered 60 pages: Palliative Care Division and Departments of Medicine and Oncology, McGill University, 18th International Congress on Palliative Care, October 5–8, 2010.

133. See Amy M. Sullivan, Nina M. Gadmer, and Susan D. Block, "The Project on Death in America Faculty Scholars Programs: A Report on Scholars' Progress," *Journal of Palliative Medicine* 12, no. 2 (2009): 155–159.

134. Anderson and Goldstein, 201–202; Joan D. Penrod, "Hospital-Based Palliative Care Consultation: Effects on Hospital Costs," *Journal of Palliative Medicine* 13, no. 8 (2010): 973–979; R. Sean Morrison et al., "Palliative Care Consultation Teams Cut Hospital Costs for Medicaid Beneficiaries," *Health Affairs* 30 (March 2011): 454–463; Meier, "Increasing Access to Palliative Care," 351; and Amy S. Kelley et al., "Hospice Enrollment Saves Money for Medicare and Improves Care Quality Across a Number of Different Lengths-of-Stay," *Health Affairs* 32 (March 2013): 552–561.

135. Stephen R. Connor et al., "Comparing Hospice and Nonhospice Patient Survival Among Patients Who Die Within a Three-Year Window," *Journal of Pain and Symptom Management* (March 3, 2007): 238–246.

136. Jennifer S. Temel et al., "Early Palliative Care for Patients with Metastatic Non-Small-Cell Lung Cancer," *New England Journal of Medicine* 363 (August 19, 2010): 733–742.

137. Connor et al., 245; Donald G. McNeil Jr., "Palliative Care Extends Life, Study Finds," *New York Times*, August 19, 2010, A15; and Areej El-Jawahri, Joseph A. Greer, and Jennifer S. Temel, "Does Palliative Care Improve Outcomes for Patients with Incurable Illness? A Review of the Evidence," *Journal of Supportive Oncology* 9 (May/June 2011): 87–94; and Byock, 107–109.

138. Robert Y. Lin, Rozalyn J. Levine, and Brian C. Scanlan, "Evolution of End-of-Life Care at United States Hospitals in the New Millennium," *Journal of Palliative Medicine* 15, no. 5 (2012): 592–601.

139. The safeguards set forth by pro–PAS caregivers are listed in the last chapter and include securing a second medical opinion, repeated requests for assistance in dying by the patient, and no physician's being forced to participate in PAS against her or his conscience.

140. For discussion of euthanasia and PAS in other nations, see Vanderpool, "Life-Sustaining Treatment and Euthanasia: II. Historical Aspects of"; and Sidney Wanzer and

Joseph Genmullen, *To Die Well* (Philadelphia, PA: Da Capo Press, 2008), 171–173.

141. For example, Kevin B. O'Reilly, "State Takes First-ever Path to Approve Assisted Suicide," *American Medical News*, May 29, 2013, at http://www.amednews.com/article/20130529/profession/1305 29952/8/ (accessed August 8, 2013); National Right to Die, "Opposition to Assisting Suicide Remains AMA Policy," at http://www.nrlc.org/arch ive/news/2003/NRL07/opposition_to_assisting_suicide_.htm (accessed August 8, 2013); Wesley J. Smith, "World Medical Association and AMA Oppose Euthanasia, Assisted Suicide," July 30, 2013, at http://www.lifenews.com/2013/07/30/world-medical-association-and-ama-oppose-euthanasia (accessed August 8, 2013); Association of Northern California Oncologists and Medical Oncology Association of Southern California, "Position Statement on Physician-Assisted Suicide and Opposition to AB 374," April 16, 2007.

142. Wanzer and Glenmullen, 150.

143. Alex Schadenberg, "Do Americans Want to Legalize Assisted Suicide? What the Polls Won't Tell You," *LifeSiteNews*, January 8, 2013, at http://www.lifesitenews.com/home/print_article/news/376 45/ (accessed August 23, 2013).

144. "Assisted Suicide Legalization Supported by Half of Americans, Poll Says," *Huffington Post*, at http://www.huffingtonpost.com/20 13/05/22/assisted-suicide-legaliza tion_n_3314849.html (accessed August 23, 2013). See also Pew Research, Religion, and Public Life Project, 2–3 and 13–14.

145. For example, Ira Brock, "Physician-Assisted Suicide is Not Progressive," *The Atlantic*, October 15, 2012, at http://www.theatlantic.com/health/archive/2012/10/physic ian-assisted-sucide-is-not-progres sive (August 8, 2013); and Barbara Rockett, "Physician-Assisted Suicide in Direct Conflict with Doctor's Role," *White Coat Notes*, July 31, 2012 (quote from 1), at http://www.boston.com/whitcoatnotes/2012–07/31/barbara-rockett-physician-assisted-suicide (accessed August 8, 2013).

146. Timothy E. Quill and Christine K. Cassel, "Professional Organizations' Position Statements on Physician-Assisted Suicide: A Case for Studied Neutrality," *Annals of Internal Medicine* 138 (February 4, 2003): 208–212, quotes from 208.

147. In keeping with the historical roots of Compassion and Choices, Wanzer also believes that euthanasia (the physician's direct administration of a lethal injection) as practiced in the Netherlands should become legal in the United States. Wanzer and Glenmullen, 90 and 152–153. For the changing names of the Hemlock Society, see Wanzer and Glenmullen, 156–158.

148. Sidney H. Wanzer et al. "The Physician's Responsibility toward Hopelessly Ill Patients: A Second Look," *New England Journal of Medicine* 320 (March 30, 1989): 844–849. For the originality of this article in the United States, see Wanzer and Glenmullen, 7.

149. Wanzer and Glenmullen, 12–13, 75–123, and 149–173, quote from 150.

150. Wanzer and Glenmullen, 12–13, quote from 12.

151. Wanzer and Glenmullen, 80–86.

152. Wanzer and Glenmullen, 87–88 and 163–170.

153. Lin et al., 600; and Meier, "Increasing Assess to Palliative Care," 343–380.

154. Gawande, 1–2, quotes from 1, 4, and 6, with my italicizing the word *new*; see also Amy S. Kelley and Diane I. Meier, "Palliative Care—A Shifting Paradigm," *New England Journal of Medicine* 363 (August 10, 2010): 781–782.

155. For Storey's career, see the last foregoing chapter under the subheading "Hospice and Palliative Care After Medical Coverage Began."

156. Teresa Brown, SR4.

157. See David B. Rivkin Jr. and Elizabeth Price Foley, "'Death Panels' Come Back to Life," *Wall Street Journal*, December 30, 2001, A15; and Harold Y. Vanderpool, "End-of-Life Talk Not Same as 'Death Panel,'" *Galveston News*, January 18, 2011, B3.

158. Meier et al., 2010, 1–4, quote from 1; and Jacqueline K. Yuen, M. Carrington Reid, and Michael D. Fetters, "Hospital Do-Not-Resuscitate Orders: Why They Have Failed and How to Fix Them," *Journal of General Internal Medicine* 26, no. 7 (2011): 791–797, esp. 795.

159. James L. Bernat, "Medical Futility: Definition, Determination, and Disputes in Critical Care," *Neurocritical Care* 2 (2005): 198–205.

160. Billings and Krakauer, 852.

161. Deborah L. Kasman, "When Is Medical Treatment Futile?" *Journal of General Internal Medicine* 19 (October 2004): 1053–1058; and Dianna A. Howard and Timothy M. Pawlik, "Withdrawing Medically Fu-

tile Treatment," *Journal of Oncology Practice* 5 (July 2009): 193–195.

162. Leslie Kane, "Exclusive Ethics Survey Results: Doctors Struggle with Tougher-Than-Ever Dilemmas," *Medscape Medical Ethics*, at http://www.medscape.com/viewar ticle/731485 (accessed October 31, 2012).

163. Frist, "How Do You Want to Die?"; see also Gloria Duke, Susan Yarbrough, and Katherine Pang, "The Patient Self-Determination Act: 20 Years Revisited," *Journal of Nursing Law* 13, no. 4 (2009): 114–123.

164. Mark D. Sullivan, "The Illusion of Patient Choice in End-of-Life Decisions," *American Journal of Geriatric Psychiatry* 10 (July–August 2002): 365–372.

165. Angela Fagerlin and Carl E. Schneider, "Enough: The Failure of the Living Will," *Hastings Center Report* 34 (March–April 2004): 30–42, quotes from 30–33.

166. Szalados, 321–322. My numerous jointly held lectures with a department chair in anesthesiology bear witness to these points.

167. Sullivan, 365–372; Karen Blank, "Respectful Decisions at the End of Life," *American Journal of Geriatric Psychiatry* 10 (July–August 2002): 362–364; and David I. Shalowitz, Elizabeth Garrett-Mayer, and David Wendler, "The Accuracy of Surrogate Decision Makers: A Systematic Review," *Archives of Internal Medicine* 166 (March 13, 2006): 493–497.

168. Yuen et al., 781–797; and Bailey et al., 751–759.

169. Susan E. Hickman et al., "Use of the Physician Order for Life-Sustaining Treatment (POLST) Paradigm Program in the Hospice Setting," *Journal of Palliative Medicine* 12, no. 2 (2009): 133–141; Diane E. Meier and Larry Beresford, "POLST Offers Next Stage in Honoring Patient Preferences," *Journal of Palliative Medicine* 12, no. 4 (April 2009): 291–295.

170. See the four levels of official POLST requirements at "POLST Program Requirements," at http://ohsu.edu/polst/developing/core-requirements.htm (accessed December 13, 2012). Some POLST-like programs designate themselves by alternative acronyms, which, for the sake of convenience, will be called POLST here. For example, North Carolina uses the acronym MOST, which refers to Medical Orders for Scope Treatment.

171. Meier and Beresford, 295.

172. Kristina Braine Newport et al., "The 'PSOST': Providers' Sign-

out for Scope Treatment," *Journal of Palliative Care* 13, no. 9 (2010): 1055–1058.

173. Susan W. Tolle et al., "A Prospective Study of the Efficacy of the Physician Order Form for Life-Sustaining Treatment," *Journal of the American Geriatrics Society* 46 (September 1998): 1097–1102; Hickman et al., 2009, 132–141; Susan E. Hickman et al., "A Comparison of Methods to Communicate Treatment Preferences in Nursing Facilities: Traditional Practices Versus the Physician Order for Life-Sustaining Treatment Program," *Journal of the American Geriatrics Society* 58 (2010): 1241–1248; Bernard J. Hammes et al., "The POLST Program: A Retrospective Review of the Demographics of Use and Outcomes in One Community Where Advance Directives Are Prevalent," *Journal of Palliative Medicine* 15, no. 1 (2012): 77–84.

174. Harrington and Smith, 2667–2678; Robert Schwartz, "End-of-Life Care: Doctors' Complaints and Legal Restraints," *Saint Louis University Law Journal* 53 (2009): 1169–1170; Ben A. Rich, "Legislating Patient-Care Protocols," UC Davis Health System, 2009, at http://www.ucdmc.ucdavis.edu/welcome/features/20090513_Medicine_Rich/index.html (accessed August 20, 2012); and Jacquelyn Baylon, "State Laws Giving Terminally Ill Patients a Right to Know about End-of-Life Options," May 18, 2011, at http://thepinkfund.org/2011/05/18/state-laws-giving-terminally-ill-patients-a-right-to-know-about-end-of-life-options/ (accessed August 17, 2012).

175. Carol Levine, "The Family Health Care Decision Act," United Hospital Fund, March 29, 2010, at http://www.uhfnyc/news/880653 (accessed August 7, 2012).

176. NY Health Access, "Family Health Care Decisions Act," at http://www.wnylc.com/health/entry/142/ (accessed August 19, 2014). Other states have official policies in place that require doctors to rely on the input of persons who were not identified in advanced directors, and they also list these decision makers in a priority ranking. See, for example, section 9.15 of the University of Texas Medical Branch's *Handbook of Operating Procedures.*

177. For a summary of the PCIA in the form of directives to physicians, a summary of the law, and questions and answers, see State of New York Department of Health, "Palliative Care Information Act—Letter to Physicians, Summary of the Law, Questions and Answers,

and Laws of New York Chapter 331," at http://www.capc.org/research-and-references-for-palliative-care/additional-resources/new-york-state-department-of-health-pallia tive-care-information-act.pdf (accessed August 7, 2012).

178. State of New York Department of Health, "Palliative Care Access Act—Dear CEO/Administrator Letter, Questions and Answers for Providers," at http://www.ny.gov/professionals/patients_rights/pallia tive_care (accessed August 12, 2012).

179. This quote is from the introduction to State of New York Department of Health, "Palliative Care Access Act (PHS Section 2997-d): Palliative Care Requirements for Hospitals, Nursing Homes, Home Care and Assisted Living Residences (Enhanced and Special Needs)," at http://www.ny.gov/professionals/patient_rights/palliative_care (accessed August 12, 2012).

180. Robert A. Milch, "New York's Palliative Care Information Act: Flawed but Needed," *Bioethics Forum* (June 23, 2011): 5–6, quotes from 5 and 6; and Alan B. Astrow and Beth Popp, "The Palliative Care Information Act in Real Life," *New England Journal of Medicine* 364 (May 19, 2011): 1885–1887.

181. Richard Smith, "A Good Death: An Important Aim for Health Services and for Us All," *British Medical Journal* 320 (January 14, 2000): 129–30.

182. Cicely Saunders, "On Dying Well," reprinted in Saunders, *Cicely Saunders: Selected Writings*, 197–202; Marilyn J. Field and Christine K. Cassel, eds., *Approaching Death: Improving Care at the End of Life* (Washington, D.C.: National Academy Press, 1997), 24–25; and Ezekiel J. Emanuel and Linda L. Emanuel, "The Promise of a Good Death," *The Lancet* 351 (May 1998): su21–su29.

183. "Decent" is viewed as an accompanying term with "good" in the Field and Cassel's *Approaching Death* (24). An "acceptable" death is the term preferred by Sarah Hales, Camilla Zimmermann, and Gary Rodin, "The Quality of Dying and Death," *Archives of Internal Medicine* 168 (May 12, 2008): 912–918, esp. 917.

184. Richard Smith, 129–130.

185. Cicely Saunders also affirmed in the 21st century that the hospice movement embodied the search for "good death." Saunders, "Foreword" [to the 2004 edition of the *Oxford Textbook of Palliative Medicine*], in *Cicely Saunders: Selected Writings*, 276.

186. James Grogono, "Sharing

Control in Death: The Role of an 'Amicus Mortis,'" *British Journal of Medicine* 320 (April 29, 2000): 1205.

187. Karen E. Steinhauser, E. C. Clipp, M. McNeilly, N. A. Christakis, L. M. McIntyre, and J. A. Tulsky, "In Search of a Good Death: Observations of Patients, Families, and Providers," *Annals of Internal Medicine* 132 (May 16, 2000): 825–832.

188. Elizabeth Tong et al., "What Is a Good Death? Minority and Nonminority Perspectives," *Journal of Palliative Care* 13 (Autumn 2003): 168–175.

189. Karen A. Kehl, "Moving toward Peace: An Analysis of the Concept of Good Death," *American Journal of Hospice and Palliative Medicine* 23 (August/September 2006): 277–286; and Hales et al., 912–918, quotes from 912.

190. The issues here are complex. At points, Chochinov briefly mentions that the term *dignity* has its problems because it was being used to justify euthanasia and physician-assisted suicide and was "an elusive concept" prior to his and his colleagues' research; they also knew of Daryl Pullman's defense of "basic dignity" as "essentially a universe concept." But the term *dignity* was widely regarded as ambiguous and useless, as denoting honor and esteem for dignitaries, as a term that had been historically co-opted by proponents of euthanasia and physician-assisted suicide and in frequently proposed (and sometimes successful) death with dignity legislation, and as shunned by most philosophers in favor of terms with far more specific moral meanings. Chochinov and his colleagues believed that they were resurrecting dignity as an overarching term for palliative care because they asked terminally ill patient-subjects of research questions about what they took dignity to mean. Upon analyzing all the answers subjects gave, they found that dignity could serve an overarching and foundational term for palliative care. They then declared that dignity was an empirically based model for palliative care. Harvey Max Chochinov, "Dignity-Conserving Care—A New Model for Palliative Care: Helping the Patient Feel Valued," *JAMA* 287 (May 1, 2002): 2253–2254; Daryl Pullman, "Death, Dignity, and Moral Nonsense," *Journal of Palliative Care* 20, no. 3 (2004): 171–178; Harvey Max Chochinov, "Dying, Dignity, and New Horizons in Palliative End-of-Life Care," *CA: A Cancer Journal for Clinicians* 56 (March/April 2006):

84–103; Ruth Macklin, "Reflections on the Human Dignity Symposium: Is Dignity a Useless Concept?" *Journal of Palliative Care* 20, no. 3 (2004): 212–216; Harvey Max Chochinov et al., "Dignity in the Terminally Ill: A Developing Empirical Model," *Social Science and Medicine* 54 (February 2002): 433–443; and Harvey M. Chochinov et al., "Dignity in the Terminally Ill: Revisited," *Journal of Palliative Medicine* 9, no. 3 [December] (2006): 662–672, quotes from 671.

191. Chochinov et al., February 2002, 433, Chochinov, May 2002, 3253; and Chochinov, March/April 2006, 92.

192. Chochinov, March/April 2006, 100–101.

193. Chochinov, May 2002, 2253; Chochinov, March/April 2006, 100–101.

194. Harvey Max Chochinov et al., "Dignity in the Terminally Ill: A Cross-Sectional, Cohort Study," *The Lancet* 360 (December 21/28, 2002): 2026–2030, quotes from 2029, emphasis mine; see also Chochinov, May 2002, 2254 and 2259.

195. These include "quality of life," as well as helping patients "feel valued," "evince self-regard," retain a "sense of worth," and believe that life has "purpose and meaning." See, for example, Chochinov, May 2002, 2253, 2257, and 2257; Harvey Max Chochinov, "Thinking Outside the Box: Depression, Hope, and Meaning at the End of Life," *Journal of Palliative Medicine* 6, no. 6 (2003): 975–976; Chochinov, March/April 2006, 89; and Chochinov et al., December 2006, 666.

196. These include symptom relief, expert and sensitive communication, respect based on patients' informed choices, and the psychological and social and spiritual concerns of patients. Chochinov et al., December 2006, 662–672, quote from 666; Chochinov et al. February 2002; Chochinov, May 2002, 2254 (which lists all the core components of 21st-century palliative care and claims that all of these prove that "dignity provides an overarching framework" for end-of-life care); Chochinov, 2003, 973–977; Chochinov et al., December 2006 (which precisely aligns "sense of dignity" with each and all of the core elements of palliative care); Chochivov, March/April 2006, with the listing in Table 2, 95; and Harvey Chochinov, "Dignity and the essence of Medicine: The A, B, C, and D of Dignity Conserving Care," *British Journal of Medicine* 335 (July 2007): 184–185 (where "dignity" is elevated to the status of

the essence of medicine and medical ethics).

197. Chochinov et al., December 2002, 2026–2030, quote from 2029. Fifty-four percent of these patients reported "no sense of loss of dignity"; 30 percent "only occasionally felt "some sense of loss of dignity," which they did not regard "as a particular concern"; 14 percent experienced mild or moderate losses of dignity; and 2 percent had a "strong" loss of dignity in that they frequently felt degraded, ashamed or embarrassed.

198. William Breitbart and Karen S. Heller, "Reframing Hope: Meaning-Centered Care for Patients Near the End of Life," *Journal of Palliative Care* 6, no. 6 (2003): 979–988.

199. Chochinov et al., February 2002, quotes from 437 and 441; Chochinov, May 2002, 2254–2257; Harvey Max Chochinov, "Dignity and the Eye of the Beholder," *Journal of Clinical Oncology* 22 (April 1, 2004): 1336–1340, esp. 1338; Chochinov, March/April 2006, esp. 93, 95–97; and Chochinov et al., December 2006, 666–672.

200. See Peabody, "The Care of the Patient"; and Chochinov's quoting from Peabody at the end of his 2007 article (187).

201. Peabody, 878.

202. Chochinov, May 2002, 2258; Chochinov, 2003, 973–974; and Chochinov, 2004, 1226–1340, esp. 1338–1339.

203. See some of the positive research findings of patients' responses to this protocol in Harvey Chochinov et al., "Dignity Therapy: A Novel Psychotherapeutic Intervention for Patients Near the End of Life," *Journal of Clinical Oncology* 23 (August 20, 2005): 5520–5525.

204. Susan McClement et al., "Dignity Therapy: Family Member Perspectives," *Journal of Palliative Medicine* 10, no. 5 (2007): 1076–1082.

205. The following is greatly abbreviated and slightly edited from Jonathan Avery, "A Story Worth Telling," *Journal of Palliative Medicine* 12, no. 3 (March 2009): 263. Skips in the story are not indicated by ellipses.

206. As late as 2011 and national poll found that 86 percent of Americans were familiar with hospice care, but only 24 percent said they had ever heard of palliative care. Victoria Colliver, "Palliative Therapy Teams Coordinate Care," *SFGate*, July 5, 2013, at http://www.sfgate.com/health/article/Palliative-therapy-teams-coordinate-care-43496 97.php (accessed July 5, 2013). As the discussion about death panels

above indicates, too many persons still associate palliative care with "giving up." For example, Heather Miller, "Maybe We Need to Redefine 'Palliative Care,'" WebMD, at http://blogs.wedmd.com/cancer/2013/08/mabye-we-need-to-redefine-palliative-care.html (accessed August 21, 2013); and Teresa Brown, SR4.

207. See Stephanie Lacefield Lewis, "What's in a Name Anyway?" *Journal of Palliative Care* 16, no. 3 (2013): 220–221.

Epilogue

1. Richard A. Parker, "Caring for Patients at the End of Life: Reflections after 12 Years of Practice," *Annals of Internal Medicine* 136 (January 1, 2002): 72–75, quote from 72.

2. Parker, 72.

3. Richard B. Balaban, "A Physician's Guide to Talking about End-of-Life Care," *Journal of General Internal Medicine* 15 (2000): 195–200, quote from 199.

4. Francis Bacon, "Of the Advancement of Learning," in *The Works of Francis Bacon*, eds. James Spedding, Robert Leslie Ellis, and Douglas Denon Heath (Boston: Taggard and Thompson, 1864), 34.

5. Francis Bacon, "The Advancement of Learning," in *Francis Bacon: The Major Works*, ed. Brian Vickers (Oxford: Oxford University Press, 2002), 175.

6. See the second stanza in Larkin's poem "Aubade," at http://www.poetryfoundation.org/poem/178058 (accessed July 15, 2014). See also the discussion of secular philosophers at the end of the discussion of the death and dying movement in Chapter 7.

7. Barney G. Glaser and Anselm L. Strauss, *Awareness of Dying* (Chicago: Aldine, 1965), 200.

8. John A. Beall, "Mercy—for the Terminally Ill Cancer Patient!" *JAMA* 249 (June 3, 1983): 2883.

9. Leslie J. Blackhall, "Must We Always Use CPR?" *New England Journal of Medicine* 317 (November 12, 1987): 1281–1285. The quote above augments Blackhall's title with his phrases on 1281 and 1284.

10. Myles H. Sheehan, "On Dying Well," *America: The National Catholic Weekly*, July 29, 2000, 1–4, quote from 2.

11. Atul Gawande, "Letting Go," *New Yorker*, August 2, 2010, 12.

12. This story is related by Gawande, 10–11.

Bibliography

Primary Sources

"About the IOM." http://iom.edu/about-IOM.aspx (accessed August 5, 2013).

Abrams, Ruth, Gertrude Jameson, Mary Poehlman, and Sylvia Snyder. "Terminal Care in Cancer." *New England Journal of Medicine* 232 (June 21, 1945): 719–724.

Adams, Andrew B. "Dilemmas of Hospice: A Critical Look at Its Problems." *CA: A Cancer Journal for Clinicians* 34 (July/August 1984): 183–190.

Agarwal, Rajeev. "Palliative Care—Hinduism." *Dolentium Hominum* 20 (2005): 91–93.

Agate, John. "Care of the Dying in Geriatric Departments." *The Lancet* (February 17, 1973): 364–366.

Aitken-Swan, Jean. "Nursing the Late Cancer Patient at Home." *Practitioner* 183 (1959): 64–69.

al-Shari, Mohammad Zafir, and Abdulla al-Khenaizan. "Palliative Care for Muslim Patients." *Journal of Supportive Oncology* 3 (November/December 2005): 432–436.

Alsofrom, Judy. "The 'Hospice' Way of Dying—At Home with Friends and Family." *American Medical News* 20 (February 21, 1977): 7–9.

Alvarez, Walter. "The Care of the Dying." *JAMA* 150 (September 13, 1952): 86–91.

_____. "Help for the Dying Patient." *Geriatrics* 18 (February 1964): 69.

_____. *Incurable Physician: An Autobiography.* Englewood Cliffs, NJ: Prentice-Hall, 1963.

"AMA Grams: The Physician and the Dying Patient." *JAMA* 227 (February 18, 1974): 728.

"AMA Passes 'Death with Dignity' Resolution." *Science News* 24 (December 15, 1973): 375.

American Heart Association. "Guidelines for Cardiopulmonary Resuscitation and Emergency Cardiac Care." *JAMA* 268 (October 28, 1992): 2172–2181.

American Heart Association Scientific Statement. "Low-Energy Biaphasic Waveform Defibrillation: Evidence-Based Review Applied to Emergency Cardiovascular Care Guidelines." *Circulation* 97 (1998): 1654–1667.

American Medical Association Council on Ethical and Judicial Affairs. "Medical Futility in End-of-Life Care." *JAMA* 281 (March 10, 1999): 937–941.

Anderson, Wendy G., and Nathan E. Goldstein. "Update in Hospice and Palliative Care." *Journal of Palliative Medicine* 13, no. 2 (2010): 197–202.

Angus, D. C., C. A. Sirio, and J. Bion. "International Comparisons of Critical Care Outcome and Resource Consumption." *Critical Care Clinics* 13 (April 1997): 389–408.

Angus, Derek C., Amber E. Barnato, Walter T. Linde-Zwirble, Lisa A. Weissfeld, R. Scott Watson, and Tim Rickert. "Use of Intensive Care at the End of Life in the United States: An Epidemiologic Study." *Critical Care Medicine* 32, no. 3 (2004): 638–643.

Annas, George J. "The Health Care Proxy and the Living Will." *New England Journal of Medicine* 324 (April 25, 1991): 1210–1213.

_____. "How We Lie." Special Supplement. *Hastings Center Report* 25 (November–December 1995): S12–S14.

Anonymous. "Physiological Nature of Death." *Boston Medical and Surgical Journal* 15 (September 21, 1836): 109.

Aring, Charles D. "Intimations of Mortality: An Appreciation of Death and Dying." *Annals of Internal Medicine* 69 (July 1968): 137–152.

Arnold, Robert. "Ambivalence and Ambiguity in Hospitalized, Critically Ill Patients and Its Relevance to Palliative Care." *Journal of Palliative Medicine* 3, no. 1 (2000): 17–22.

Aronson, Gerald J. "Treatment of the Dying Person." In *The Meaning of Death*, edited by Herman Feifel, 251–258. New York: McGraw-Hill, 1959.

Association of Northern California Oncologists and Medical Oncology. "Position Statement on Physician-Assisted Suicide and Opposition to AB 374." April 16, 2007.

Astrow, Alan B., and Beth Popp. "The Palliative Care Information Act in Real Life." *The New England Journal of Medicine* 364 (May 19, 2011): 1885–1887.

Audino, Felicity, and Kathleen Foley. "Professional Education in End-of-Life Care: A U.S. Perspective." *Journal of the Royal Society of Medicine* 94 (September 2001): 472–476.

Avery, Jonathan. "A Story Worth Telling." *Journal of Palliative Medicine* 12, no. 3 (March 2009): 263.

Ayd, Frank J., Jr. "The Hopeless Case." *JAMA* 181 (September 29, 1962): 1099–1103.

Back, Anthony L., Jessica P. Young, Ellen Mc-Cown, Ruth A. Engelberg, Elizabeth K. Vig, Lynn F. Reinke, Marjorie D. Wenrich, Barbara B. McGrath, and J. Randall Curtis. "Abandonment at the End of Life from Patient, Caregiver, Nurse, and Physician Perspectives." *Archives of Internal Medicine* 169 (March 9, 2009): 474–479.

Bacon, Francis. *Advancement of Learning*. Edited by Joseph Devey. New York: P.F. Collier and Son, 1902.

_____. *The Great Instauration in New Atlantis and the Great Instauration*. Edited by Jerry Weinberger. Wheeling, IL: Harlan Davidson, 1989.

_____. *The Historie of Life and Death*. 1638. Reprint, New York: Arno Press, 1977.

_____. *The Major Works: Oxford World's Classics*. Edited with introduction and notes by Brian Vickers. Oxford: Oxford University Press, 2002.

_____. *Of the Advancement and Proficiencie of Learning: Or the Partitions of Sciences Nine Books*. Translated by Gilbert Wats. London: Thomas Williams, 1674.

_____. *The Works of Francis Bacon*. Vol. IX. Edited by James Speeding, Robert Leslie Ellis, and Douglas Denon Heath. Boston: Taggard and Thompson, 1864.

Baggs, Judith Gedney, Sally A. Norton, Madeline H. Schmitt, and Craig R. Sellers. "The Dying Patient in the ICU: The Role of the Interdisciplinary Team." *Critical Care Clinics* 20 (2004): 525–540.

Bailey, F. Amos, Rebecca S. Allen, Beverly R. Williams, Patricia S. Goode, Shanette Granstaff, David T. Redden, and Kathryn L. Burgio. "Do-Not-Resuscitate Orders in the Last Days of Life." *Journal of Palliative Medicine* 15, no. 7 (2012): 751–759.

Baker, Joan M., and Karen C. Sorensen. "A Patient's Concern with Death." *American Journal of Nursing* 63 (1963): 90–92.

Balaban, Richard B. "A Physician's Guide to Talking about End-of-Life Care." *Journal of General Internal Medicine* 15 (2000): 195–200.

Baldwin, Simeon. "The Natural Right to a Natural Death." *St. Paul Medical Journal* 1 (December 1899): 875–889.

Bard, Samuel. *A Discourse Upon the Duties of a Physician*. Bedford, MA: Applewood Books, 1996 [1769].

Barsteiner, Jane H. "Death and Dying." *Journal of Practical Nursing* 24 (1974): 28–30.

Barton, David, John M. Flexner, Jan Van Eys, and Charles E. Scott. "Death and Dying: A Course for Medical Students." *Journal of Medical Education* 47 (December 1972): 945–951.

Barzansky, Barbara, J. J. Veloski, R. Miller, and H. S. Jonas. "Education in End-of-Life Care during Medical School and Residency Training." *Academic Medicine* 7 (October Supplement 1999): S102–S104.

Baxter, Richard. *The Saint's Everlasting Rest*. New York: American Tract Society, n.d.

Beall, John A. "Mercy—for the Terminally Ill Cancer Patient!" *JAMA* 249 (June 3, 1983): 2883.

Bean, William B. "On Death." *Annals of Internal Medicine* 101 (February 1958): 199–202.

Beatty, Donald C. "Shall We Talk About Death?" *Pastoral Psychology* 6 (1955): 11–14.

Beck, Claude S. "Reminiscences of Cardiac Resuscitation." *Review of Surgery* (March–April 1970): 77–86.

Berger, Jeffrey T. "Rethinking Guidelines for the Use of Palliative Sedation." *Hasting Center Report* (May–June 2010): 32–38.

Bernat, James L. "Medical Futility: Definition, Determination, and Disputes in Critical Care." *Neurocritical Care* 2 (2005): 198–205.

Billings, J. Andrew. "What Is Palliative Care?" *Journal of Palliative Medicine* 1, no. 1 (1998): 73–81.

Billings, J. Andrew, and Susan Block. "Palliative Care in Undergraduate Medical Education." *JAMA* 278 (September 3, 1997): 733–738.

Billings, J. Andrew, and Eric L. Krakauer. "On Patient Autonomy and Physician Responsibility in End-of-Life Care." *Archives of Internal Medicine* 171 (May 9, 2011): 849–853.

Billings, Martha E., Ruth Engelberg, J. Randall Curtis, Susan Block, and Amy M. Sullivan. "Determinants of Medical Students' Perceived Preparation to Perform End-of-Life Care, Quality of End-of-Life Care Education, and Attitudes toward End-of-Life Care." *Journal of Palliative Medicine* 13, no. 3 (2010): 319–326.

Blackhall, Leslie J. "Must We Always Use CPR?" *New England Journal of Medicine* 317 (November 12, 1987): 1281–1285.

Blank, Karen. "Respectful Decisions at the End of Life." *American Journal of Geriatric Psychiatry* 10 (July–August 2002): 362–364.

Blank, Linda L. "Defining and Evaluating Physician Competence in End-of-Life Patient Care." *Western Journal of Medicine* 163 (September 1995): 297–301.

Bluestone, E. M. "On the Significance of Death in Hospital Practice." *The Modern Hospital* 78 (March 1952): 86–88.

Boerhaave, Herman. *Dr. Boerhaave's Academical Lectures of the Theory of Physic*. Vol. VI. London: J. Rivington, 1757.

_____. "The Palliative Cure, or Treatment of Symptoms." In *Dr. Boerhaave's Academical Lectures of the Theory of Physic*, 432–440. London: W. Innys, 1751.

Bonet, Theophile. *A Guide to the Practical Physician*. London: Thomas Flesher, 1688.

Book Notices. "*Book on the Physician Himself*, by D. W. Cathell." *JAMA* 62 (January 24, 1914): 318.

Book Notices. "*The Care of the Aged, the Dying, and the Dead*, by Alfred Worcester." *JAMA* 105, no. 3 (July 20, 1935): 225.

Breitbart, William, and Karen S. Heller. "Reframing Hope: Meaning-Centered Care for Patients Near the End of Life." *Journal of Palliative Care* 6, no. 6 (2003): 979–988.

Brock, Ira. "Physician-Assisted Suicide Is Not Progressive." *The Atlantic*. http://www.theatlantic.com/health/archive/2012/10/physician-assisted-suicide-is-not-progressive (accessed August 8, 2013).

Brockopp, Dorothy. "Palliative Care: Essential Concepts in the Education of Health Professionals." *Journal of Palliative Care* 2 (1987): 18–23.

Brodie, Benjamin Collins. *The Works of Sir Benjamin Collins Brodie*. Edited by Charles Hawkins. London, 1865.

Brody, Howard. "Assisted Death—A Compassionate Response to a Medical Failure." *New England Journal of Medicine* 327 (November 5, 1992): 1384–1388.

Brody, Howard, Margaret L. Campbell, Kathy Faber-Langendoen, and Karen S. Ogle. "Withdrawing Intensive Life-Sustaining Treatment—Recommendations of Compassionate Clinical Management." *New England Journal of Medicine* 336 (February 27, 1997): 652–657.

Brody, Howard, and Joanne Lynn. "The Physician's Responsibility Under the New Medicare Reimbursement for Hospice Care." *New England Journal of Medicine* 310 (April 5, 1984): 920–922.

Brown, Norman K., Roger J. Bulger, Harold Laws, and Donovan J. Thompson. "The Preservation of Life." *JAMA* 211 (January 5, 1970): 76–82.

Brown, Teresa. "When It's the Doctor Who Can't Let Go." *New York Times*, September 7, 2014.

Browne, Oswald. *On the Care of the Dying: A Lecture to Nurses*. London: George Allen, 1894.

Browne, Thomas. "A Letter to a Friend." http://penelope.uchicago.edu/letter.html (accessed June 10, 2010).

_____. *Pseudodoxia Epidemica: or, Enquiries into vary many received Tenants and commonly presumed Truths*. 1672. http://penelope.uchicago.edu/pseudodoxia.shtml (accessed January 13, 2013).

_____. *Religio Medici*. Edited by Jean-Jacques Denonain. Cambridge: Cambridge University Press, 1955.

Buchan, T., and T. Page. "Teaching the Management of Terminal Illness in Zimbabwe." *Central African Journal of Medicine* 31 (April 1985): 82–85.

Buffett, E. P. "Euthanasia: The Pleasures of Dying." *New Englander and Yale Review* 55 (August 1891): 231–242.

Burt, Robert A. "The Supreme Court Speaks: Not Assisted Suicide But a Constitutional Right to Palliative Care." *New England Journal of Medicine* 337 (October 23, 1997): 1234–1236.

Byock, Ira R. *The Best Care Possible*. New York: Avery, 2012.

_____. "Hospice and the Family Physician." *Journal of Family Practice* 18 (1984): 781–784.

_____. "Hospice and Palliative Care: A Parting of Ways or a Path to the Future?" *Journal of Palliative Medicine* 2, no. 2 (1998): 170–172.

_____. "Physician-Assisted Suicide Is *Not* an Acceptable Practice for Physicians." In *Physician-Assisted Suicide*, edited by Robert F. Weir. Bloomington: Indiana University Press, 1997.

Cabot, Hugh. "Avoiding Psychological Damage in the Care of Hospital Patients." *The Modern Hospital* 17 (September 1921): 184–186.

Cabot, Richard C., and Russell L. Dicks. *The Art of Ministering to the Sick*. New York: Macmillan, 1936.

Callahan, Daniel. "Bioethics as a Discipline." *Hastings Center Studies* 1, no. 1 (1973): 66–73.

_____. *The Troubled Dream of Life: Living with Mortality*. New York: Simon & Schuster, 1993.

Calman, Kenneth C. "Palliative Medicine: On the Way to Becoming a Recognized Discipline." *Journal of Palliative Care* 4 (1988): 12–14.

Cameron, C. S. *The Truth About Cancer*. Englewood Cliffs, NJ: Prentice Hall, 1956.

Campbell, Margaret L., and Robert R. Frank. "Experience with an End-of-Life Practice at a University Hospital." *Critical Care Medicine* 25 (1997): 197–202.

"Cancer and Conscience." *Time*, November 3, 1961, 60.

Cantor, Norman L. "A Patient's Decision to Decline Lifesaving Medical Treatment: Bodily Integrity versus the Preservation of Life." *Rutgers Law Review* 26 (Winter 1973): 228–264.

Caralis, Panagiota V., and Jeffrey S. Hammond. "Attitudes of Medical Students, House Staff, and Faculty Physicians toward Euthanasia and Termination of Life-Sustaining Treatment." *Critical Care Medicine* 20 (May 1992): 683–690.

Carlson, R. W., E. E. Weiland, and K. Srivathsan. "Does a Full-time, 24 Hour Intensivist Improve Care and Efficiency?" *Critical Care Clinics* 12 (July 1996): 525–551.

Carlton, Rodger, and Elaine Ford. "Medical Education in Palliative Care." *Academic Medicine* 70 (April 1995): 258–259.

Cassarett, David J. "The Future of the Palliative Medicine Fellowship." *Journal of Palliative Medicine* 3, no. 2 (2000): 151–155.

_____. "Rethinking Hospice Eligibility Criteria." *JAMA* 305 (March 9, 2011): 1031–1032.

Cassarett, David J., and Timothy Quill. "'I'm Not

Ready for Hospice': Strategies for Timely and Effective Hospice Discussions." *Annals of Internal Medicine* 146 (March 20, 2007): 443–449.

Cassel, Christine K., and Kathleen M. Foley. *Principles for Care of Patients at the End of Life: An Emerging Consensus among the Specialties of Medicine*. New York: Milbank Memorial Fund, 1999.

Cassel, Christine K., and Diane E. Meier. "Morals and Moralism in the Debate Over Euthanasia and Assisted Suicide." *New England Journal of Medicine* 323 (September 13, 1990): 750–752.

Cassileth, Barrie R., Christine Brown, Carla Liberatore, John Lovejoy, Scott A. Parry, Catherine Streeto, Kate Watkins, and Deborah Berlyne. "Medical Students' Reactions to a Hospice Preceptorship." *Journal of Cancer Education* 4 (1989): 261–263.

Cathell, D. W. *Book on the Physician Himself*. Philadelphia: F. A. Davis, 1903.

_____. *The Physician Himself*. Baltimore: Cushings and Bailey, 1882.

Center for Bioethics, University of Minnesota. *End of Life Care: An Ethical Overview*. Minneapolis: University of Minnesota's Center for Bioethics, 2005.

Chapman, Earle M. "He Was in the Prime of Life." *Rhode Island Medical Journal* 39 (September 1956): 494–497

Chase, Peter Pineo, and Irving A. Beck. "Making a Graceful Exit." *Rhode Island Medical Journal* 39 (September 1956): 497–499 and 516–525.

Chochinov, Harvey Max. "Dignity-Conserving Care—A New Model for Palliative Care: Helping the Patient Feel Valued." *JAMA* 287 (May 1, 2002): 2253–2254.

_____. "Dignity and the Essence of Medicine: The A, B, C, and D of Dignity Conserving Care." *British Journal of Medicine* 335 (July 2007): 184–185.

_____. "Dignity and the Eye of the Beholder." *Journal of Clinical Oncology* 22 (April 1, 2004): 1336–1340.

_____. "Dying, Dignity, and New Horizons in Palliative End-of-Life Care." *CA: A Cancer Journal for Clinicians* 56 (March/April 2006): 84–183.

_____. "Thinking Outside the Box: Depression, Hope, and Meaning at the End of Life." *Journal of Palliative Medicine* 6, no. 6 (2003): 975–976.

Chochinov, Harvey Max, Thomas Hack, Linda J. Kristjanson, Susan McClement, and Mike Harlos. "Dignity in the Terminally Ill: A Cross-Sectional, Cohort Study." *The Lancet* 360 (December 21/28, 2002): 2026–2030.

_____. "Dignity Therapy: A Novel Psychotherapeutic Intervention for Patients Near the End of Life." *Journal of Clinical Oncology* 23 (August 20, 2005): 5520–5525. Chochinov, Harvey Max, Thomas Hack, Susan McClement, Linda Kristjanson, and Mike Harlos. "Dignity in the Terminally Ill: A Developing Empirical Model." *Social Science and Medicine* 54 (February 2002): 433–443.

Chochinov, Harvey M., Linda J. Kristjanson, Thomas F. Hack, T. Hassard, Susan McClement, and Mike Harlos. "Dignity in the Terminally Ill: Revisited." *Journal of Palliative Medicine* 9, no. 3 [December] (2006): 662–672.

Chodoff, Paul. "The Dying Patient." *Medical Annals of the District of Columbia* 29 (August 1960): 447–450.

Christakis, Nicholas A. *Death Foretold: Prophecy and Prognosis in Medical Care*. Chicago: University of Chicago Press, 1999.

_____. "Timing of Referral of Terminally Ill Patients to an Outpatient Hospice." *Journal of General Internal Medicine* 9 (June 1994): 314–320.

Christian, Henry A. "The Medical Profession's Obligation to the Patient." *The Modern Hospital* 7 (1916): 9–12.

Clark, David. "End-of-Life Care Around the World: Achievements to Date and Challenges Remaining." *OMEGA* 56, no. 1 (2007–2008): 101–110.

Clarke, L. Pierce. "The Injection of Stimulants into the Heart-Walls." *Boston Medical and Surgical Journal* 82 (April 18, 1895): 395.

Code of Ethics of the American Medical Association: Adopted May 1847. San Francisco: Jos. Winterburn, 1867.

Cohen, Jordan J. "Dying Patients Need Better Doctoring." *Academic Medicine* 72 (August 1997): 704.

Collins, Vincent J. "Limits of Medical Responsibility in Prolonging Life." *JAMA* 206 (October 7, 1968): 389–392.

Connor, Stephen R. "New Initiatives Transforming Hospice Care." *Hospice Journal* 14 (1999): 199–200.

Connor, Stephen R., Bruce Pyenson, Kathryn Fitch, Carol Spence, and Kosuke Iwasake. "Comparing Hospice and Nonhospice Patient Survival Among Patients Who Die Within a Three-Year Window." *Journal of Pain and Symptom Management* (March 3, 2007): 238–246.

Coolican, Margaret B., June Stark, Kenneth J. Doka, and Charles A. Carr. "Education about Death, Dying, and Bereavement in Nursing Programs." *Nurse Educator* 19 (November/December 1994): 35–40.

COPD International. "COPD Statistical Information." http://www.copd-international.com/library/statistics.htm (accessed March 25, 2012).

Corless, Inge B. "Implications of the New Hospice Legislation and the Accompanying Regulations." *Nursing Clinics of North America* 20 (June 1985): 281–298.

Cowley, L. Tad, Ernle Young, and Thomas A. Raffin. "Care of the Dying: An Ethical and Historical Perspective." *Critical Care Medicine* 20, no. 10 (October 1992): 1473–1482.

Culhane-Pera, Kathleen A., Dorothy E. Vawter,

Phua Xiong, Barbara Babbitt, and Mary M. Solberg, eds. *Healing by Heart: Clinical and Ethical Case Stories of Hmong Families and Western Providers.* Nashville: Vanderbilt University Press, 2003.

Curtis, J. Randall, and R. Sean Morrison. "The Future of Funding for Palliative Care Research: Suggestions for Our Field." *Journal of Palliative Medicine* 12, no. 1 (2009): 26–28.

Cushing, Harvey. *Consecratio Medici and Other Papers.* Boston: Little, Brown, 1928.

Daaleman, Timothy P., and Larry VandeCreek. "Placing Religion and Spirituality in End-of-Life Care." *JAMA* 284 (November 15, 2000): 2514–2517.

Dana, Richard Henry, Jr. *Two Years Before the Mast.* New York: New American Library, 1964 [1869].

Darves, Bonnie. "Palliative Medicine Career Paths." NEJM Career Center (October 2008). http://www.nejmjobs.org/career-resources/palliative-medicine.aspx (accessed September 2).

Davidson, Ramona Powell. "Let's Talk about Death: To Give Care in Terminal Illness." *American Journal of Nursing* 64 (January 1966): 74–75.

Deim, Susan, John D. Lantos, and James A. Tulsky. "Cardiopulmonary Resuscitation on Television: Miracles and Misinformation." *New England Journal of Medicine* 334 (June 13, 1996): 1578–1582.

Dember, Laura M. "Critical Care Issues in the Patient with Chronic Renal Failure." *Critical Care Clinics* 18 (2000): 421–440.

Department of Health and Human Services: Medicare Program; Hospice Care, Final Rule. *Federal Register* 48 (December 16, 1983): 56008–56036.

DePorte, J. V. "Where Do People Die—at Home or in Hospitals?" *The Modern Hospital* 33 (August 1929): 73–80.

Descharnais, Susan, Rickey E. Carter, Winnie Hennessy, Jerome E. Kurent, and Cindy Carter. "Lack of Concordance between Physician and Patient: Reports on End-of-Life Care Discussions." *Journal of Palliative Medicine* 10, no. 3 (2007): 728–740.

Dickinson, George E. "Death Education in U.S. Medical Schools: 1975–1980." *Journal of Medical Education* 56 (February 1981): 111–114.

Dobb, G. J. "Intensive Care in Australia and New Zealand: No Nonsense 'Down Under.'" *Critical Care Clinics* 13 (April 1997): 299–316.

Dobratz, Marjorie C. "Hospice Nursing: Present Perspectives and Future Directives." *Cancer Nursing* 13 (1990): 116–122.

"The Doctor." *Medical Review of Reviews* 20 (January 1914): 76–77.

Dowler, Bennet. "Researches on the Natural History of Death." *New Orleans Medical and Surgical Journal* 6 (January 1850): 594–615.

Doyle, D. "Palliative Medicine: The First 18 Years of a New Sub-specialty of General Medicine." *Journal of the Royal College of Physicians of Edinburgh* 35 (2005): 199–205.

Doyle, Derek. "Education and Training in Palliative Care." *Journal of Palliative Care* 2 (1987): 5–7.

Ducachet, Henry W. "On the Signs of Death, and the Manner of Distinguishing Real from Apparent Death." *American Medical Recorder* 5 (1822): 39–52.

Duke, Gloria, Susan Yarbrough, and Katherine Pang. "The Patient Self-Determination Act: 20 Years Revisited." *Journal of Nursing Law* 13, no. 4 (2009): 114–123.

Dukes, Carol S., B. A. Turpin, and J. R. Atwood. "Hospice Education about People with AIDS as Terminally Ill Patients: Coping with a New Epidemic of Death." *American Journal of Hospice and Palliative Care* 12 (January/February 1995): 25–31.

Dunglison, Robley. *Address to the Medical Graduates of the Jefferson Medical College.* Philadelphia: Printed by Adam Waldie, 1837.

Dunn, Geoffrey. "Palliative Medicine and the Surgeon." *Journal of Palliative Medicine* 13, no. 5 (2011): 538.

Dupree, Richard M. "Hospice—Compassionate, Comprehensive, Approach to Terminal Care." *Postgraduate Medicine* 72 (1982): 239–246.

el-Jawahri, Areej, Joseph A. Greer, and Jennifer S. Temel. "Does Palliative Care Improve Outcomes for Patients with Incurable Illness? A Review of the Evidence." *Journal of Supportive Oncology* 9 (May/June 2011): 87–94.

Ellershaw, John, and Chris Ward. "Care of the Dying Patient: The Last Hours or Days of Life." *British Medical Journal* 326 (January 4, 2003): 30–34.

Emanuel, Ezekiel J., and Linda L. Emanuel. "The Promise of a Good Death." *The Lancet* 351 (May 1998): su21–su29.

Emanuel, Ezekiel J., Diane L. Fairclugh, Pam Wolfe, and Linda L. Emanuel. "Talking with Terminally Ill Patients and Their Caregivers about Death, Dying, and Bereavement: Is It Stressful? Is It Helpful?" *Archives of Internal Medicine* 164 (October 11, 2004): 1999–2004.

Emanuel, Ezekiel J., David Weinberg, Rene Gonin, Lacinda R. Hummel, and Linda L. Emanuel. "How Well Is the Patient Self-Determination Act Working? An Early Assessment." *American Journal of Medicine* 95 (December 1993): 619–628.

Epstein, F. H. "The Role of the Physician in the Preservation of Life." *QJM* 100 (2007): 585–589.

"Euthanasia." *Spectator Archive* (March 18, 1871): 10ff.

Evans, Andrew L., and Baruch A. Brody. "The Do-Not-Resuscitate Order in Teaching Hospitals." *JAMA* 253 (April 19, 1985): 2236–2239.

Faber-Langendoen, Kathy. "A Multi-Institution Study of Care Given to Patients Dying in Hospitals." *Archives of Internal Medicine* 156 (October 14, 1996): 2130–2136.

Faber-Langendoen, Kathy, and Paul N. Lanken. "Dying Patients in the Intensive Care Unit: Foregoing Treatment, Maintaining Care." *Annals of Internal Medicine* 133 (December 5, 2000): 886–893.

Fade, Ann, and Karen Kaplan. "Managed Care and End of Life Decisions." *Trends in Health Care, Law, & Ethics* 10 (Winter/Spring 1995): 97–100.

Fadiman, Anne. *The Spirit Catches You and You Fall Down: A Hmong Child, Her American Doctors, and the Collision of Two Cultures.* New York: Farrar, Strauss and Giroux, 1997.

Fagerlin, Angela, and Carl E. Schneider. "Enough: The Failure of the Living Will." *Hastings Center Report* 34 (March–April 2004): 30–42.

Fairbanks, Rollin J. "Ministering to the Dying." *Journal of Pastoral Care* 2 (1948): 6–14.

Farrell, John J. "The Right of a Patient to Die." *Journal of the South Carolina Medical Association* 54 (July 1958): 231–233.

Ferrell, Betty R., and Nessa Coyle, eds. *Oxford Textbook of Palliative Nursing.* 3rd ed. Oxford: Oxford University Press, 2010.

Ferriar, John. *Medical Histories and Reflections.* 4 vols. Philadelphia: Thomas Dobson, 1816.

Field, Marilyn J., and Christine K. Cassel, eds. *Approaching Death: Improving Care at the End of Life.* Washington, D.C.: National Academy Press, 1997.

Finlay, I. G. "Palliative Medicine Overtakes Euthanasia." *Palliative Medicine* 8 (1994): 271–272.

Finlay, Llora. "UK Strategies for Palliative Care." *Journal of the Royal Society of Medicine* 94 (September 2001): 437–441.

Fins, Joseph J. *A Palliative Ethics of Care.* Sudbury, MA: Jones and Bartlett, 2006.

Fins, Joseph J., and Elizabeth G. Nilson. "An Approach to Education Residents about Palliative Care and Clinical Ethics." *Academic Medicine* (June 2000): 662–665.

Fitts, William T., and I. S. Ravdin. "What Philadelphia Physicians Tell Patients with Cancer." *JAMA* 153 (November 7, 1953): 901–904.

Fletcher, Joseph. "The Patient's Right to Die." *Harper's* 221 (October 1960): 139–143.

Flint, Austin. *A Treatise on the Principles and Practice of Medicine.* 3rd Edition. Philadelphia: Henry C. Lea, 1868.

Flory, James, Yinong Young-Xu, Ipek Gurol, Norman Levinsky, Arlene Ash, and Ezekiel Emanuel. "Place of Death: U.S. Trends Since 1980." *Health Affairs* 23 (2004): 194–200.

Foley, Frank J., J. Flannery, D. Graydon, G. Flintoft, and D. Cook. "AIDS Palliative Care—Challenging the Palliative Paradigm." *Journal of Palliative Care* 11 (1995): 19–22.

Foster, Daniel W. "Religion and Medicine: The Physician's Perspective." In *Health/Medicine and the Faith Traditions,* edited by Martin E. Marty and Kenneth L. Vaux, 245–270. Philadelphia: Fortress Press, 1982.

Fox, Ellen. "Predominance of the Curative Model of Medical Care." *JAMA* 278 (September 3, 1997): 761–763.

Fraser, Heather C., Jean S. Kutner, and Mark P. Pfeifer. "Senior Medical Students' Perception of the Adequacy of Education on End-of-Life Issues." *Journal of Palliative Medicine* 4, no. 3 (2001): 337–343.

Fraser, Marcy A., and Jerilyn Hesse. "AIDS Homecare and Hospice in San Francisco: A Model for Compassionate Care." *Journal of Palliative Care* 4 (1988): 116–118.

Frist, Bill. "How Do You Want to Die?" http://theweek.com/bullpen/column/33111/how-do-you-want-to-die (accessed September 14, 2012).

Furlow, Thomas W., Jr. "Tyranny of Technology." *The Humanist* (July–August 1974): 6–9.

Fusgen, I., and J. D. Summa. "How Much Sense Is There in an Attempt to Resuscitate an Aged Person?" *Gerontology* 24 (1978): 37–45.

Gardner, Karen. "The Hospice Response to AIDS." *Quality Review Bulletin* 14 (June 1988): 198–200.

Gauderer, M. W. L., J. L. Ponsky, and R. J. Izant Jr. "Gastrostomy Without Labarotomy: A Percutaneous Endoscopic Technique." *Journal of Pediatric Surgery* 15 (1980): 872–875.

Gauderer, Michael W. L. "Percutaneous Endoscopic Gastrostomy—20 Years Later: A Historical Perspective." *Journal of Pediatric Surgery* 36 (January 2001): 217–219.

Gavey, C. J. *The Management of the "Hopeless" Case.* London: H. K. Lewis, 1952.

Gawande, Atul. "Letting Go." *New Yorker,* August 2, 2010, 1–12.

George, Tom M. "The Next Frontier in End-of-Life Care." *Michigan Medicine* 98 (November 1999): 24–26.

Gibson, Christopher A., W. Lichtenthal, A. Berg, and W. Breitbart. "Psychologic Issues in Palliative Care." *Anesthesiology Clinics of North America* 24 (2006): 61–80.

Gibson, Rosemary. "The Robert Wood Foundation Grant-making Strategies to Improve Care at the End of Life." *Journal of Palliative Care* 1 (1998): 415–417.

Gilmore, Anne. "Treating the Terminal Patient: 'Ignorance Is Rife.'" *Canadian Medical Association Journal* 135 (August 1, 1986): 235–236.

Gisborne, Rev. Thomas. *On the Duties of Physicians, Resulting from Their Profession.* Oxford: John Henry Parker, 1847.

Glaister, J. Norman. "Phantasies of the Dying: Some Remarks on the Management of Death." *The Lancet* (August 6, 1921): 315–317.

Glaser, Barney G., and Anselm L. Strauss. *Awareness of Dying.* Chicago: Aldine, 1965.

_____. *Time for Dying*. Chicago: Aldine, 1968.

Gleckman, Howard. "Palliative Care Expanding In Hospitals." *Forbes*. http://www.forbes.com/sites/howardgleckman2011/10/15/palliative-care-expanding (accessed August 29, 2012).

Goffnett, Carol. "Your Patient's Dying—Now What?" *Nursing* 9 (November 1979): 31–33.

Goldberg, Gabrielle R., and Diane E. Meier. "A Swinging Pendulum." *Archives of Internal Medicine* 171 (May 9, 2011): 854.

Goldsmith, Benjamin, Jessica Dietrich, Qingling Du, and R. Sean Morrison. "Variability in Access to Hospital Palliative Care in the United States." *Journal of Palliative Medicine* 11, no. 8 (2008): 1094–1099.

Goldwater, S. S. "The Hospital and the Surgeon." *The Modern Hospital* 7 (October 1916): 273–277 and (November 1916): 371–377.

Gordon, Michael. "Resuscitation of the Terminally Ill." *Canadian Medical Association Journal* 142 (1990): 531.

Gorer, Goeffrey. *Death, Grief and Mourning*. New York: Doubleday, 1965.

_____. "The Pornography of Death." *Modern Writing* (1965): 56–62.

Gottesman, Julius. "Resuscitation by the Intra-Cardiac Injection of Epinephrin." *JAMA* 79 (October 14, 1922): 1334–1335.

Grant, Frederick C., ed. *Hellenistic Religions: The Age of Syncretism*. New York: Liberal Arts Press, 1953.

Grant, Ian. "Care for the Dying." *British Medical Journal* 2 (December 28, 1957): 1539–1540.

Gregory, John. *Lectures on the Duties and Qualifications of a Physician*. London: W. Strahan and P. Cadell, 1772.

Greshake, Gisbert. "Towards a Theology of Dying." In *The Experience of Dying*, edited by Norbert Greenacher and Alios Muller, 80–98. New York: Herder and Herder, 1974.

Grogono, James. "Sharing Control in Death: The Role of an 'Amicus Mortis.'" *British Journal of Medicine* 320 (April 29, 2000): 1205.

Gunten, Charles F. von. "Oncologists and End-of-Life Care." *Journal of Palliative Medicine* 11, no. 6 (2008): 813.

Hackett, Thomas P., and Avery D. Weisman. "The Treatment of the Dying." *Current Psychiatric Therapies* 2 (1962): 121–126.

Hales, Sarah, Camilla Zimmermann, and Gary Rodin. "The Quality of Dying and Death." *Archives of Internal Medicine* 168 (May 12, 2008): 912–918.

Halford, Sir Henry. *Essays and Orations Read and Delivered at the Royal College of Physicians*. 3rd ed. London: John Murray, Albemarle Street, 1833.

Hammes, Bernard J., Brenda L. Rooney, Jacob D. Gundrum, Susan E. Hickman, and Nickijo Hager. "The POLST Program: A Retrospective Review of the Demographics of Use and Outcomes in One Community Where Advance Directives Are Prevalent." *Journal of Palliative Medicine* 15, no. 1 (2012): 77–84.

Hanks, Geoffrey W. "The Mainstreaming of Palliative Care." *Journal of Palliative Medicine* 11, no. 8 (2008): 1063–1064.

Hanson, Laura C. "Communication Is Our Procedure." *Journal of Palliative Medicine* 14, no. 10 (2011): 1084–1085.

Harman, Eloise M. "Acute Respiratory Distress Syndrome: Prognosis." *Medscape*. http://emedicine.medscape.com/article/165139-overview (accessed February 18, 2014).

Harrington, Sarah Elizabeth, and Thomas J. Smith. "The Role of Chemotherapy at the End of Life: When Is Enough, Enough?" *JAMA* 299 (June 22, 2008): 2667–2677.

Hardwig, John. "Families and Futility: Forestalling Demands for Futile Treatment." *Journal of Clinical Ethics* 16 (Winter 2005): 335–344.

Hastings Center. *Guidelines on the Termination of Life-Sustaining Treatment and the Care of the Dying*. Bloomington: Indiana University Press, 1987.

Hebb, Frank. "The Care of the Dying." *Canadian Medical Association* 65 (1951): 261–263.

Hegland, Kennedy F. "Unauthorized Rendition of Lifesaving Medical Treatment." *California Law Review* 53 (August 1965): 860–877.

"Help the Hospices: Facts and Figures." http://www.helpthehospices.org.ud/about-hospice-care/facts-figures/ (accessed August 25, 2013).

Hickman, Susan E., Christine A. Nelson, Nancy A. Perrin, Alvin H. Moss, Bernard J. Hammes, and Susan W. Tolle. "A Comparison of Methods to Communicate Treatment Preferences in Nursing Facilities: Traditional Practices Versus the Physician Order for Life-Sustaining Treatment Program." *Journal of the American Geriatrics Society* 58 (2010): 1241–1248.

Hickman, Susan E., Christine A. Nelson, Alvin H. Moss, Bernard J. Hammes, Allison Terwilliger, Ann Jackson, and Susan W. Tolle. "Use of the Physician Order for Life-Sustaining Treatment (POLST) Paradigm Program in the Hospice Setting." *Journal of Palliative Medicine* 12, no. 2 (2009): 133–141.

Hill, T. Patrick. "Treating the Dying Patient: The Challenge for Medical Education." *Archives of Internal Medicine* 155 (June 26, 1995): 1265–1269.

Hinton, J. M. "Facing Death." *Journal of Psychosomatic Research* 10 (1966): 22–28.

"The History of COPD." *International Journal of Chronic Obstructive Pulmonary Disease* 1 (March 2006): 3–14.

Holder, Angela Roddey. "Informed Consent: Its Evolution." *JAMA* 214 (November 9, 1970): 1181–1182.

_____. "Informed Consent: The Obligation." *JAMA* 214 (November 16, 1970): 1383–1384.

_____. "Informed Consent: Limitations." *JAMA* 214 (November 23, 1970): 1611–1612.

Holford, J. M. "Terminal Care." *Nursing Times* 69 (January 25, 1973): 113–115.

Hollingsworth, J. H. "The Results of Cardiopulmonary Resuscitation: A 3-Year University Hospital Experience." *Annals of Internal Medicine* 71 (September 1969): 459–460.

Hooker, Claire, and Hans Pols. "Health, Medicine and the Media." *Health and History* 8 (2006): 1–13.

Hooker, Worthington. *Physician and Patient: or, A Practical View of the Mutual Duties, Relations and Interests of the Medical Profession and the Community.* New York: Baker and Scribner, 1849.

A Hospital Nurse. "Some Notes on How to Nurse the Dying." *The Trained Nurse* 5 (July–December 1890): 17–21.

Howard, Dianna A., and Timothy M. Pawlik. "Withdrawing Medically Futile Treatment." *Journal of Oncology Practice* 5 (July 2009): 193–195.

Hoyle, Clifford. "The Care of the Dying." *Post-Graduate Medical Journal* 20 (April 1944): 120.

Hufeland, Christopher W. M. *The Art of Prolonging Human Life.* London: Simpkin and Marshall, 1829.

_____. *Enchiridion Medicum, or The Practice of Medicine.* 2nd ed. New York and London: William Badde, 1844.

Jaquoa, Suleida. "Life, Interrupted: A Test of Faith." *Well* (blog), August 22, 2013. http://well.blogs.nytimes.com/2013/08/22/life-interrupted-a-test-of-faith/?_php=true&_type=blogs&_r=1 (accessed August 28, 2013).

Jecker, Nancy S. "Calling It Quits: Stopping Futile Treatment and Caring for Patients." *Journal of Clinical Ethics* 5 (Summer 1994): 138–142.

Jennings, Bruce. "Preface" to *Improving End of Life Care: Why Has It Been So Difficult? A Hastings Center Special Report* 35, no. 6 (2005): S2–S4

Johnson, A. L., Paul H. Tanser, Ray A. Ulan, and Thomas E. Wood. "Results of Cardiac Resuscitation in 552 Patients." *American Journal of Cardiology* 20 (1967): 831–835.

Joffe, Steven, and Franklin G. Miller. "Rethinking Risk-Benefit Assessment for Phase 1 Cancer Trials." *Journal of Clinical Oncology* 24 (July 1, 2006): 2987–2990.

Jones, T. T. "The Right to Live and the Right to Die." *Medical Times* 95 (November 1967): 1176–1177.

Jury, Mark, and Dan Jury. Gramp. New York: Grossman, 1976.

Kahn, Sigmund Benham, and Vincent Zarro. "The Management of the Dying Patient." *Seminars in Drug Treatment* 3 (Summer 1973): 37–44.

Kane, Hermine. "The End." *American Mercury* 19 (April 1930): 458–461.

Karnofsky, David A. "Why Prolong the Life of a Patient with Advanced Cancer?" *CA: A Cancer Journal for Clinicians* 10 (January–February 1960): 9–11.

Kasley, Virginia. "As Life Ebbs: The Art of Giving Understanding Care and Emotional Tranquility to the Dying Patient." *American Journal of Nursing* 48 (March 1948): 170–173.

Kasman, Deborah L. "When Is Medical Treatment Futile?" *Journal of General Internal Medicine* 19 (October 2004): 1053–1058.

Kasper, August M. "The Doctor and Death." In *The Meaning of Death*, edited by Herman Feifel, 259–270. New York: McGraw-Hill, 1959.

Kass, Leon R. "Averting One's Eyes or Facing the Music?—On Dignity and Death." In *Death Inside Out*, edited by Peter Steinfels and Robert M. Veatch, 101–114. New York: Harper and Row, 1974.

Kavanaugh, Robert E. "Helping Patients Who Are Facing Death." *Nursing* 4 (May 1974): 35–42.

Kehl, Karen A. "Moving toward Peace: An Analysis of the Concept of Good Death." *American Journal of Hospice and Palliative Medicine* 23 (August/September 2006): 277–286.

Kelley, Amy S., and Diane I. Meier. "Palliative Care—A Shifting Paradigm." *New England Journal of Medicine* 363 (August 10, 2010): 781–782.

Kelley, Amy S., Partha Deb, Qingling Du, Melissa D. Aldridge Carlson, and R. Sean Morrison. "Hospice Enrollment Saves Money for Medicare and Improves Care Quality Across a Number of Different Lengths-of-Stay." *Health Affairs* 32 (March 2013): 552–561.

Keywood, Olive. "Care of the Dying in Their Own Home." *Nursing Times* 70 (September 26, 1974): 1516–1517.

Kline, Nathan S., and Julius Sobin. "The Psychological Management of Cancer Cases." *JAMA* 146 (August 25, 1951): 1547–1551.

Koch, Kathryn A. "The Language of Death: Euthanatos Et Mors." *Critical Care Clinics* 12 (January 1996): 1–14.

Kouwenhoven, W. B., J. R. Jude, and G. G. Knickervocker. "Closed Chest Cardiac Massage." *JAMA* 173 (1960): 1064–1967.

Krant, Melvin J. "The Organized Care of the Dying Patient." *Hospital Practice* (January 1972): 101–108.

Krant, Melvin J., and Alan Sheldon. "The Dying Patient—Medicine's Responsibility." *Journal of Thanatology* 1 (February 1971): 1–24.

Kristjanson, Linda J., and Samar Aoun. "Palliative Care for Families: Remembering the Hidden Patients." *Canadian Journal of Psychiatry* 49 (June 2004): 359–365.

Kübler-Ross, Elisabeth. *On Death and Dying.* New York: Macmillan, 1969.

_____. "The Right to Die with Dignity." *Bulletin of the Menniger Clinic* 36 (May 1972): 302–312.

Laforet, Eugene G. "The 'Hopeless' Case." *Archives of Internal Medicine* 112 (September 1963): 314–326.

Lamas, Daniela, and Lisa Resenbaum. "Freedom from the Tyranny of Choice: Teaching the End-of-Life Conversation." *New England Journal of Medicine* 366 (May 3, 2012): 1655–1657.

Lands, Ronald. "Natural Death." *Journal of Palliative Medicine* 12, no. 10 (2009): 959.

Lantos, John D., P. A. Singer, R. M. Walker, G. P. Gramelspacher, G. R. Shapiro, M. A. Sanchez-Gonzalez, C. B. Stocking, S. H. Miles, and M. Siegler. "The Illusion of Futility in Clinical Practice." *American Journal of Medicine* 87 (July 1989): 81–84.

Larkin, Phillip. "Aubade." http://www.poetryfoundation.org/poem/178058 (accessed July 15, 2014).

Larson, Dale G., and Daniel R. Tobin. "End-of-Life Conversations Evolving Practice and Theory." *JAMA* 284 (September 27, 2000): 1573–1574.

Last Acts. *Means to a Better End: A Report on Dying in America Today.* Princeton, NJ: Last Acts, 2002.

Leak, W. N. "The Care of the Dying." *Practitioner* 161 (1948): 80–87.

Lemier, Jean G., and Arnold L. Johnson. "Is Cardiac Resuscitation Worthwhile? A Decade of Experience." *New England Journal of Medicine* 286 (May 4, 1972): 970–972.

Leuf, A. H. P. "Resuscitation After Apparent Death." *Medical News* 54 (January 26, 1889): 97–99.

Levine, Carol. "The Family Health Care Decisions Act." United Hospital Fund (March 29, 2010). http://www.uhfnyc/news/880653 (accessed August 7, 2012).

Lewin, Tamar. "Nancy Cruzan Dies, Outlived by a Debate Over the Right to Die." *New York Times,* December 27, 1990. http://www.nytimes.com/1990/12/27/US/nancy-cruzon-dies-outlived-by-a-debate-over-the-right-to-die (accessed April 17, 2012).

Lewis, Stephanie Lacefield. "What's in a Name Anyway?" *Journal of Palliative Care* 16, no. 3 (2013): 220–221.

"Life in Death." *New England Journal of Medicine* 256 (1957): 760.

Lin, Robert Y., Rozalyn J. Levine, and Brian C. Scanlan. "Evolution of End-of-Life Care at United States Hospitals in the New Millennium." *Journal of Palliative Medicine* 15, no. 5 (2012): 592–601.

Liston, Edward H. "Education on Death and Dying: A Survey of American Medical Schools." *Journal of Medical Education* 48 (June 1973): 577–578.

Lo, Bernard. "End-of-Life Care after Termination of SUPPORT." Special Supplement. *Hastings Center Report* 25 (November–December 1995): S6–S8.

Love, Elizabeth Ford. "Do All Hands Help Ease the Sting of Death by Tact and Kindliness?" *Hospitals* 18 (December 1944): 47–48.

Lund, Charles C. "The Doctor, the Patient, and the Truth." *Annals of Internal Medicine* 24 (June 1946): 955–959.

Lundberg, George D. "American Health Care System Management Objectives." *JAMA* 269 (May 19, 1993): 2554–2555.

Lynn, Joanne. "An 88-Year-Old Woman Facing the End of Life." *JAMA* 277 (May 28, 1997): 1633–1640.

MacDonald, Arthur. "Death in Man." *Medical Times* 49 (July 1921): 149–180.

_____. "Human Death." *Medical Times* 56 (August and September 1928): 206–216.

MacGregor, Ann. "Hospice: A Special Kind of Caring." *Iowa Medicine* 78 (August 1988): 362–364.

Macklin, Ruth. "Reflections on the Human Dignity Symposium: Is Dignity a Useless Concept?" *Journal of Palliative Care* 20, no. 3 (2004): 212–216.

Mackness, James. *The Moral Aspects of Medical Life.* London: John Churchill, Princes Street, Solo, 1846.

Magno, Josefina B. "USA Hospice Care in the 1990s." *Palliative Medicine* 6 (1992): 158–196.

Mahoney, John J. "The Medicare Hospice Benefit—15 Years of Success." *Journal of Palliative Medicine* 1, no. 2 (1998): 139–146.

Maisel, Alan and Mark Kuczewski. "Legal and Ethical Myths about Informed Consent." *Archives of Internal Medicine* 156 (December 9/23, 1996): 2521–2526.

Malloy, Pam, Betty R. Ferrell, Rose Virani, Gwen Uman, Anne M. Rhome, Barbara Whitlatch, and Geraldine Bednash. "Evaluation of End-of-Life Nursing Education for Continuing Education and Clinical Staff Development Educators." *Journal for Nurses in Staff Development* 22, no. 1 (January/February 2006): 31–36.

Malloy, Pam, Judith Paice, Rose Virani, Betty R. Ferrell, and Geraldine "Polly" Bednash. "End-of-Life Nursing Educational Consortium: 5 Years of Educating Graduate Nursing Faculty in Excellent Palliative Care." *Journal of Professional Nursing* 24, no. 6 (October–November 2008): 352–357.

Marshall, Patricia A. "The SUPPORT Study: Who's Talking?" Special Supplement. *Hastings Center Report* 25 (November–December 1995): S9–S11.

Martinson, Ida M. "Why Don't We Let Them Die at Home?" *RN* (January 1976): 58–65.

Marx, Carl Friedrich Heinrich. "Medical Euthanasia" (1826). Translated by Walter Cane. *Journal of the History of Medicine and Allied Sciences* 7 (1952): 401–416.

Mather, Cotton. *Euthanasia: A Sudden Death Made Happy and Easy.* Boston: S. Kneeland, 1723.

May, William. "The Metaphysical Plight of the Family." In *Death Inside Out,* edited by Peter

Steinfels and Robert M. Veatch, 49–60. New York: Harper and Row, 1974.

Mayer-Scheu, Josef. "Compassion and Death." In *The Experience of Dying*, edited by Norbert Grienackez and Alois Muller, 111–113. New York: Herder and Herder, 1974.

McClanahan, John B. "The Patient's Right to Die." *Memphis Medical Journal* 38 (August 1963): 303–316.

McClement, Susan, Harvey Max Chochinov, Thomas Hack, Thomas Hassard, Linda Joan Kristjanson, and Mike Harlos. "Dignity Therapy: Family Member Perspectives." *Journal of Palliative Medicine* 10, no. 5 (2007): 1076–1082.

McCullough. Laurence B. *John Gregory's Writings on Medical Ethics and Philosophy of Medicine.* Dordrecht/Boston/London: Kluwer Academic Publishers, 1998.

McNeil, Donald G., Jr. "Palliative Care Extends Life, Study Finds." *New York Times*, August 19, 2010, A15.

Meekin, Sharon Abele, Jason E. Klein, Alan R. Fleischman, and Joseph J. Fins. "Development of a Palliative Education Assessment Tool for Medical Student Education." *Academic Medicine* 75 (October 2000): 986–992.

Meier, Diane E. "Book Review: *The Troubled Dream of Life: Living with Mortality.*" *New England Journal of Medicine* 329 (1993): 2042–2043.

_____. "Finding My Place." *Journal of Palliative Medicine* 12, no. 4 (2009): 331–335.

_____. "'I Don't Want Jenny to Think I'm Abandoning Her': Views on Overtreatment." *Health Affairs* 33, no. 5 (May 2014): 895–898.

_____. "Increased Access to Palliative Care and Hospice Services: Opportunities to Improve Value in Health Care." *Milbank Quarterly* 89, no. 3 (2011): 343–380.

Meier, Diane E., and Larry Beresford. "POLST Offers Next Stage in Honoring Patient Preferences." *Journal of Palliative Medicine* 12, no. 4 (April 2009): 291–295.

Meier, Diane E., D. J. Casarett, C. F. von Gunten, W. J. Smith, and C. P. Storey. "Palliative Medicine: Politics and Policy." *Journal of Palliative Medicine* 13, no. 2 (2010): 141–46.

Meier, Diane E., Carol-Ann Emmons, Sylvan Wallenstein, Timothy Quill, R. Sean Morrison, and Christine K. Cassell. "A National Survey of Physician-Assisted Suicide and Euthanasia in the United States." *New England Journal of Medicine* 338 (April 23, 1998): 1193–1200.

Menefee, E. E. "The Right to Live and the Right to Die." *Medical Times* 95 (November 1967): 1178–1179.

Mengert, William F. "Terminal Care." *Illinois Medical Journal* 122 (September 1957): 99–104.

Menon, Venu, Robert A. Harrington, Judith S. Hochman, Shaun D. Goodman, Holger J. Schunemann, and E. Magnus Ohman. "Thrombolysis and Adjunctive Therapy in Acute Myocardial Infarction." *Chest* 126 (September 2004, Supplement): 549S–575S.

Mermann, Alan C., Darlene B. Gunn, and George E. Dickinson. "Learning to Care for the Dying: A Survey of Medical Schools and a Model Course." *Academic Medicine* 66 (January 1991): 35–38.

Mervyn, Frances. "The Plight of Dying Patients in Hospitals." *American Journal of Nursing* 71 (October 1971): 1988–1990.

Messert, Bernard, and Charles E. Quaglieri. "Cardiopulmonary Resuscitation: Perspectives and Problems." *The Lancet* (August 21, 1976): 410–411.

Milch, Robert A. "New York's Palliative Care Information Act: Flawed But Needed." *Bioethics Forum* (June 23, 2011): 5–6.

Miles, Steven H. "Medical Futility." *Law, Medicine & Health Care* 20 (1992): 310–315.

Miller, Lois Mattox. "Neither Life nor Death." *Reader's Digest* (December 1960): 55–59.

Mireles-Cabodevila, Eduardo, Enrique Diaz-Guzman, Gustavo A. Heresi, and Robert L. Chatburn. "Alternative Modes of Mechanical Ventilation: A Review for the Hospitalist." *Cleveland Clinic Journal of Medicine* 76 (July 2009): 417–430.

Montagnini, Marcos, Basil Varkey, and Edmund Duthie, Jr. "Palliative Care Education Integrated into a Geriatrics Rotation for Resident Physicians." *Journal of Palliative Medicine* 7, no. 5 (2004): 652–653.

Mor, Vincent, and David Kidder. "Cost Savings in Hospice. Final Results of the National Hospice Study." *HSR: Health Services Research* 20 (October 1985): 407–422.

Moratti, S. "The Development of 'Medical Futility.'" *Journal of Medical Ethics* 35 (2009): 369–372.

More, Thomas. *Utopia.* Translated by Clarence H. Miller. New Haven, CT: Yale University Press, 2001.

_____. *Utopia: Latin Text and English Translation.* Edited by George M. Logan et al. Cambridge: Cambridge University Press, 1995.

Morrison, R. Sean, Jessica Dietrich, Susan Ladwig, Timothy Quill, Joseph Sacco, John Tangeman, and Diane E. Meier. "Palliative Care Consultation Teams Cut Hospital Costs for Medicaid Beneficiaries." *Health Affairs* 30 (March 2011): 454–463.

Morrison, R. Sean, and Diane E. Meyer. "Palliative Care." *New England Journal of Medicine* 350 (June 17, 2004): 2582–2590.

Morrison, R. Sean, Elizabeth Morrison, and Denise Glickman. "Physician Reluctance to Discuss Advance Directives." *Archives of Internal Medicine* 154 (October 24, 1994): 2311–2318.

Mount, Belfour M. "The Problem of Caring for

the Dying in a General Hospital: The Palliative Care Unit as a Possible Solution." *CMA Journal* 115 (June 17, 1976): 119–121.

Munk, William. *Euthanasia or, Medical Treatment in Aid of an Easy Death.* London and New York: Longmans, Green, 1887.

_____. *The Life of Sir Henry Halford.* London: Longmans, Green, 1895.

Murphy, Bradford J. "Psychological Management of the Patient with Incurable Cancer." *Geriatrics* 9 (1953): 130–134.

Murphy, Donald J., and Thomas E. Finucane. "New Do-Not-Resuscitate Policies: A First Step in Cost Control." *Archives of Internal Medicine* 153 (July 26, 1993): 1641–1648.

Mutto, Eduardo Mario, Carlos Cavazzoli, Josepmaria Argemi Ballbe, Villoradolfo Tambone, Carlos Ceneno, and Marcelo Jose Villar. "Teaching Dying Patient Care in Three Universities in Argentina, Spain, and Italy." *Journal of Palliative Medicine* 12, no. 7 (2009): 603–607.

National Consensus Project. *Clinical Practice Guidelines for Quality Palliative Care.* 2nd ed. Pittsburgh, PA: National Consensus Project for Quality Palliative Care, 2009.

National Right to Die. "Opposition to Assisting Suicide Remains AMA Policy." http://www.nrlc.org/archive/news/2003/NRL07/opposition_to_assisting_suicide_.htm (accessed August 8, 2013).

Nelson, Judith E., moderator. "Palliative Care in the ICU." *Journal of Palliative Medicine* 15, no. 2 (2012): 168–174.

Newport, Kristina Braine, Shejal Patel, Laurie Lyckholm, Barton Bobb, Patrick Coyne, and Thomas J. Smith. "The 'POLST': Providers' Signout for Scope Treatment." *Journal of Palliative Care* 13, no. 9 (2010): 1055–1058.

New York Academy of Medicine. "Joint Subcommittee on the Care of Patients with Terminal Illness." *Bulletin of the New York Academy of Medicine* 63 (May 1987): 417–422.

Nightingale, Florence. *Notes on Nursing.* New York: D. Appleton, 1860 [1859].

Noble, Hugh. *Euthanasia.* University of Edinburgh, 1854.

Novack, Dennis H., Robin Plumer, Raymond L. Smith, Herbert Ochitill, Gary R. Morrow, and John M. Bennett. "Changes in Physician's Attitudes toward Telling the Cancer Patient." *JAMA* 241 (March 2, 1979): 897–900.

Noyes, Russel, Jr., and Terry A. Travis. "The Care of Terminally Ill Patients." *Archives of Internal Medicine* 132 (October 1973): 607–611.

Nuland, Sherwin B. *How We Die.* New York: Vintage Books, 1993.

NY Health Access. "Family Health Care Decisions Act." http://www.wnylc.com/health/entry/142/ (accessed August 19, 2014).

Oken, Donald. "What to Tell Cancer Patients." *JAMA* 175 (April 1, 1961): 1120–1128.

Okon, Tomasz R. "Palliative Care Review: Spiritual, Religious, and Existential Aspects of Palliative Care." *Journal of Palliative Medicine* 8, no. 2 (2005): 392–414.

Oschner, A. J. "Hospital Growth Marks Dawn of New Era." *The Modern Hospital* 1 (September 1913): 1–5.

Osler, William. "Man's Redemption of Man." In *Osler's "A Way of Life" and Other Addresses,* 355–370. Durham, NC: Duke University Press, 2001.

_____. "Notes and Comments." *Canada Medical and Surgical Journal* 16 (March 1888): 510–511.

_____. *The Principles and Practice of Medicine.* New York: D. Appleton, 1892.

_____. "Treatment of Disease." *British Medical Journal* (July 24, 1909): 185–189.

Page, T. "Teaching the Management of Terminal Illness in Zimbabwe." *Central African Journal of Medicine* 31 (April 1985): 82–85.

"Palliative Medicine: Meeting a Critical Need." http://www.cfps.ca/archive/communic/news releases/nr05october1999.asp (accessed February 20, 2003).

Pan, Cynthia X., R. Sean Morrison, Diane E. Meier, Dana K. Natale, Suzy L. Goldhirsch, Peter Kralovec, and Christine K. Cassel. "How Prevalent Are Hospital-Based Palliative Care Programs? Status Report and Future Directions." *Journal of Palliative Medicine* 4, no. 3 (2001): 315–324.

Paradis, Lenora Finn, ed. *Hospice Handbook: A Guide for Managers and Planners.* Rockville, MD: Aspen Systems Corporation, 1985.

Parker, Richard A. "Caring for Patients at the End of Life: Reflections after 12 Years of Practice." *Annals of Internal Medicine* 136 (January 1, 2002): 72–75.

"The Patient's Philosophy, His Heart, and His Bill." *JAMA* 185 (July 13, 1963): 29–30.

Peabody, Francis Weld. "The Care of the Patient." *JAMA* 88 (1927): 877–882.

Peatfield, R. C., Deanna Taylor, R. W. Sillett, and M. W. McNicol. "Survival After Cardiac Arrest in Hospital." *The Lancet* (June 11, 1977): 1223–1225.

Penrod, Joan D. "Hospital-Based Palliative Care Consultation: Effects on Hospital Costs." *Journal of Palliative Medicine* 13, no. 8 (2010): 973–979.

Percival, Thomas. *Medical Ethics.* Manchester: S. Russell, 1803.

_____. *Medical Ethics; or, A Code of Institutes and Precepts, Adapted to the Professional Conduct of Physicians and Surgeons.* In *Percival's Medical Ethics,* edited by Chauncey D. Leake. Huntington, NY: Robert E. Krieger, 1975.

Perkins, William. *A Salve for a Sicke Man, or a Treatise Containing the Nature, Differences, and Kindes of Death: As Also the Right Manner of Dying.* In *The Workes of that Famous and*

Worthie Divine in the University of Cambridge, vol. 1, edited by J. Legatt. Cambridge: M.W. Perkins, 1608.

Petty, Thomas L. "The History of COPD." *International Journal of Chronic Obstructive Pulmonary Disease* 1 (March 2006): 3–14.

_____. "The Modern Evolution of Mechanical Ventilation." *Clinics in Chest Medicine* 9 (March 1988): 1–10.

Pew Research, Religion and Public Life Project. "Views on End-of-Life Medical Treatments." November 21, 2013. http://www.pewforum.org/2013/11/21/views-on-end-of-life-medical-treatments (accessed November 25, 2013).

Pfeiffer, Mildred C. J., and Eloise M. Lemon. "A Pilot Study of Home Care of Terminal Cancer Patients." *American Journal of Public Health* 43 (1953): 909–914.

Philip, A. P. W. *An Inquiry into the Nature of Sleep and Death*. London: Henry Renshaw, 1834.

"Physician and Patient, Personal Care." *American Journal of Nursing* 29 (June 1929): 756.

Podell, Lynn B. "Medicare Coverage of Hospice Care." *American Journal of Hospital Pharmacy* 41 (May 1984): 942–944.

"POLST Program Requirements." http://www.ohsu.edu/polst/developing/core-requirements.htm (accessed December 13, 2012).

"Pope Pius XII: The Prolongation of Life." In *Ethics in Medicine: Historical Perspectives and Contemporary Concerns*, edited by Stanley Joel Reiser, Arthur J. Dyck, and William J. Curran, 501–504. Cambridge, MA: MIT Press, 1977.

"Porter Storey, MD." http://www.reachmd.com/xmradioguest.aspx?pid-70632 (accessed September 29, 2011).

Prendergast, Thomas J., and John M. Luce. "Increasing Incidence of Withholding and Withdrawal of Life Support from the Critically Ill." *American Journal of Respiratory and Critical Care Medicine* 155 (1997): 15–20.

President's Commission for the Study of Ethical Problems in Medicine and Biomedical and Behavioral Research. *Deciding to Forego Life-Sustaining Treatment*. Honolulu, HI: University Press of the Pacific, 2006 [1983].

Prince-Paul, Maryjo. "Understanding the Meaning of Social Well-Being at the End of Life." *Oncology Nursing Forum* 35, no. 3 (2008): 365–371.

Provonsha, Jack W. "The Prolongation of Life." *Bulletin of the American Protestant Hospital Association* 35 (Spring 1971): 14–16.

Puchalski, Christina. "Spirituality in Health: The Role of Spirituality in Critical Care." *Critical Care Clinics* 20 (2004): 487–504.

Puchalski, Christina, B. Ferrell, R. Virani, S. Otis-Green, P. Baird, J. Bull, H. Chochinov, G. Handzo, H. Nelson-Becker, M. Prince-Paul, K. Pugliese, and D. Sulmasy. "Improving the Quality of Spiritual Care as a Dimension of Palliative Care: The Report of the Consensus Conference." *Journal of Palliative Medicine* 12, no. 19 (2009): 885–904.

Pullman, Daryl. "Death, Dignity, and Moral Nonsense." *Journal of Palliative Care* 20, no. 3 (2004): 171–178.

Puri, Nitin, Vinod Puri, and R. P. Dellinger. "History of Technology in the Intensive Care Unit." *Critical Care Clinics* 25 (2009): 185–200.

Quill, Timothy E. "Death with Dignity: A Case of Individualized Decision Making." *New England Journal of Medicine* 324 (March 7, 1991): 691–694.

_____. "Initiating End-of-Life Discussions with Seriously Ill Patients: Addressing the 'Elephant in the Room.'" *JAMA* 284 (November 15, 2000): 2502–2507.

_____. *A Midwife Through the Dying Process*. Baltimore: Johns Hopkins University Press, 1996.

Quill, Timothy E., et al. *Primer of Palliative Care*. 5th ed. Glenview, IL: American Academy of Hospice and Palliative Medicine, 2010.

Quill, Timothy E., and J. Andrews Billings. "Palliative Care Textbooks Come of Age." *Annals of Internal Medicine* 129 (October 1998): 590–594.

Quill, Timothy E., and Howard Brody. "Physician Recommendations and Patient Autonomy: Finding a Balance between Physician Power and Patient Choices." *Annals of Internal Medicine* 125 (November 1, 1996): 763–769.

Quill, Timothy, and Christine K. Cassel. "Professional Organizations' Position Statements on Physician-Assisted Suicide: A Case for Studied Neutrality." *Annals of Internal Medicine* 138 (February 4, 2003): 208–212.

Quill, Timothy E., Christine K. Cassel, and Diane E. Meier. "Care of the Hopelessly Ill: Proposed Clinical Criteria for Physician-Assisted Suicide." *New England Journal of Medicine* 327 (November 5, 1992): 1380–1384.

Quint, Jeanne C., Anselm L. Strauss, and Barney G. Glaser. "Improving Nursing Care of the Dying." *Nursing Forum* 6 (1967): 369–378.

Rabow, Michael W., Stephen J. McPhee, Joan M. Fair, and Grace E. Hardie. "A Failing Grade for End-of-Life Content in Textbooks: What Is to Be Done?" *Journal of Palliative Medicine* 2, no. 2 (1999): 153–155.

Raghavan, Mythili, Alexander K. Smith, and Robert M. Arnold. "African Americans and End-of-Life Care." *Journal of Palliative Medicine* 13, no. 9 (2008): 1384–1385.

Raich, Peter C., Richard John C. Pearson, and Richard M. Iammarino. "Hospices Are Developing in West Virginia: What Physicians Need to Know." *West Virginia Medical Journal* 79 (June 1983): 116–119.

Ramsey, Paul. *The Patient as Person: Explorations in Medical Ethics*. 2nd edition. New Haven, CT: Yale University Press, 2002.

Randall, Fiona, and R. S. Downie. *Palliative Care Ethics*. Oxford: Oxford University Press, 1999.

Ranney, George E. "Death, a Universal Law." *Transactions of the Michigan State Medical Society* 16 (1982): 9–29.

Raphael, Carol, Joann Ahrens, and Nicole Fowler. "Financing End-of-Life Care in the USA." *Journal of the Royal Society of Medicine* 94 (September 2001): 458–461.

Ravitch, Mark M. "Let Your Patient Die with Dignity." *Medical Times* 93 (June 1965): 594–595.

Reilly, Thomas F. "Signs and Symptoms of Impending Death." *JAMA* 66 (January 18, 1916): 160–164.

Review: Medical Ethics. "*Physician and Patient*, by Worthington Hooker." *American Journal of Medical Sciences* 23 (January 1852): 149–177.

Reviews. "*Principia Therapeutica*, by Harrington Sainsbury." *Journal of Mental Sciences* 52 (1906): 788–789.

Reviews and Notices of Books. "*Euthanasia, or Medical Treatment in Aid of an Easy Death*, by William Munk, M.D." *The Lancet* 7 (January 7, 1888): 21–22.

Rhymes, Jill. "Hospice Care in America." *JAMA* 264 (July 18, 1990): 369–372.

Rich, Ben A. "Legislating Patient-Care Protocols." UC Davis Health System, 2009. http://www.ucdmc.ucdavis.edu/welcome/features/20090513_Medicine_Rich/index.html (accessed August 20, 2012).

Richardson, B. W., MD. "Natural Euthanasia." *Popular Science Monthly* 13 (1875): 612–620.

Rickles, Frederick R. "Thrombolytic (Fibrinolytic) Drugs and Progress in Treating Cardiovascular Disease." *FASEB Journal* 19, no. 6 (2005). http://www.fasej.org/content/19/6/671.full (accessed November 1, 2012).

Rinaldo, Matthew J. "Medicare to Cover Hospice Services." *Journal of the Medical Society of New Jersey* 79 (December 1982): 1015–1016.

Ritchie, Christine S., Lyn Ceronsky, Todd R. Cote, Sharol Herr, Steven Z. Pantilat, Thomas J. Smith, and Lori Yosick. "Palliative Care Programs: The Challenges of Growth." *Journal of Palliative Medicine* 13, no. 9 (2010): 1065–1070.

Rivkin, David B., Jr., and Elizabeth Price Foley. "'Death Panels' Come Back to Life." *Wall Street Journal*, December 30, 2001, A15.

Roberts, Thomas G., Bernardo H. Goulart, Lee Squitieri, Sarah C. Stallings, Elkan F. Halpern, Bruce A. Chabner, G. Scott Gazelle, Stan N. Finkelstein, and Jeffrey W. Clark. "Trends in the Risks and Benefits of Patients with Cancer Participating in Phase 1 Cancer Trials." *JAMA* 292 (November 3, 2004): 2130–2140.

Robinson, Katya, Sharyn Sutton, Charles F. Von Guten, Frank D. Ferris, Nicholas Molodyko, Jeanne Martinez, and Linda L. Emanuel. "Assessment of the Education for Physicians on End-of-Life Care (EPEC) Project." *Journal of Palliative Medicine* 7, no. 5 (2004): 637–645.

Robynson, Ralphe. *More's Utopia*. Edited with introduction by J. Rawson Lumby. Cambridge: Cambridge University Press, 1892.

Rocket, Barbara. "Physician-Assisted Suicide in Direct Conflict with Doctor's Role." *White Coat Notes*, July 31, 2012. http://www.boston.com/whitecoatnotes/2012–07/31/barbara-rockett-physician-assisted-suicide (accessed August 8, 2013).

Rosenberg, Andrew L., and Ravi S. Tripathi. "Perioperative Management for Patients Receiving Ventricular Assist Devices and Mechanical Circulatory Support: A Systems-Oriented Approach." *Contemporary Critical Care* 7, no. 12 (May 2010): 1–12.

Ross, Douglas, Heather C. Fraser, and Jean S. Kutner. "Institutionalization of a Palliative and End-of-Life Care Educational Program in a Medical School Curriculum." *Journal of Palliative Medicine* 4, no. 4 (2001): 512–518.

Rousseau, Paul. "The Ethical Validity and Clinical Experience of Palliative Sedation." *Mayo Clinic Proceedings* 75 (October 2000): 1064–1069.

Rubenfield, Gordon D. "Principles and Practice of Withdrawing Life-Sustaining Treatments." *Critical Care Clinics* 20 (2004): 435–451.

Rubsamen, David S. "Doctor and the Law: What Every Doctor Needs to Know about Changes in 'Informed Consent.'" *Medical World News* 14 (February 9, 1973): 66–67.

Rudd, T. N. "Family Doctor at the Death-Bed." *Medical World* 85 (July 1956): 50–52.

Ruff, R. "Have We the Right to Prolong Dying?" *Medical Economics* 37 (1960): 39–44.

Rush, Benjamin. *The Selected Writings of Benjamin Rush*. Edited by Gagobert D. Runes. New York: Philosophical Library, 1947.

Rutledge, Thomas A. "Informed Consent for the Terminal Patient." *Baylor Law Review* 27 (1975): 111–121.

Ryder, Claire F., and Diane M. Ross. "Terminal Care—Issues and Alternatives." *Public Health Reports* 92 (January–February 1977): 20–29.

Rynearson, Edward H. "You Are Standing at the Bedside of a Patient Dying of Untreatable Cancer." *CA: A Cancer Journal for Clinicians* 9 (1958): 85–87.

Sachdeva, Ramesh C., and Kalpalatha K. Guntupalli. "Acute Respiratory Distress Syndrome." *Critical Care Clinics* 13 (July 1997): 502–521.

Sadick, Barbara. "What Is Palliative Care? And Why Is It So Rare?" *Wall Street Journal*, September 15, 2014, R2.

Safar, Peter, ed. *Advances in Cardiopulmonary Resuscitation*. New York: Springer-Verlag, 1975.

_____. "History of Cardiopulmonary-Cerebral Resuscitation." In *Cardiopulmonary Resuscitation*, edited by William Kaye and Nicholas G Bircher, 1–53. New York: Churchill Livingstone, 1989.

_____. "On the History of Modern Resuscitation." *Critical Care Medicine* 24 (Supplement, February 1996): 35–115.

Sainsbury, Harrison. *Principia Theapeutica.* London: Methuen, 1906.

St. Christopher's Hospice: Annual Report, 1976–1977 (December 1977): 2–73.

Saraiya, Biren. "Oncologists and End-of-Life Care: Letter to the Editor." *Journal of Palliative Medicine* 12, no. 2 (2009): 116.

Saunders, Cicely. *Cicely Saunders: Selected Writings.* Edited with introduction by David Clark. Oxford: Oxford University Press, 2006.

_____. "Dimensions of Death." In *Religion and Medicine,* edited by M. A. H. Melinsky, 113–116. London: SCM Press, 1975.

_____. "Evaluation of Hospice Activities." *Journal of Chronic Diseases* 37 (1984): 871.

_____. "The Last Stages of Life." *American Journal of Nursing* 65 (March 1956): 70–75.

_____. "On Dying Well." *Cambridge Review* (February 27, 1984): 49–52.

_____. "A Place to Die." *Crux* 11 (1973–1974): 24–27.

_____. "St. Christopher's Hospice." *British Hospital Journal and Social Service Review* 77 (November 10, 1967): 2127–2130.

_____. "Working at St. Joseph's Hospice in Hackney." *Annual Report of St. Vincent's Dublin* (1962): 37.

Schiessl, Christine, Maria Walshe, Svenja Wildfeuer, Philip Larkin, Raymond Voltz, and Jana Juenger. "Undergraduate Curricula in Palliative Medicine: A Systematic Analysis Based on the Palliative Education Assessment Tool." *Journal of Palliative Medicine* 16, no. 1 (2013): 20–30.

Schnaper, Nathan. "Death and Dying: Has the Topic Been Beaten to Death?" *Journal of Nervous and Mental Disease* 160 (March 1975): 157–158.

Schnaper, Nathan, and Peter H. Wiernick. "The Hospice: New Wine in Old Bottles?" *Maryland State Medical Journal* 32 (1983): 102–104.

Schneiderman, Lawrence J., Nancy S. Jecker, and Albert R. Jonsen. "Medical Futility: Its Meaning and Ethical Implication." *Annals of Internal Medicine* 112 (June 15, 1990): 949–954.

Schonwetter, Ronald. "Hospice and Palliative Medicine Goes Mainstream." *Journal of Palliative Medicine* 9, no. 8 (2006): 1240–1242.

Schulz, Richard, and David Aderman. "Clinical Research and the Stages of Dying." *Omega* 5 (Summer 1974): 137–143.

Schwartz, Robert. "End-of-Life Care: Doctors' Complaints and Legal Restraints." *Saint Louis University Law Journal* 53 (2009): 1169–1170.

Sepulveda, Cecilia, Amanda Martin, Tokuo Yoshida, and Andreas Ullrich. "Palliative Care: The World Health Organization's Global Perspective." *Journal of Pain and Symptom Management* 24 (August 2002): 91–95.

Shalowitz, David I., Elizabeth Garrett-Mayer, and David Wendler. "The Accuracy of Surrogate Decision Makers: A Systematic Review." *Archives of Internal Medicine* 166 (March 13, 2006): 493–497.

Sheehan, Miles H. "On Dying Well." *America: The National Catholic Weekly,* July 29, 2000. 1–4.

Shindell, S. "Editorials: Home Medical Care—A Pilot Study." *Medical Annals of the District of Columbia* 19 (1950): 89–90.

Sibbald, W. J., and T. Singh. "Critical Care in Canada: The North American Difference." *Critical Care Clinics* 13 (April 1997): 347–362.

Sigwart, Ulrich, Jacques Puel, Velimir Mirkovitch, Francis Joffre, and Lucas Kappenberger. "Intravascular Stents to Prevent Occlusion and Restenosis after Transluminal Angioplasty." *New England Journal of Medicine* 316 (March 19, 1987): 701–706.

Simonaitis, Joseph E. "Law and Medicine: More About Informed Consent." *JAMA* 224 (June 25, 1973): 1831–1832.

Skolnick, Andrew A. "End-of-Life Care Movement Growing." *JAMA* 278 (September 24, 1997): 967–969.

Smith, Anthony M. "Palliative Care Services in Britain and Ireland 1990—An Overview." *Palliative Medicine* 6 (1992): 277–291.

Smith, H. Shelton, Robert T. Handy, and Lefferts A. Loetscher. *American Christianity: An Historical Interpretation with Representative Documents.* Vol. 1. New York: Scribner's, 1960.

Smith, Richard. "A Good Death: An Important Aim for Health Services and for Us All." *British Medical Journal* 320 (January 14, 2000): 129–130.

Smith, Thomas J., and Lowell J. Schnipper. "The American Society of Clinical Oncology Program to Improve End-of-Life Care." *Journal of Palliative Medicine* 1, no. 2 (1998): 221–230.

Spaeth, George L. "Letters: Telling the Cancer Patient." *JAMA* 242 (October 26, 1979): 1847–1848.

Speeding, James, Robert Leslie Ellis, and Douglas Denon Heath. *The Works of Francis Bacon.* Volume IX. Boston: Taggard and Thompson, 1864.

Spettell, Claire M., Wayne S. Rawlins, Randall Krakauer, Joaquim Fernandes, Mary E. S. Breton, Wayne Gowdy, Sharon Brodeur, Maureen MacCoy, and Troyen A. Brennan. "A Comprehensive Case Management Program to Improve Palliative Care." *Journal of Palliative Medicine* 12, no. 9 (2009): 827–832.

State of New York Department of Health. "Palliative Care Access Act (PHS Section 2997-d): Palliative Care Requirements for Hospitals, Nursing Homes, Home Care and Assisted Living Residences (Enhanced and Special Needs)." http://www.ny.gov/professionals/patient_rights/palliative_care (accessed August 12, 2012).

_____. "Palliative Care Access Act—Dear CEO/

Administrator Letter, Questions and Answers for Providers." http://www.ny.gov/professionals/patient_rights/palliative_care (accessed August 12, 2012).

_____. "Palliative Care Information Act—Letter to Physicians, Summary of the Law, Questions and Answers, and Laws of New York Chapter 331." http://www.capc.org/research-and-refer ences-for-palliative-care/additional-resources/new-york-state-department-of-health-pallia tive-care-information-act.pdf (accessed August 7, 2012).

Steinhauser, Karen E., C. I. Voils, E. C. Clipp, H. B. Bosworth, N. A. Christakis, and J. A. Tulsky. "'Are You At Peace?' One Item to Probe Spiritual Concerns at the End of Life." *Archives of Internal Medicine* 166 (January 9, 2006): 101–105.

Steinhauser, Karen E., E. C. Clipp, M. McNeilly, N. A. Christakis, L. M. McIntyre, and J. A. Tulsky. "In Search of a Good Death: Observations of Patients, Families, and Providers." *Annals of Internal Medicine* 132 (May 16, 2000): 825–832.

Stevenson, David G. "Growing Pains for the Medicare Hospital Benefit." *New England Journal of Medicine* 367 (November 1, 2012): 1683–1685.

"Steve's *Strategic* Guide to Phase 1 Cancer Clinical Trials." http://canceerguide.org/trials_phase1.html (accessed September 27, 2012).

Stoddard, Sandol. "Hospice in the United States: An Overview." *Journal of Palliative Care* 5 (1989): 10–19.

Storey, Porter. "Goals of Hospice Care." *Texas Medicine* 86 (February 1990): 50–54.

_____. "Hospice and Palliative Medicine (HPM)." *Academic Medicine* 87 (September 2012): 1305.

Strauss, Anselm L. "Reforms Needed in Providing Terminal Care in Hospitals." *Archives of the Foundation of Thanatology* 1 (1969): 21–22.

Strauss, Anselm L., Barney Glaser, and Jeanne Quint. "The Nonaccountability of Terminal Care." *Hospitals, J.A.H.A.* 38 (January 16, 1964): 73–87.

Suetonius. *Suetonius in Two Volumes.* Translated by J.C. Rolfe. Cambridge, MA: Harvard University Press, 1944.

Sullivan, Mark D. "The Illusion of Patient Choice in End-of-Life Decisions." *American Journal of Geriatric Psychiatry* 10 (July–August 2002): 365–372.

The SUPPORT Principle Investigators. "A Controlled Trial to Improve Care for Seriously Ill Hospitalized Patients: The Study to Understand Prognoses and Preferences for Outcomes and Risks of Treatments (SUPPORT)." *Journal of the American Medical Association* 274 (November 22/29, 1995): 1591–1598.

Symmers, W. S. "Not Allowed to Die." *British Medical Journal* 1 (February 1968): 442.

"Symposium on Terminal Care." *CA: A Cancer Journal for Clinicians* 10 (1960): 12–24.

Szalados, James E. "Discontinuation of Mechanical Ventilation at End-of-Life: The Ethical and Legal Boundaries of Physician Conduct in Termination of Life Support." *Critical Care Clinics* 23 (2007): 317–337.

Taffet, George E., Thomas A. Teasdale, and Robert Luchi. "In-Hospital Cardiopulmonary Resuscitation." *JAMA* 260 (October 14, 1988): 2069–2072.

Temel, Jennifer S., Joseph A. Greer, Alona Muzikansky, Emily R. Gallagher, Sonal Admane, Vicki A. Jackson, Constance M. Dahlin, Craig D. Blinderman, Juliet Jacobsen, William F. Pirl, J. Andrew Billings, and Thomas J. Lynch. "Early Palliative Care for Patients with Metastatic Non-Small-Cell Lung Cancer." *New England Journal of Medicine* 363 (August 19, 2010): 733–742.

Teno, Joan M., and Stephen R. Connor. "Referring a Patient and Family to High-Quality Palliative Care at the Close of Life." *JAMA* 301 (February 11, 2009): 651–659.

Thalhuber, Wayne H. "Overcoming Physician Barriers to Hospice Care." *Minnesota Medicine* 78 (February 1995): 18–22.

Tolle, Susan W., Virginia P. Tilden, Christine A. Nelson, and Patrick M. Dunn. "A Prospective Study of the Efficacy of the Physician Order Form for Life-Sustaining Treatment." *Journal of the American Geriatrics Society* 46 (September 1998): 1097–1102.

Tomlinson, Tom, and Howard Brody. "Futility and the Ethics of Resuscitation." *JAMA* 264 (September 12, 1990): 1276–1280.

Tong, Elizabeth, Susan A. McGraw, Edward Dobihal, Rosemary Baggish, Emily Cherlin, and Elizabeth H. Bradley. "What Is a Good Death? Minority and Non-minority Perspectives." *Journal of Palliative Care* 13 (Autumn 2003): 168–175.

Tong, Rosemarie. "Towards a Just, Courageous, and Honest Resolution of the Futility Debate." *Journal of Medicine and Philosophy* 20 (1955): 165–189.

Torrens, Paul R. "Hospice Care: What Have We Learned?" *American Review of Public Health* 5 (1985): 65–83.

Towns, Kathryn, Elizabeth Dougherty, Nanor Kevork, David Wiljer, Dori Seccareccia, Gary Rodin, Lisa W. Le, and Camilla Zimmermann. "Availability of Services in Ontario Hospices and Hospitals Providing Inpatient Palliative Care." *Journal of Palliative Medicine* 15, no. 5 (2012): 527–534.

Truog, Robert D. "The Problem with Futility." *New England Journal of Medicine* 326 (June 4, 1992): 1560–1563.

Tucker, Kathryn L. "Ensuring Informed End-of-Life Decisions." *Journal of Palliative Medicine* 12, no. 2 (2009): 119–120.

Tulsky, James A., Margaret A. Chesney, and Bernard Lo. "How Do Medical Residents Discuss Resuscitation with Patients?" *Journal of General Internal Medicine* 10 (1995): 436–442.

VanAalst-Cohen, Emily S., Raine Riggs, Ira R. Byock. "Palliative Care in Medical School Curricula: A Survey of United States Medical Schools." *Journal of Palliative Medicine* 11, no. 9 (2008): 1200–1202.

Vanderpool, Harold Y. "Caring for People with Cancer." *Philosophical Society of Texas Proceedings* 55 (1992): 85–92.

_____. "Changing Concepts of Disease and the Shaping of Contemporary Preventative Medicine." In *Preventative Medicine and Community Health*, edited by Anne W. Domeck, 7–34. Galveston: University of Texas Medical Branch, 1982.

_____. "Doctors and the Dying of Patients in American History." In *Physician-Assisted Suicide*, edited by Robert F. Weir, 33–66. Bloomington: Indiana University Press, 1997.

_____. "End-of-Life Talk Not Same as 'Death Panel.'" *Galveston News*, January 18, 2011, B3.

_____. "The Ethics of Clinical Experimentation with Anticancer Drugs." In *Cancer Treatment and Research in Humanistic Perspective*, edited by Steven C. Gross and Soloman Garb, 16–46. New York: Springer, 1985.

_____. "The Ethics of Terminal Care." *JAMA* 239 (February 27, 1978): 850–852.

_____. "Introduction and Overview: Ethics, Historical Case Studies, and the Research Enterprise." In *The Ethics of Research Involving Human Subjects*, 1–30. Frederick, MD: University Publishing Group, 1996.

_____. "Life-Sustaining Treatment and Euthanasia: II. Historical Aspects of." In *Encyclopedia of Bioethics*, vol. 4, 4th ed., edited by Bruce Jennings, 1849–1863. Farmington Hills, MI: Macmillan Reference USA, 2014.

_____. "The Religious Features of Scientific Medicine." *Kennedy Institute of Ethics Journal* 18 (2008): 203–234.

_____. "The Responsibilities of Physicians toward Dying Patients." In *Medical Complications in Cancer Patients*, edited by J. Klastersky and M. J. Staquet, 117–133. New York: Raven Press, 1981.

Veatch, Robert M. "The Birth of Bioethics: Autobiographical Reflections of a Patient Person." *Cambridge Quarterly of Healthcare Ethics* 11, no. 4 (2002): 344–352.

_____. "Choosing Not to Prolong Dying." *Medical Dimensions Magazine* (December 1972: 8–10 and 40.

_____. "Death and Dying: The Legislative Options." *Medical Communications* 6 (Winter 1977/Spring 1978): 23–29.

_____. *Death, Dying, and the Biological Revolution.* New Haven, CT: Yale University Press, 1976.

_____. *Disrupted Dialogue.* Oxford: Oxford University Press, 2005.

Wagner, Bernice M. "Teaching Students to Work with the Dying." *American Journal of Nursing* 64 (November 1964): 128–131.

Walling, Anne M., Steven M. Asch, Karl A. Lorenz, Carol P. Roth, Tod Barry, Katherine L. Kahn, and Neil S. Wenger. "The Quality of Care Provided to Hospitalized Patients at the End of Life." *Archives of Internal Medicine* 170 (June 28, 2010): 1057–1063.

Wanzer, Sidney H., Daniel D. Federman, S. James Adelstein, Christine K. Cassel, Edwin H. Cassem, Ronald E. Cranford, Edward W. Hook, Bernard Lo, Charles G. Moertel, Peter Safar, Alan Stone, and Jan Van Eys. "The Physician's Responsibility toward Hopelessly Ill Patients: A Second Look." *New England Journal of Medicine* 320 (March 30, 1989): 844–849.

Wanzer, Sidney, and Joseph Genmullen. *To Die Well.* Philadelphia, PA: Da Capo Press, 2008.

"A Way of Dying." *Atlantic Monthly* (January 1957): 53–55.

Weissman, David E. "End-of-Life Physician Education: Is Change Possible?" *Journal of Palliative Care* 1 (1998): 401–407.

_____. "The Growth of Hospital-Based Palliative Care." *Journal of Palliative Medicine* 4, no. 3 (2001): 307–308.

_____. "A New Journal." *Journal of Palliative Medicine* 1, no. 1 (1998): 1–2.

_____. "Next Gen Palliative Care." *Journal of Palliative Medicine* 15, no. 1 (2012): 2–4.

_____. "Talking about Dying: A Clash of Cultures." *Journal of Palliative Medicine* 3, no. 2 (2000): 134–147.

Werner, Paul T. "Hospice Care—An Alternative." *Journal of the Medical Association of Georgia* 71 (1982): 693–694.

"What Others Say in Opposition to Dr. Ruff." *Medical Economics* 37 (1960): 40.

"When Do We Let the Patient Die?" *Annals of Internal Medicine* 68 (March 1968): 695–700.

White, Kenneth R., Patrick J. Coyne, and Urvashi B. Patel. "Are Nurses Adequately Prepared for End-of-Life Care?" *Journal of Nursing Scholarship* 33 (Second Quarter 2001): 147–151.

Williams, C. J. B. "On the Success and Failures of Medicine." *The Lancet* 5 (April 5, 1862): 345–347.

Williams, Charles B. "Euthanasia." *Medical and Surgical Reporter* 70 (June 30, 1894): 909–911.

Williams, S. D. "Euthanasia." In *Essays by Members of the Birmingham Speculative Club*, 210–237. London: Williams and Norgate, 1870.

Williams, Sharon W., Larua C. Hanson, Carlton Boyd, Melissa Green, Moses Goldman, Gratia Wright, and Giselle Corbie-Smith. "Communication, Decision Making, and Cancer: What African Americans Want Physicians to Know." *Journal of Palliative Medicine* 11, no. 9 (2008): 1211–1226.

Willison, John. *The Afflicted Man's Companion.* New York: J. C. Totten, 1806.

Wilson, Dottie, Ina Ajemian, and Balfour Mount. "Montreal (1975)—The Royal Victoria Hospital Palliative Care Service." In *The Hospice: Development and Administration*, edited by Glen W. Davidson, 3–19. Washington: Hemisphere Publishing Corporation, 1978.

Worcester, Alfred. *The Care of the Aged, the Dying, and the Dead.* Springfield, IL: Charles C. Thomas, 1935.

_____. "The Care of the Dying." In *Physician and Patient*, edited by L. Eugene Emerson, 200–224. Cambridge, MA: Harvard University Press, 1929.

_____. "Past and Present Methods in the Practice of medicine." *Boston Medical and Surgical Journal* 166 (February 1, 1912): 159–164.

_____. "A Word with the Authors: Primer Tracks Growth in the Field." http://aahpm.org/apps/blog/?tag=primer (accessed September 29, 2011).

"Working with Families." http://www.caresearch.com.au/caresearch/tabid/1445/Default.aspx (accessed January 11, 2013).

World Health Organization. *National Cancer Control Programmes.* Geneva, Switzerland: World Health Organization, 2002.

Wright, Alexi A., and Ingrid T. Katz. "Letting Go of the Rope—Aggressive Treatment, Hospice Care and Open Access." *New England Journal of Medicine* 357 (July 26, 2007): 324–327.

Wright, Michael, Justin Wood, Thomas Lynch, and David Clark. "Mapping Levels of Palliative Care Development: A Global View." *Journal of Pain Symptom Management* 35, no. 5 (May 2008): 469–485.

Yale New Haven Hospital: Committee on Policy for DNR Decisions. "Report on Do Not Resuscitate Decisions." *Connecticut Medicine* 47 (August 1983): 477–483.

Young, J. D., and M. K. Sykes. "Artificial Ventilation: History, Equipment, and Techniques." *Thorax* 14 (1990): 753–758.

Yuen, Jacqueline K., M. Carrington Reid, and Michael D. Fetters. "Hospital Do-Not-Resuscitate Orders: Why They Have Failed and How to Fix Them." *Journal of General Internal Medicine* 26, no. 7 (2011): 791–797.

Zafar, S. Yousuf, Jennifer L. Malin, Steen C. Grambow, David H. Abbott, Jane T. Kolimaga, Leah L. Zullig, Jane C. Weeks, John Z. Ayanian, Katherine L. Kahn, Patricia A. Ganz, Paul J. Catalano, Dee W. West, and Dawn Provenzale. "Chemotherapy Use and Patient Treatment Preferences in Advanced Colorectal Cancer." *Cancer* (September 12, 2012): 1–28. http://onlinelibrary.wiley.com.libux.utmb.edu/doi/10.1002/cncr.27815/full (accessed September 12, 2012).

Secondary Sources

Abel, Emily K. *The Inevitable Hour: A History of Caring for Dying Patients in America.* Baltimore: Johns Hopkins University Press, 2013.

Abt, I. A. "Christopher Wilhelm Hufeland." *Annals of Medical History* (1931): 27–38.

Ackerknecht, Erwin H. *Therapeutics from the Primitives to the 20th Century.* New York: Hafner Press, 1973.

Albury, W. R. "Ideas of Life and Death." In *Companion Encyclopedia of the History of Medicine*, vol. 1, edited by W. F. Bynum and Roy Porter, 249–280. New York: Routledge, 1993.

Andrews, Corey E. "'Ev'ry Heart Can Feel': Scottish Poetic Responses to Slavery in the West Indies, from Blair to Burns." *International Journal of Scottish Literature* 4 (Spring/Summer 2008).

Androutsos, G.M., M. Karamanou, and A. Kostakis. "Baron Gullaume Dupuytren (1777–1835): One of the Most Outstanding Surgeons of the 19th Century." *Hellenic Journal of Surgery* 83 (2011): 239–243.

"Assisted Suicide Legalization Supported by Half of Americans, Poll Says." *Huffington Post.* http://www.huffingtonpost.com/2013/05/22/assisted-suicide-legalization_n_3314849.html (accessed August 23, 2013).

Atkinson, David W. "The English Ars Morendi: Its Protestant Transformation." *Renaissance and Reformation* XVIII (1982): 1–10.

Bains, Jatinder. "From Reviving the Living to Raising the Dead: The Making of Cardiac Resuscitation." *Social Science of Medicine* 47, no. 9 (1998): 1341–1349.

Baker, Robert, and Laurence McCullough. "Medical Ethics' Appropriation of Moral Philosophy: The Case of the Sympathetic and Unsympathetic Physician." *Kennedy Institute of Ethics Journal* 17, no. 1 (2007): 3–22.

Baylon, Jacquelyn. "State Laws Giving Terminally Ill Patients a Right to Know about End-of-Life Options." May 18, 2011. http://thepinkfund.org/2011/05/18/state-laws-giving-terminally-ill-patients-a-right-to-know-about-end-of-life-options/ (accessed August 17, 2012).

Beaty, Nancy Lee. *The Craft of Dying: A Study of the Literary Tradition of the "Ars Moriendi" in England.* New Haven, CT: Yale University Press, 1970.

Beauchamp, Tom L. "Worthington Hooker on Ethics in Clinical Medicine." In *The Codification of Medical Morality*, vol. 2, edited by Robert Baker, 105–119. Dordrecht: Kluwer Academic Publishers, 1995.

Beauchamp, Tom L., and James F. Childress. *Principles of Biomedical Ethics.* New York: Oxford University Press, 1976.

_____. *Principles of Biomedical Ethics.* 4th edition. New York: Oxford University Press, 1994.

_____. *Principles of Biomedical Ethics*. 6th edition. New York: Oxford University Press, 2009.

Becker, Ernest. *The Denial of Death*. New York: Free Press, 1973.

Bennett, P.N. "Alexander Gordon (1752–99) and His Writing: Insights into Medical Thinking in the Late Eighteenth Century." *Journal of the Royal College of Physicians of Edinburgh* 42 (2012): 165–171.

Berman, Alex. "The Heroic Approach in 19th-Century Therapeutics." In *Sickness and Health in America*, edited by Judith Walzer Leavitt and Ronald L. Numbers, 81–83. Madison: University of Wisconsin Press, 1978.

Bliss, Michael. "Cushing, James Harvey." In *Dictionary of Medical Biography*, edited by W. F. Bynum and Helen Bynum, 388–392. Westport, CT: Greenwood Press, 2007.

Bordley, James, III, and A. McGehee Harvey. *Two Centuries of American Medicine*. Philadelphia: W. B. Saunders, 1976.

Brandt, Allan M. "Bioethics: Then and Now." *Lahey Clinic Medical Ethics* (Spring 2000). http://www.bucklin.org/bioethics-history.html (accessed July 18, 2013).

Broman, Thomas H. *The Transformation of German Academic Medicine, 1750–1820*. Cambridge and New York: Cambridge University Press, 1996.

Bryant, E. E. *The Reign of Antoninus Pius*. Cambridge: Cambridge University Press, 1895.

Campbell, Debra. "Catholicism from Independence to World War I." In *Encyclopedia of the American Religious Experience*, vol. 1, edited by Charles H. Lippy and Peter W. Williams, 357–374. New York: Scribner's, 1988.

Campbell, Larna Jane. "Principle and Practice: An Analysis of Nineteenth and Twentieth Century Euthanasia Debates." PhD dissertation, University of Edinburgh, 2003.

Carlin, David. "Sir Thomas Browne's *Religio Medici* and the Publishing House of Ticknor and Fields." *Osler Library Newsletter*, no. 89 (October 1998): 1–4.

Choron, Jacques. *Death and Western Thought*. New York: Collier Books, 1963.

_____. *Death and the Modern Man*. New York: Collier Books, 1964.

Clark, David. "From Margins to Centre: A Review of the History of Palliative Care in Cancer." *Lancet Oncology* 8 (May 2007): 430–438.

_____. "The International Observatory on End of Life Care: A New Initiative to Support Palliative Care Development Around the World." *Journal of Pain and Palliative Care Pharmacotherapy* 17, no. 3/4 (2003): 231–238.

_____. "Introduction" to *Cicely Saunders: Selected Writings*, edited with introduction by David Clark. Oxford: Oxford University Press, 2006.

Clark, David, and Carlos Centeno. "Palliative Care in Europe: An Emerging Approach to Compar-ative Analysis." *Clinical Medicine* 6 (March/April 2006): 197–201.

Clymer, Meredith. *Dr. Benjamin Rush: The Annual Oration*. Philadelphia: Collins Printer, 1876.

Cohen, Bernard. "Florence Nightingale." *Scientific American* 250 (March 1984): 128–137.

Colliver, Victoria. "Palliative Therapy Teams Co-ordinate Care." *SFGate*, July 5, 2013. http://www.sfgate.com/health/article/Palliative-thera py-teams-coordinate-care-4349697.php (accessed July 5, 2013).

Cox, Lauren. "The Top 10 Medical Advances of the Decade." ABC News Unit, December 17, 2009. http://www.medpagetoday.com/Intecti ousDisease/PublicHealth/17594 (accessed November 1, 2012).

Coyle, Nessa. "Introduction of Palliative Nursing Care." In *Oxford Textbook of Palliative Nursing*, 3rd ed., edited by Betty R. Ferrell and Nessa Coyle, 3. Oxford: Oxford University Press, 2010.

Crellin, John. "Theophile Bonet (1620–1689)." *American Journal of Pathology* 98 (January 1980): 212.

Crenner, Christopher. *Private Practice*. Baltimore: Johns Hopkins University Press, 2005.

Cromwell, Judith Lissauer. *Florence Nightingale, Feminist*. Jefferson, NC, and London: McFarland, 2013.

Dowbiggin, Ian. *A Concise History of Euthanasia: Life, Death, God, and Medicine*. New York: Rowman & Littlefield, 2005.

Duffy, John. *The Healers*. New York: McGraw-Hill, 1976.

"E. H. Rynearson of Mayo Clinic." *New York Times*, February 20, 1987. http://nytimes/1987/02/20/obituaries/eh-rynearson-of-mayo-clinic.html (accessed February 7, 2013).

Emanuel, Ezekiel. "Euthanasia: Historical, Ethical, and Empiric Perspectives." *Archives of Internal Medicine* 154 (September 12, 1994): 1890–1900.

_____. "The History of Euthanasia Debates in the United States and Britain." *Annals of Internal Medicine* 121, no. 10 (November 15, 1994): 793–802.

Engstrom, Joakim, Erik Bruno, Birgitta Holm, and Ove Hellzen. "Palliative Sedation at the End of Life—A Systematic Literature Review." *European Journal of Oncology Nursing* 11 (2007): 26–35.

Faden, Ruth R., and Tom L. Beauchamp. *A History and Theory of Informed Consent*. New York: Oxford University Press, 1986.

Feifel, Herman, ed. *The Meaning of Death*. New York: McGraw-Hill, 1959.

Flexner, Simon, and James Thomas Flexner. *William Henry Welch and the Heroic Age of American Medicine*. Baltimore: Johns Hopkins University Press, 1993 [1941].

"Florence Nightingale." http://www-history.mes.st-and.ac.uk/Biographies/Nightingale.html (accessed July 9, 2014).

Foley, Kathleen M. "The Past and Future of Palliative Care." *Hastings Center Special Report* 35, no. 6 (2005): S42–S46.

Ford, John M. T. "John Ferriar." Wellcome Institute for the History of Medicine, 1987. http://www.thornber.net/cheshire/ideasmen/ferriar.html (accessed October 29, 2009).

"Four Temperaments." http://en.wikipedia.org/wiki/Four temperaments (accessed May 22, 2013).

Franki, Richard. "More Hospitals House Palliative Care Teams." *Oncology Report*, August 30, 2012. http://www.oncologypractice.com/single-view/more-hospitals-house-palliative-care-teams/b92d4063830dcdb16e0f56da16c1f21c.html (accessed September 5, 2012).

_____. "More Hospitals Providing Palliative Care." *Oncology Report*. http://www.oncologypractice.com/index.php?id=6016&type=98&tx_ttnews[tt_news]=2142 (accessed August 6, 2012).

Fye, W. Bruce. "Profiles in Cardiology: John Ferriar." *Clinical Cardiology* 21 (1998): 533–534.

Garrison, Fielding H. *An Introduction to the History of Medicine*. 4th edition. Philadelphia: W.B. Saunders, 1929.

_____. "Samuel Bard and the King's College School." *New York Academy of Medicine* 1 (May 1935).

Gotay, Carolyn Cook. "Models of Terminal Care: A Review of the Research Literature." *Clinical and Investigative Medicine* 6 (1983): 131–141.

Granshaw, Lindsay. "The Hospital." In *Companion Encyclopedia of the History of Medicine*, vol. 2, edited by W. F. Bynum and Roy Porter, 1180–1203. London: Routledge, 1993.

Hallenbeck, James L. *Palliative Care Perspectives*. Oxford: Oxford University Press, 2003.

Haller, John S., Jr. *American Medicine in Transition, 1840–1910*. Chicago: University of Illinois Press, 1981.

Hannaway, Caroline. "Dunglison, Robley." In *Dictionary of Medical Biography*, vol. 2, edited by W.F. Bynum and Helen Bynum, 440–441. Westport, CT: Greenwood Press, 2007.

Hawkins, Clifford. "Writing the MD Thesis." *British Medical Journal* (November 6, 1976): 1121–1124.

Hermreck, Arlo S. "The History of Cardiopulmonary Resuscitation." *American Journal of Surgery* 156 (December 1988): 433–435.

"History: Liver and Ascites." http://depts.washington.edu/physdx/liver/history.html (accessed May 20, 2013).

Holden, Constance. "The Hospice Movement and Its Implication." *Annals of the American Academy of Political and Social Sciences* 447 (January 1980): 59–63.

Hughes, Nic, and David Clark. "'A Thoughtful and Experienced Physician': William Munk and the Care of the Dying in Late Victorian England." *Journal of Palliative Medicine* 7 (2004): 703–710.

Imber, Gerald. *Genius on the Edge: The Bizarre Double Life of Dr. William Steward Halstead*. New York: Kaplan, 2010.

Institute of Medicine. *Xenotransplantation: Science, Ethics, and Public Policy*. Washington, D.C.: National Academy Press, 1996.

Irons, Ernest E. "Theophile Bonet 1620–1689: His Influence on the Science and Practice of Medicine." *Bulletin of the History of Medicine* XII, no. 5 (December 1942): 623–665.

"John Norman Glaister." http://www.braziers.org.uk/research-and-publications/john-norman-glaister (accessed August 12, 2013).

Jonsen, Albert R. *The Birth of Bioethics*. New York: Oxford University Press, 1998.

Kane, Leslie. "Exclusive Ethics Survey Results: Doctors Struggle with Tougher-Than-Ever Dilemmas." *Medscape Medical Ethics*. http://www.medscape.com/viewarticle/731485 (accessed October 30, 2012).

Kelly, David F. *The Emergence of Roman Catholic Medical Ethics in America*. New York: Edwin Mellen Press, 1979.

Kerr, Derek. "Alfred Worcester: A Pioneer in Palliative Care." *American Journal of Hospice and Palliative Care* 9 (May/June 1992): 13–14 and 36–38.

King, Lester. *The Medical World of the Eighteenth Century*. Huntington, NY: Robert E. Krieger, 1971 [1958].

Koenig, Harold, Dana King, and Verna B. Carson. *Handbook of Religion and Health*. New York: Oxford University Press, 2001.

Lavi, Shai J. *The Modern Art of Dying: A History of Euthanasia in the United States*. Princeton, NJ: Princeton University Press, 2005.

Lee, Richard V. "Cardiopulmonary Resuscitation in the Eighteenth Century." *Journal of the History of Medicine and Allied Sciences* 27 (1972): 418–433.

Leviton, Daniel. "Death Education." In *New Meanings of Death*, edited by Herman Feifel, 254–272. New York: McGraw-Hill, 1977.

Lewis, Milton J. *Medicine and Care of the Dying: A Modern History*. Oxford and New York: Oxford University Press, 2007.

Ludmerer, Kenneth M. *Time to Heal*. Oxford: Oxford University Press, 1999.

Marchan, Ed, Jack Jallo, Fred Rincon, and Matthew Vibbert. "The Intensivist." *JHN Journal* 5 (2010): 20–22.

McCullough, Laurence. "Hooker, Worthington." In *Dictionary of Medical Biography*, edited by W.F. Bynum and Helen Bynum, vol. 3, 664. Westport, CT: Greenwood Press, 2007.

McKnight, Stephen A. *The Religious Foundations of Francis Bacon's Thought*. Columbia: University of Missouri Press, 2006.

McNeil, Donald G., Jr. "Palliative Care Extends Life, Study Finds." *New York Times*, August 19, 2010, A15.

MD Anderson Cancer Center. "What Are the Phases of Clinical Trials?" http://www.mdanderson.org/patient-and-cancer-information/cancer-information/clinical-trials (accessed September 27, 2012).

Miller, Albert Jay, and Michael James Acri. *Death: A Bibliographical Guide*. Metuchen, NJ: Scarecrow Press, 1977.

Miller, Heather. "Maybe We Need to Redefine 'Palliative Care.'" WebMD. http://blogs.webmd.com/cancer/2013/08/maybe-we-need-to-redefine-palliative-care.html (accessed August 21, 2013).

Mohee, Kevin. "Cardiac Pacing: A Brief History in the Development of Pacemakers." http://ssct.org/HistoryPacemakers.aspx (accessed November 28, 2011).

Morrell, J. B. "The University of Edinburgh in the Late Eighteenth Century: Its Scientific Eminence and Academic Structure." *Isis* 62 (Summer 1971): 158–171.

Morris, John S. "Sir Henry Halford, President of the Royal College of Physicians, with a Note on his Involvement in the Exhumation of King Charles I." *Postgraduate Medical Journal* 83 (June 2007): 431–433.

Mortimer, Ian. *The Dying and the Doctors: The Medical Revolution in Seventeenth-Century England*. Rochester, NY: Boydell Press, Royal Historical Society, 2009.

Mouton, Johann. "Reformation and Restoration in Francis Bacon's Early Philosophy." *The Modern Schoolman* 60 (1983): 101–120.

Neuhauser, D. "Public Opinion Is Our Supreme Court: D. W. Cathell MD, *The Physician Himself*." *Quality and Safe Health Care* 14 (2005): 389–390.

Numbers, Ronald L. "Do-It-Yourself the Sectarian Way." In *Sickness and Health in America*, edited by Judith Walzer Leavitt and Ronald L. Numbers, 87–97. Madison: University of Wisconsin Press, 1978.

"Opium in Medical Practice." http://www.drugtext.org/library/books/opiumpeople/opiummedprac.html (accessed September 19, 2010).

O'Reilly, Kevin B. "State Takes First-ever Path to Approve Assisted Suicide." *American Medical News*, May 29, 2013. http://www.amednews.com/article/20130529/profession/1305 29952/8 (accessed August 8, 2013).

Oshinsky, David M. *Polio: An American Story*. New York: Oxford University Press, 2005.

Patterson, James T. *The Dread Disease: Cancer and Modern American Culture*. Cambridge, MA: Harvard University Press, 1987.

Pelligrino, Edmund D. "The Sociocultural Impact of Twentieth-Century Therapeutics." In *The Therapeutic Revolution*, edited by Morris J. Vogel and Charles E. Rosenberg, 246–253. Philadelphia: University of Pennsylvania Press, 1979.

Pernick, Martin S. *A Calculus of Suffering*. New York: Columbia University Press, 1985.

Pickstone, J. V., and S. V. F. Butler. "The Politics of Medicine in Manchester, 1788–1792: Hospital Reform and Public Health Services in the Early Industrial City." *Medical History* 28 (1984): 227–249.

Porter, Dorothy, and Roy Porter. *Patient's Progress: Doctors and Doctoring in Eighteenth-century England*. Stanford, CA: Stanford University Press, 1989.

Reider, Philip. "Bonet, Theophile." *Dictionary of Medical Biography*. Vol. I. Westport, CT: Greenwood Press, 2007.

Reiser, Stanley Joel, Arthur J. Dyck, and William J. Curran, eds. *Ethics in Medicine*. Cambridge, MA: MIT Press, 1977.

"Review of Cathell, D.W., *Book on the Physician Himself*." *Journal of Laryngology* 6 (1892): 594–595.

Ristagno, Giuseppe, Wanchun Tang, and Max Harry Weil. "Cardiopulmonary Resuscitation: From the Beginning to the Present Day." *Critical Care Clinics* 25 (2009): 133–151.

Robert Woods Johnson Foundation Surgeons Palliative Care Workgroup. "Office of Promoting Excellence in End of Life Care: Surgeons' Palliative Care Workgroup Report from the Field." *Journal of American College of Surgery* 197 (October 2003): 661–686.

Rothman, David J. *Strangers at the Bedside: A History of How Law and Bioethics Transformed Medical Decision Making*. New York: Basic Books, 1991.

Rothstein, William G. *American Physicians in the Nineteenth Century: From Sects to Science*. Baltimore and London: Johns Hopkins University Press, 1972.

Rutkow, Ira. *Seeking the Cure: A History of Medicine in America*. New York: Scribner's, 2010.

_____. "A Selective History of Groin Hernia Surgery in the Early 19th Century." *Surgical Clinics of North America* 78 (December 1998): 921–940.

"St. Joseph's Hospice." *American Journal of Nursing* 65 (March 1965): 7.

Samuel, Lawrence R. *Death, American Style: A Cultural History of Dying in America*. New York: Rowman & Littlefield, 2013.

"Samuel Bard (1742–1821) Colonial Physician." *JAMA* 205, no. 8 (August 19, 1968): 586–587.

Schadenberg, Alex. "Do Americans Want to Legalize Assisted Suicide? What the Polls Won't Tell You." *LifeSiteNews*, January 8, 2013. http://www.lifesitenews.com/home/print_article/news/37645 (accessed August 23, 2013).

Shryock, Richard Harrison. "Nursing Emerges as a Profession: The American Experience." In *Sickness and Health in America*, edited by Judith Walzer Leavitt and Ronald L. Numbers, 203–215. Madison: University of Wisconsin Press, 1978.

Smith, Wesley J. "World Medical Association and AMA Oppose Euthanasia, Assisted Suicide." July 30, 2013. http://www.lifenews.com/2013/07/30/world-medical-association-and-ama-oppose-euthanasia (accessed August 8, 2013).

Sokol, Daniel K. "How The Doctor's Nose Has Shortened Over Time: A Historical Overview of the Truth-Telling Debate in the Doctor-Patient Relationship." *Journal of the Royal Society of Medicine* 99 (December 2008): 632–633.

Soniak, Matt. "'Time Me, Gentlemen': The Fastest Surgeon of the 19th Century." http://www.theatlantic.com/health/archive/2012/10/time-me-gentlemen (accessed May 21, 2013).

Starr, Paul. *The Social Transformation of American Medicine*. New York: Basic Books, 1982.

Steinfels, Peter. "Introduction." In *Death Inside Out*, edited by Peter Steinfels and Robert M. Veatch. New York: Harper and Row, 1974.

Stoddard, Sandol. *The Hospice Movement*. New York: Stein and Day, 1978.

Stolberg, Michael. "Active Euthanasia in Pre-Modern Society, 1500–1880: Learned Debates and Popular Practices." *Social History of Medicine* 20 (July 7, 2007): 205–221.

Sullivan, Amy M. Nina M. Gadmer, and Susan D. Block. "The Project on Death in America Faculty Scholars Programs: A Report on Scholars' Progress." *Journal of Palliative Medicine* 12, no. 2 (2009): 155–159.

Tercier, John Anthony. *The Contemporary Deathbed: The Ultimate Rush*. New York: Palgrave Macmillan, 2005.

Wainwright, Loudon. "A Profound Lesson for the Living." *LIFE*, November 21, 1969, 34–43.

Wawersik, J. "History of Chloroform Anesthesia." *Anaesthesiologie und Reanimation* 22 (1997): 144–152.

Winslow, Ron, Amy Dockser Marcus, and Christopher Weaver. "The Future of Medicine Is *Now*." *Wall Street Journal*, December 29, 2012, C1 and C2.

Zagorin, Perez. *Francis Bacon*. Princeton, NJ: Princeton University Press, 1998.

Zuraw, Lydia. "As Palliative Care Need Grows, Specialists Are Scarce." *New America Media*. http://www.npr.org/blogs/health/2013/or/o3/176121004/as-palliative-need-grows (accessed July 5, 2013).

Index